Diagnostic Applications of Health Intelligence and Surveillance Systems

Divakar Yadav
National Institute of Technology, Hamirpur, India

Abhay Bansal
Amity University, India

Madhulika Bhatia
Amity University, India

Madhurima Hooda
Amity University, India

Jorge Morato
Universidad Carlos III de Madrid, Spain

IGI Global
PUBLISHER of TIMELY KNOWLEDGE

A volume in the Advances in Medical Technologies and Clinical Practice (AMTCP) Book Series

Published in the United States of America by
IGI Global
Medical Information Science Reference (an imprint of IGI Global)
701 E. Chocolate Avenue
Hershey PA, USA 17033
Tel: 717-533-8845
Fax: 717-533-8661
E-mail: cust@igi-global.com
Web site: http://www.igi-global.com

Library of Congress Cataloging-in-Publication Data

Names: Yadav, Divakar, 1976- editor. | Bansal, Abhay, editor. | Bhatia, Madhulika, 1984- editor. | Hooda, Madhurima, 1985- editor. | Morato, Jorge, 1967- editor.
Title: Diagnostic applications of health intelligence and surveillance systems / [edited by] Divakar Yadav, Abhay Bansal, Madhulika Bhatia, Madhurima Hooda, Jorge Morato.
Description: Hershey, PA : Medical Information Science Reference, [2021] | Includes bibliographical references and index. | Summary: "The book is a great reference about the various application and scientific work going on in this area of how AI is driving the Health sector and helping health practitioners to predict disease intensity using the latest technology"-- Provided by publisher.
Identifiers: LCCN 2020023875 (print) | LCCN 2020023876 (ebook) | ISBN 9781799865278 (h/c) | ISBN 9781799865285 (eISBN)
Subjects: MESH: Artificial Intelligence | Diagnostic Techniques and Procedures | Medical Informatics Applications | Public Health Surveillance
Classification: LCC R859.7.A78 (print) | LCC R859.7.A78 (ebook) | NLM W 26.55.A7 | DDC 616.07/50028563--dc23
LC record available at https://lccn.loc.gov/2020023875
LC ebook record available at https://lccn.loc.gov/2020023876

This book is published in the IGI Global book series Advances in Medical Technologies and Clinical Practice (AMTCP) (ISSN: 2327-9354; eISSN: 2327-9370)

British Cataloguing in Publication Data
A Cataloguing in Publication record for this book is available from the British Library.

Advances in Medical Technologies and Clinical Practice (AMTCP) Book Series

Srikanta Patnaik
SOA University, India
Priti Das
S.C.B. Medical College, India

ISSN:2327-9354
EISSN:2327-9370

Mission

Medical technological innovation continues to provide avenues of research for faster and safer diagnosis and treatments for patients. Practitioners must stay up to date with these latest advancements to provide the best care for nursing and clinical practices.

The **Advances in Medical Technologies and Clinical Practice (AMTCP) Book Series** brings together the most recent research on the latest technology used in areas of nursing informatics, clinical technology, biomedicine, diagnostic technologies, and more. Researchers, students, and practitioners in this field will benefit from this fundamental coverage on the use of technology in clinical practices.

Coverage

- Nutrition
- Nursing Informatics
- Medical Imaging
- Diagnostic Technologies
- Clinical Nutrition
- Clinical High-Performance Computing
- Biomedical Applications
- Medical Informatics
- Biometrics
- Clinical Studies

IGI Global is currently accepting manuscripts for publication within this series. To submit a proposal for a volume in this series, please contact our Acquisition Editors at Acquisitions@igi-global.com or visit: http://www.igi-global.com/publish/.

The Advances in Medical Technologies and Clinical Practice (AMTCP) Book Series (ISSN 2327-9354) is published by IGI Global, 701 E. Chocolate Avenue, Hershey, PA 17033-1240, USA, www.igi-global.com. This series is composed of titles available for purchase individually; each title is edited to be contextually exclusive from any other title within the series. For pricing and ordering information please visit http://www.igi-global.com/book-series/advances-medical-technologies-clinical-practice/73682. Postmaster: Send all address changes to above address.

Titles in this Series

For a list of additional titles in this series, please visit: http://www.igi-global.com/book-series/advances-medical-technologies-clinical-practice/73682

AI Innovation in Medical Imaging Diagnostics
Kalaivani Anbarasan (Saveetha School of Engineering, India)
Medical Information Science Reference • © 2021 • 300pp • H/C (ISBN: 9781799830924) • US $345.00

Deep Learning Applications in Medical Imaging
Sanjay Saxena (International Institute of Information Technology, India) and Sudip Paul (North-Eastern Hill University, India)
Medical Information Science Reference • © 2021 • 274pp • H/C (ISBN: 9781799850717) • US $245.00

Design and Quality Considerations for Developing Mobile Apps for Medication Management Emerging Research and Opportunities
Kevin Yap (La Trobe University, Australia) Eskinder Eshetu Ali (Addis Ababa University, Ethiopia) and Lita Chew (National University of Singapore, Singapore)
Medical Information Science Reference • © 2021 • 256pp • H/C (ISBN: 9781799838326) • US $225.00

Expert Approaches to Health IT Tools in Clinical Practice
Ramgopal Kashyap (Amity University, Raipur, India)
Medical Information Science Reference • © 2021 • 300pp • H/C (ISBN: 9781799840510) • US $245.00

Opportunities and Challenges in Digital Healthcare Innovation
Kamaljeet Sandhu (University of New England, Australia)
Medical Information Science Reference • © 2020 • 261pp • H/C (ISBN: 9781799832744) • US $285.00

Mathematical Models of Infectious Diseases and Social Issues
Nita H. Shah (Department of Mathematics, Gujarat University, Ahmedabad, India) and Mandeep Mittal (Department of Mathematics, Amity Institute of Applied Sciences, Amity University, Noida, India)
Medical Information Science Reference • © 2020 • 316pp • H/C (ISBN: 9781799837411) • US $245.00

Nano-Strategies for Combatting Antimicrobial Resistance and Cancer
Muthupandian Saravanan (Mekelle University, Ethiopia) Venkatraman Gopinath (University of Malaya, Malaysia) and Karthik Deekonda (Monash University, Sunway Campus, India)
Medical Information Science Reference • © 2020 • 300pp • H/C (ISBN: 9781799850496) • US $285.00

IGI Global
PUBLISHER of TIMELY KNOWLEDGE

701 East Chocolate Avenue, Hershey, PA 17033, USA
Tel: 717-533-8845 x100 • Fax: 717-533-8661
E-Mail: cust@igi-global.com • www.igi-global.com

Editorial Advisory Board

Table of Contents

Detailed Table of Contents

Data mining plays a vital role in converting the medical data like text, image, and graphs into meaningful new data, which helps to take the better decision. In this chapter, an overview of the current research is discussed using the data mining techniques for the finding, analysis, and prediction of various diseases. The focus of this study is to identify the well-performing data mining algorithms used on medical and clinical databases. Multiple algorithms have been identified: text-based mining, association rule-based mining, pattern-based mining, keyword-based mining, machine learning, neural network support vector machine, apriori algorithm, k-means clustering, and natural language. Analyses of the algorithm show that there is no single algorithm or model more suitable for diagnosing or predicting diseases. In some scenarios, some algorithms work very well but not in another data set. There are many examples in clinical or medical research where the combination of different algorithms gives good results.

High glucose level disrupts the structure of the retinal layer in the eyes and causes diabetic retinopathy which is characterized with new pathologic blood vessels in the eyes. Although diabetic retinopathy is not clear at the beginning of the disease, it is the most common problem in people who have diabetes and causes blindness or cloudy vision if it is not diagnosed at the beginning of the disease. For early diagnosis of diabetic retinopathy, regular fundus controls and examination of the edema in the vessels of the retina are made periodically by ophthalmologists. With in the scope of this study, it is made possible to provide the early diagnosis and the level of diabetic retinopathy by using deep learning, image processing methods, and convolutional neural networks of the retina. In order to provide ease and rapid of diagnosis of the diabetic retinopathy in daily life, the diagnosis protocol has been turned into a mobile application. With the mobile application, both the diagnosis and more regular results of the diabetic retinopathy can be obtained easily and practically.

given for the development and efficient use of mobile health applications by prostate cancer patients and healthcare providers.

The purpose of this chapter is to examine the incautious usage of social media and its impact on emotional intelligence and health. After a brief introduction to the emotional intelligence and the conceptualisation and evaluation of this construct, this chapter discusses a variety of studies that shed light on the social media, emotional intelligence and health relationships. The idea of emotional intelligence (EI) is of unmatched enthusiasm for both the literature and inside scholarly world. This chapter discusses emotional intelligence and focuses on the evolution of EI by examining the different models. This chapter lists some applications of emotional intelligence in our daily life. The chapter also discusses how the abilities correlate with emotional intelligence and helps individuals cope with unsettling emotions effectively and encourage pleasurable emotions to facilitate personal development and well-being.

Epilepsy is a brain disorder that can be defined as a short-time and temporary occurrence of symptoms because of abnormal extreme or synchronous neuronal activity of the brain. Almost one percent of the world's population is struggling with epilepsy illness. The detection of epileptic seizures is mainly realized with reading the electroencephalogram (EEG) recordings by medical doctors due to the unpredictable and complex nature of the disease. This process takes much time and depends on the expert's experience. For this reason, automatic seizure detection using EEG recordings is necessary and of great importance for the comfort of medical doctors and patients. While detecting epileptic seizure automatically, machine learning techniques are used in the field of computer science. This chapter deals with the methods, approaches, models, and techniques which are utilized to detect epileptic seizures.

To guard people against some grave infectious disease, the surveillance system is a key performance measure of global public health threats and vulnerability. The diseases surveillance system helps in public health monitor, control, and prevent infectious diseases. Infectious diseases remain major causes of death. It's important to monitor and surveillance worldwide for developing a framework for risk assessment and health regulation. Surveillance systems help us in understanding the factors driving infectious disease and developing new technological aptitudes with modeling, pathogen determination, characterization, diagnostics, and communications. This chapter discussed surveillance system working, progress toward global public healthy society considering perspectives for the future and improvement of infectious disease surveillance without limited and fragmented capabilities, and making even global coverage.

Nanoparticles (NPs) are tiny particles having dimensions ranging from 1 nm to 100 nm. Nanoparticles are field of profound scientific interest, on account of diverse conceivable applications in various fields such as electronic, optical, agriculture, biomedical, etc. Many of the interesting properties of nanoparticles are intimately linked on shape and size of nanomaterials. In nanoparticles, percentage of surface atoms are high; nanoparticles show properties dependent on shape which are utilized in catalysis, optics, data storage, etc. Further, the physical properties of nanoparticles such as melting point, density, optical properties, electrical conductivity, chemical stability, etc. make them suitable candidates to be utilized in several fields. Many of the nanoparticles have been widely studied and many applications explored for example gold and silver nanoparticles, while research is being carried out to investigate the probable applications in several other fields. This review provides the readers a summary of the applications of various nanoparticles.

The recent decade has seen considerable changes in the way the technology interacts with human lives and almost all the aspects of life be it personal or professional has been touched by technology. Many smart devices have also started playing a vital role in many fields and domains and the internet of things (IoT) has been the harbinger of the advent of IoT devices. IoT devices have proven to be monumental in imparting 'smartness' in the otherwise static machines. The ability of the devices to interact and transfer the data to the internet and ultimately to the end-user has revolutionized the technological world and has brought many seemingly disparate fields in the technological purview. Out of the many fields where IoT has started gaining momentum, one of the most important ones is the healthcare sector. Many wearable smart devices have been developed over time capable to transmit real-time data to hospitals and doctors. It is essential for tracking the progress of the critically ill patients and has opened the horizon for attending patients remotely using these smart devices.

Preface

AN OVERVIEW OF THE SUBJECT MATTER

Health surveillance and health intelligence are crucial components of progressive health systems. Health surveillance fits to the premeditated progression of collecting statistics of connotation from health systems, populaces, channels, and numerous additional resources, specially the data which is epidemiological. Health surveillance is staged in a methodical way, agreeing to a perfectly specified strategy linked with an obvious necessity to gather the required data. This surveillance relies on automated systems for data gathering by entities and entail substantial disbursement of resources. There are countless old-style data-points poised by health surveillance, some of which are, disease meeting a investigative instance definition (in number of cases), folks who have customary certain intercessions (in numbers), health resources being utilized (the sorts and their numbers), encompassing their diminution, sentinel or perilous clinical actions (their occurrence), clinical hitches, deaths related to a particular disease (their numbers and details) and topographical dispersal and spell progression of collected data.

Health intelligence implies understanding, investigation, dispensation, and cohort of valuable products that assist civic health experts, clinicians, responders, decision creators, policy creators etc. Their primary intent is to make health surveillance data prudent and utilizing it to attain advanced objectives. It is developed through an organized process that encompasses recurrent review of vital information or specific bits of info. The cohort of health intelligence is typically managed by a tinier cluster of related connoisseurs even if assemblage of health surveillance data entails the joint work of various individuals. This helps in determining superiority, veracity, and inevitability of the information required for health surveillance.

Administering health surveillance data is a specialized task carried out across wide-ranging organizations. Health intelligence activities in a military organization may, for example, be dedicated on the appraisal of the risks to deploy personnel to a remote or tropical location. But, in a key corporation this may build and use health intelligence products to aid in preparation and erecting a major risk facility such as a power station, chemical plant, or mine. Health intelligence activities in a state health department may be concentrated on gauging the advent of epidemic diseases, rare diseases, and the day to day operation of a health system. Health intelligence specialists, reliant on the protagonists they are undertaking, develop specific proficiency in specialized areas as delineated above and work meticulously with decision and policy makers to unceasingly restructure and enhance the health surveillance and intelligence structure to improve operation.

A DESCRIPTION OF WHERE THIS TOPIC FITS IN THE WORLD TODAY

Health surveillance provides and illuminates data to expedite the deterrence and influence of diseases. This is a means to assess the health condition and comportment of the people. As surveillance can immediately quantify the activities of population, it could be an aid for evaluating the necessity for interventions and for precisely measuring the effects of intercessions. The purpose is to galvanize decision makers to lead and cope more successfully by providing timely, valuable evidence. This offers the scientific and factual database crucial to apprised decision making and appropriate public health action. To prevent the spread of epidemics of acute infectious diseases, such as COVID19 there is a need to intercede promptly to stop the spread of disease. Thus, a surveillance system offers swift untimely alerting information from clinics and laboratories.

A DESCRIPTION OF THE TARGET AUDIENCE

Primary Audience: Undergraduate, Post graduate students; Ph.D and Research Scholars as well as Faculty of various Universities.

Secondary Audience: Any one part of scientific community or General Readers who want to explore this Topic.

Review of Data Mining Techniques Used in Health Care

Data mining play a very vital role to convert the medical data like text, image, and graphs in to meaningful new data which helps to take the better decision. In this paper an overview of the current research being discussed out using the data mining techniques for the finding, analysis and prediction of various diseases. The focus of this study is to identify the well-performing data mining algorithms used on medical and clinical databases. There are multiple algorithms have been identified: Text based mining, Association rule based mining, Pattern based mining, Keyword based mining, Machine learning, Neural network Support vector machine, Apriori algorithm, k-means clustering and Natural language. Analyses of the algorithm show that there is no single algorithm or model which are more suitable for diagnose or predict the diseases. In some scenarios some algorithms work very well but not in another data set. There are lots many example in clinical or medical research where the combination of different algorithms gives good results.

Detection of Diabetic Retinopathy With Mobile Application Using Deep Learning

High glucose level disrupts the structure of the retinal layer in the eyes and causes diabetic retinopathy which is characterized with new pathologic blood vessels in the eyes. Although diabetic retinopathy is not clear at the beginning of the disease, it is the most common problem in people who have diabetes. It causes blindness or cloudy vision if it is not diagnosed at the beginning of the disease. For early diagnosis of diabetic retinopathy, regular fundus controls and examination of the edema in the vessels of the retina are made periodically by ophthalmologists. Within the scope of this study, it is made possible to provide the early diagnosis and the level of diabetic retinopathy by using deep learning, image processing methods, and convolutional neural networks of the retina. In order to provide ease and rapid of diagnosis of diabetic retinopathy in daily life, the diagnosis protocol has been turned into a mobile application. With the mobile application, both the diagnosis and more regular results of the diabetic retinopathy can be obtained easily and practically.

Android-Based Skin Cancer Recognition System Using Convolutional Neural Network

Skin Cancer which is one of the most common types of cancer in the world is a malignant growth seen on the skin due to various reasons. There was an increase in the number of the cases of skin cancer nearly 200% between 2004-2009. Since the ozone layer is depleting, harmful rays reflected from the sun cannot be filtered. In this case, the likelihood of skin cancer will increase over the years and pose more risks for human beings. Early diagnosis is very significant as in all types of cancers in skin cancer. In this study, a mobile application is developed in order to detect whether the skin spots photographed by using the machine learning technique for early diagnosis have a suspicion of skin cancer. Thus, an auxiliary decision support system is developed that can be used both by the clinicians and individuals. For cases that are predicted to have a risk higher than a certain rate by the machine learning algorithm, Early diagnosis could be initiated for the patients by consulting a physician when the case is considered to have a higher risk by machine learning algorithm.

mHealth: A Resolution in Improving Global Health

mHealth or Mobile health care has become an increasingly important issue in several disciplines such as health communication, public health, and health promotion. This enables the users to use portable devices such as smartphones, smart bands or tablets for health monitoring purpose. The users have the ability to utilize software applications to interact with mobile devices and store relevant data for further classification and diagnosis. The apps then process the gathered data using the given algorithms and provide the user with personalized diagnosis, and further recommendations for treatment and even suggestive measures to improve general health and fitness. Another benefit of mobile technology is that the data and health statistics of a single patient can be compared with large data sets to facilitate treatment and proper guidance. Doctors, nurses, and other health professionals use mobile devices to access patient information, databases, and resources. Help in today's world is just a click away.

Computational Studies in Breast Cancer

Early detection of breast cancer is a world-wide need as many hospitals have appeared in commitment of research pathway. As per who (world health organisation), early detection of breast cancer boosts the choice of making corrective judgement on medication plan. This corrective choice helps women to save themselves from expensive and unwanted medical test and treatment. Physical observation and medical history play an important role in diagnosing this disease; however, for detailed understanding some reliable and accurate methods are still required. This paper reviews existing computational methods and need of novel algorithms that can help in accurately diagnosing this disease. Correct diagnosis and yield results devising treatment strategy. For correct diagnosis micro-array gene expression data is widely used, this paper highlights various computational studies done on breast cancer microarray data. This review highlights the benefit of computational model being an impressive tool for discovery of cancer along with devising its therapies.

The Role of Genetic Data Analysis for Precision Therapy in Cancer: Personalized Medicine Concept in Cancer Treatment

Cancer has been known as a devastating disease which takes thousands of lives every year. And since this is a heterogenous disease, therefore standard treatments, like chemotherapy, radiation & chemo-radio therapy are effective in specific patient population subset only. Genetic differences play a very crucial role in defining cancer susceptibility and also in determining the drug's efficacy by affecting regulation, expression & activity of drug metabolizing enzymes, drug transporters & drug receptors. This genetic variability of the disease lends itself to the emerging field of precision or personalized medicine. There are some specific ways of acquiring data for precision or personalized medicine approach like genome wide association scan (GWAS). This is basically identification and scanning of biomarkers throughout the complete DNA/genome of several individuals to study any type of genetic variations which are linked with any form of cancer.

The Role of eHealth Interventions in Improving Clinical Outcomes and Overall Health for Prostate Cancer Patients: A Review

Globally, prostate cancer is a major health care problem. It is among the most frequently diagnosed malignancies and is the primary cancer in males in North America and the Caribbean, Europe and some parts of Africa. Mobile health interventions afford prostate cancer patients in following prostate specific antigen results including trends, getting a better understanding of the severity of their disease and evaluate carefully the benefits and risks of the available treatment options. This review will examine the use of mobile health applications in prostate cancer research particularly in (i) clinical decision of selecting best treatment option or active surveillance, (ii) monitoring disease- and treatment-related symptoms, (iii) oncological and supportive care, (iv) treatment decisions, and (v) health literacy and promotion of physical exercise. The benefits of telemedicine are discussed. Challenges will be examined and recommendations given for the development and efficient use of mobile health applications by prostate cancer patients and healthcare providers.

Incautious Usage of Social Media: Impact on Emotional Intelligence and Health Concerns

The purpose of this chapter is to examine the Incautious Usage of Social Media and its Impact on Emotional Intelligence and Health. After a brief introduction to the emotional intelligence and the conceptualisation and evaluation of this construct, this chapter discusses a variety of studies that shed light on the social media, emotional intelligence and health relationships. The idea of Emotional Intelligence (EI) is of unmatched enthusiasm for both the literature and inside scholarly world. This chapter discusses "Emotional Intelligence" and focuses on the evolution of EI by examining the different models. This chapter lists some applications of emotional intelligence in our daily life. The chapter also discusses how the abilities correlate with emotional intelligence and helps individuals cope with unsettling emotions effectively and encourage pleasurable emotions to facilitate personal development and well-being.

Epileptic Seizure Detection Using Machine Learning Techniques

Epilepsy is a brain disorder which can be defined as a short-time and temporary occurrence of symptoms because of abnormal extreme or synchronous neuronal activity of the brain. Almost one percent of the world's population is struggling with epilepsy illness. The detection of epileptic seizures is mainly realized with reading the electroencephalogram (EEG) recordings by medical doctors due to the unpredictable and complex nature of the disease. This process takes much time and depends on the expert's experience. For this reason, automatic seizure detection using EEG recordings is necessary and of great importance for the comfort of medical doctors and patients. While detecting epileptic seizure automatically, machine learning techniques are used in the field of computer science. This chapter deals with the methods, approaches, models and techniques which are utilized to detect epileptic seizures.

Public Health Surveillance System-Infectious Diseases: Surveillance System

To guard people against some grave infectious disease, the surveillance system is a key performance measure of global public health threats and vulnerability. The diseases surveillance system helps in public health monitor, control, and prevent infectious diseases. Infectious diseases remain major causes of death all-inclusive, novel rapid increase emerging infections in the rate of diseases or geographic range it's important to monitor and surveillance worldwide for developing a framework for risk assessment and health regulation. Surveillance system helps us in understanding the factors driving infectious disease and developing new technological aptitudes with modeling, pathogen determination, characterization, diagnostics, and communications. This chapter discussed surveillance system working, progress toward global public healthy society considering perspectives for the future and improvement of infectious disease surveillance without limited and fragmented capabilities, and making even global coverage.

Applications of Nanoparticles in Various Fields

Nanoparticles (NPs) are tiny particles having dimensions ranging from 1 nm to 100 nm. Nanoparticles are field of profound scientific interest, on account of diverse conceivable applications in various fields such as electronic, optical, agriculture, biomedical etc. Many of the interesting properties of nanoparticles are intimately linked on shape and size of nanomaterials. In nanoparticles percentage of surface atoms are high, nanoparticles show properties dependent on shape which are utilized in catalysis, optics, data storage etc. Further, the physical properties of nanoparticles such as melting point, density, optical properties, electrical conductivity, chemical stability etc. make them suitable candidates to be utilized in several fields. Many of the nanoparticles have been widely studied and many applications explored for example gold and silver nanoparticles, while research is being carried out to investigate the probable applications in several other fields. This review provides the readers a summary of the applications of various nanoparticles.

Internet of Things (IoT) in Healthcare

The recent decade has seen considerable changes in the way the technology interacts with human lives and almost all the aspects of life be it personal or professional has been touched by technology. Many Smart devices have also started playing a vital role in many fields and domains and the Internet of Things

(IoT) has been the harbinger of the advent of IoT devices. IoT devices have proven to be monumental in imparting 'smartness' in the otherwise static machines. The ability of the devices to interact and transfer the data to the internet and ultimately to the end-user has revolutionized the technological world and has brought many seemingly disparate fields in the technological purview. Out of the many fields where IoT has started gaining momentum, one of the most important ones is the Healthcare sector. Many wearable smart devices has been developed over time capable to transmit real-time data to hospitals and doctors. It is essential for tracking the progress of the critically ill patients and has opened the horizon for attending patients remotely using these smart devices.

IoT in Healthcare Using Clinical Decision Support System

Most of the developing countries face major problems in providing quality healthcare. It is very essential to move the health stream to a higher level with more effective. Though medical care is improving, due to the enormous amount of data, making the decisions is more complex. The technology already links patients, providers, and customers in many ways that are converting the patient experience and delivery of care. This chapter reveals the importance of healthcare by using CDSS along with IoT. By combining connected devices with CDSS will help the clinicians to take decisions immediately for any disease. It provides an efficient, effective quality measurement, and enhancement because of its ability to get the data of any patient at any time anywhere.

CONCLUSION

In modern health system, health surveillance and health intelligence may play an important role to it. There are many informal sources useful for gathering data related to health system. So, there is a need and challenge of interpreting and analyzing these data so that useful findings can be utilized, directly and indirectly related to them.

Objective of this Book is to identify data-points, collected by health surveillance activities to meet diagnostic definition of cases. Time series analysis of geographic distribution of data as well as prediction of number of survival and non-survival cases from some particular diseases. The book has included chapters on and related to health intelligence which may help readers to know how health surveillance data can be made useful and meaning full value can be added to it. Health intelligence uses health surveillance data to make it valuable and easy to extract information. The number of cases of disease meeting a diagnostic case definition. Health intelligence prediction about clinical complications can be used for prediction of reoccurrences of deaths from a particular disease or so. The book will prove very useful reading for those who are working in area of Health Intelligence.

This book can also be useful for those who needs reference about various contribution done by many experts. The contents of the book is really challenging and lot of research going on which will help readers to increase their knowledge about the Topic. This will help the scholars, students and industry people to really get an idea of what are the various application and scientific work going on in this area of driving how AI is deriving Health sector and helping health practitioners to predict disease intensity and which in turn gives grip of the latest technology and give a wide plot which keeps the readers engaged.

Chapter 1
Review of Data Mining Techniques Used in Healthcare

Usha Gupta
https://orcid.org/0000-0002-2886-7859
Manav Rachna International Institute of Research and Studies, India

Kamlesh Sharma
https://orcid.org/0000-0002-6000-5933
Manav Rachna International Institute of Research and Studies, India

ABSTRACT

Data mining plays a vital role in converting the medical data like text, image, and graphs into meaningful new data, which helps to take the better decision. In this chapter, an overview of the current research is discussed using the data mining techniques for the finding, analysis, and prediction of various diseases. The focus of this study is to identify the well-performing data mining algorithms used on medical and clinical databases. Multiple algorithms have been identified: text-based mining, association rule-based mining, pattern-based mining, keyword-based mining, machine learning, neural network support vector machine, apriori algorithm, k-means clustering, and natural language. Analyses of the algorithm show that there is no single algorithm or model more suitable for diagnosing or predicting diseases. In some scenarios, some algorithms work very well but not in another data set. There are many examples in clinical or medical research where the combination of different algorithms gives good results.

BACKGROUND

Over the past years, people are more inclined towards the research on data that is being used in health care field. Researchers are rapidly using the medical data for evaluating the health care provided to patients and are also evaluating the healthcare feedback from patients and health divisions. The quality of this kind of evaluation is totally dependent on the quality of data they are using and also the completeness of data gathered from such units.

DOI: 10.4018/978-1-7998-6527-8.ch001

During recent years, the healthcare professionals like hospitals, Clinics; medical practioners uses technologies for maintaining the records of patients as well as the treatments provided. Such records can be in the form of hospital information systems (HIS's), electronic health records (EHR's), electronic medical records (EMR's), clinical decision support systems (CDSS's), laboratory information systems (LIS's).

Currently, medical health care givers uses Electronic medical records for recording the condition of patient's health, like data related to the diagnosis of disease, prescriptions given, results of treatments, and procedures performed. This electronic based medical record system has become a valuable source for analysis performed at large-scale by health professionals. However, these records are diverse in nature, and there is a sense of incompleteness, redundancy, and privacy of the data records being stored in EMR's, due to these features it becomes tough to perform analysis of data directly. Hence, it requires to pre-processed data sources for improving the quality of data and also the analysis part. As the data stored is vast and vigorous so it needs to be processed differently with different technologies.

Here the data stored in EMR systems can be categorized in three different categories as given below:

1. Structured data
2. Semi-structured data
3. Un-structured data.

Here, the structured form of data contains data information of patients like birth date and related information, medicinal drugs given, any sort of allergies if exist, vital information of patient like height and weight, blood group, blood pressure etc, all these information gets stored in the form of fixed mode data bases.

Whereas the Semi-structured data is consists of the patient's information to be stored in the form of flow chart format, like that of RDF (resource description files), comprises of value, name and timestamp. And the Un-structured data contains the narrative form of data, like notes of clinical records, records of surgical data, summaries related to discharge of any patient from hospitals or medical unit, reports like radiology and pathology. Unstructured data stores very essential medical information but there is a drawback of common structural frameworks, and also chances of errors do exist in such form of data, like no proper use of grammar, errors in spelling, local dialects, and semantic ambiguities, all these results in increase of complexity of processing and analysis of data.

As for structured data, preprocessing technologies such as data cleaning, integration of data, transforming data, and reduction in data are required. And for semi-structured or unstructured data, which contains health and medical related information and data, needs more complex and challenging processing methods.

As per study in medical field, the data around medical and health division is either unstructured or semi-structured. So it becomes very difficult to manage such data. So there arises a need for handling such data to perform required functions. Hence data mining is one of the applications to perform operations on medical data. The adoption of data mining technique in healthcare field brings medical information technology into action and health practitioners believes in such technologies for improving the healthcare services and hence therefore can further helps in systematic innovations. However the resources required for managing such data in a mining process is a big challenge.

There are several benefits which are provided when data mining is used in healthcare related prediction (Jain et.al 2019) such as adequate diagnosis to patients, detection of drug abuse, proper provision for treatments to patients, prior detection of diseases, and rate of survivability patients from disease etc.

There are various data mining methodologies that have been used and applied on health care data by various researchers like, classification, association, clustering etc. All these techniques or methodologies proved to be having a very important role in the healthcare sector for supporting process of decision making, in providing proper diagnosis, in selecting treatments and also predicting the diseases etc. (Tomari et.al 2015).

In paper, the author have reviewed data mining techniques that can be used in healthcare for improving the performance and efficiency thus by reducing the patient's request processing time, optimized storage requirements for storing the patients data thereby providing a real time data extraction and retrieval mechanism for such application.

INTRODUCTION

In early 1970's, cost of storing the data was very high. But with the advancements in the field related to data gathering tools and Web in the last 25 to 30 years, one has seen a very large amount of data or information is being available in the form of electronic record format. And for storing such a huge amount of data, the size of database repository is increasing at a rapid rate. Such type of database repository contains very useful and valuable data. All this data may be very useful in process of taking decisions in any area. This all is possible just by data mining or by having process of Knowledge Discovery in Databases (KDD).

A healthcare industry requires data mining for discovering the knowledge and also finding patterns for making the decisions to make healthcare effective.

Data mining as per its definition, is nothing but the process of extraction of valuable or useful data or information from a voluminous and large source of data which was not known previously (Varghese and Tintu,2015).

In such large source of data, there lies a hidden number of relationships among such data, like relationship between patient information and data and total number of days spent in hospital during the stay (Daliri, 2017).

Data mining requires the functionality of finding useful yet meaningful patterns, details, information from the large source of data.

Data mining technique is used in healthcare sector for the sake of classifying the diseases a patient is suffering from and also by assisting the health providers in giving the required treatments and thus managing the diseases. It also assists in prediction of duration of stay of a patient in the hospital, the diagnosis process, and accurate management information systems. All these data mining techniques and technologies helps in reducing the total expenditure made by patient for disease diagnosis and its cure and also for evaluating the symptoms that are responsible for diseases (Daliri, 2017). So the mining applications are having a pivotal role in healthcare. It is thereby necessary to perform collection, storing the healthcare data, preparing it and also mining this data for making it clean and right. Clinical practices of healthcare professionals and the standardization of distributing data all across the medical organizations for helping healthcare related data mining (Tomari et.al 2015). Thus mining greatly improves the data analysis process in health care sector. The enhancements in technologies and complexities in voluminous data make implementation of these mining strategies a bit difficult. Mining techniques had been used so far are, Neural Networks, decision trees, Support Vector machine, Naïve Bayes, Association rule generation, text based mining, pattern based data mining, keyword based mining, Natural language processing, and genetic algorithm. All these techniques help the academicians in writing and publishing research papers. The process of data mining can be automated partially or fully, for analyzing uncertain volume of data such as data clusters, outlier detection and data dependencies. The patient's records are extracted and stored, merged into a database on the basis of dataset selected which is used for the analysis purposes in diagnosis for obtaining more precise prediction results for making further decisions.

DATA MINING PROCES

The data related to healthcare industry is voluminous and vast, so there arise a need for transforming such data into meaningful information for making decisions. Mining such data provides a way in analyzing the complexity of data for generating further information. This mining process includes, collecting data, preparing data, then preprocessing the data and finally transforming the data in to desired result. This process of mining helps in discovering knowledge (Garg and Sharma, 2020) comprises of 7 stages that starts from selection to discovery of knowledge.

Figure 1. Data mining application

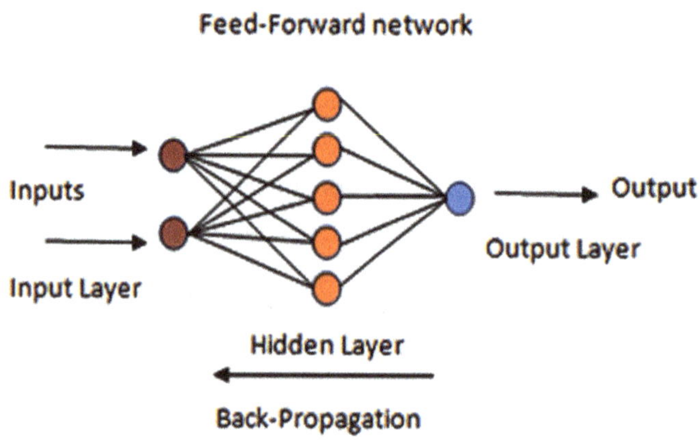

This figure elaborates the five stages that are used in discovering knowledge from large source of data [Tomari et.al, 2015, Sharma et.al, 2014, and Han, Pei and Kamber, 2011). Starting with the row data, data is selected then preprocessing, transformation, mining, interpretation takes place for extracting the knowledge captured as an outcome of all these above stages as shown in figure 1 are explained below:

Selection

The selection of data took place on the basis of some criteria. Like, all the people who are diagnosed with diabetes and thus we can find out the subsets of data with this criteria.

Preprocessing

In this stage, the removal of extra data took place which is not required as per the criteria given in previous stage. Like, when pregnancy test is conducted on patient then sex of patient is not required to note down. This is also referred to as data cleansing stage.

Transformation

In this step, data required for the research purpose is transformed, like data related to a specific demographical area is useful in research related to market in context of healthcare.

Data Mining

This is used for fetching out the meaningful patterns from data.

Interpretation and Evaluation

In this stage, the patterns discovered from mining step are interpreted into knowledge. This knowledge is then used for making required decisions.

MINING TECHNIQUES OF DATA IN HEALTH CARE INDUSTRY:

The mining techniques are applied in the large complex voluminous data for discovering knowledge. The different data mining techniques used in healthcare are given below in figure 2 and also used analysis related to various diseases. The brief description of all these techniques is also explained in the further section.

Text Based Mining Technique

Text mining technique also known as mining text data is used get the knowledge that is hidden in healthcare industry's unstructured form data. Through text mining unstructured data can be transformed in to valuable structured data. It handles heterogeneous data formats like text docs, emails, multimedia text, misspelled words, abbreviations, and multilingual posts. (Sun et.al, 2018)

Through text mining, new different topics can be easily detected in the same sentence. Its process starts with taxonomy creation, which helps in extraction of information and metadata association. Through text mining, further detailed information about the text itself can be achieved and can also helps in revealing patterns across thousands of documents in the data set.

The figure 3 given below explains the process of text mining briefly.

There are 4 stages in text mining process:

1. Information retrieval
2. Information extraction
3. Knowledge discovery

4. Knowledge application.

Figure 2. Mining techniques of data used in healthcare

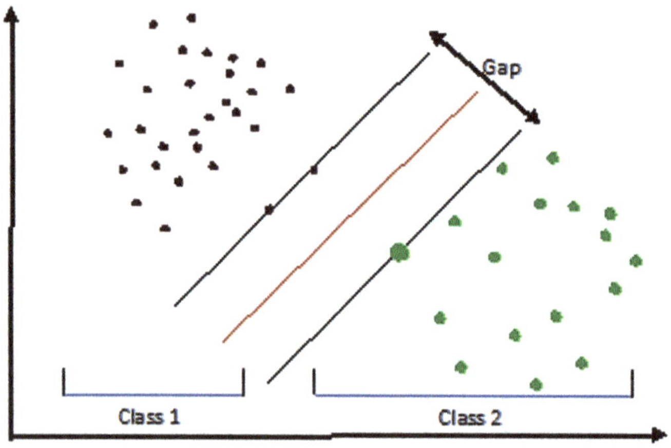

Figure 3. Process of text mining

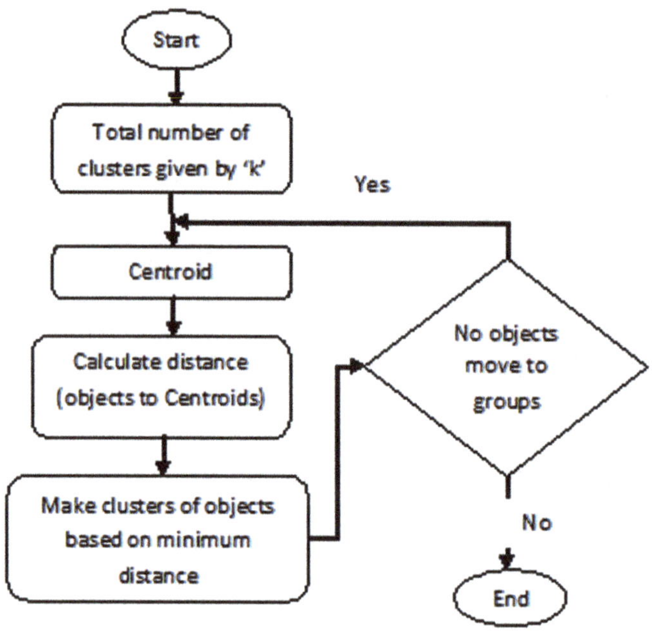

Information retrieval phase is used for collecting desired text or data. Information extraction is used for extracting predefined data or text. The information extraction can be done by named-entity recognition (NER) and relation extraction (RE).

Knowledge discovery is used for the extraction of brand new knowledge from the text. And finally this Knowledge is applied as the unknown facts inferred from texts to practice.

Association Rule Based Mining

Mining based on association rules is used for finding out the patterns which are frequent also helps in finding associations, and correlations present amongst the item sets or objects in information repositories. Rule based mining is very popular in discovering frequent and interesting relations existing amongst the data in a given database. Different measures of interestingness (Kulkarni et.al, 2017) are used for discovering frequent item sets among data by generating strong rules.

For example, discovering the symptoms of particular {Corona}, if the symptoms for this disease in healthcare are as {Fever, Dry cough, Tiredness} then a person is having Corona disease.

This sort of knowledge is useful for making better decisions and also giving proper treatments by healthcare professionals or medical experts to patients.

These mining rules works with two major important properties: Support and Confidence, here Support property indicates the frequency of appearance of any item set in database.

And Confidence is an indication that the association rule is true, and how often it is found to be true..

This value of Confidence for any association rule, with respect to a set of transactions, is the proportion of the transactions that contains having Confidence can be further defined as:

The correlation between Support and Confidence is given as:

Confidence (AB) = Probability of (B|A)

= Support_ count (AUB)/Support_ count (A) Support_ count (AUB)

: giving the number of transaction containing the item sets A U B,
Support_ count (A): number of transactions containing the item set A. (M.Inbava LLi, 2015)

Association rule based mining process works in two steps:

1. First, find all the frequent item sets, by keeping a count of total number of frequencies of occurrence of the item-sets in the database as a predetermined min. support count;
2. Secondly, generate strong association rules from these frequent item sets by satisfying the min. Support and min. Confidence value.

Pattern Based Mining

Pattern based mining methods use templates, inference rules, and algorithms. Through pattern mining, frequent patterns can be mined or extracted from large databases (Metsker et.al, 2017). A **frequent pattern** is defined as a pattern (or item set) satisfying criteria of min. Support threshold. A frequent pattern can be in the form of a simple frequent pattern, a closed pattern, or a max-pattern. Here pattern that exist frequently are called frequent patterns. And closed pattern means that there is no super patterns exist among data. And max pattern means that there is no frequent super pattern present in data.

Through pattern mining, association rules can also be generated for extracting the meaningful data or information as per requirement from database. These patterns can be in the form of multilevel or multidimensional. Pattern mining helps in finding sequential, time series, structural, spatial, temporal, multimedia, image, text, and network patterns from large databases.

Keyword Based Mining

This is referred as mining the data on the basis of keywords present in the given database. It is the process of finding for a list of keywords or phrases that are relevant for a specific task. This process uses tools related to mining keywords. These tools are basically search words from the given databases and retrieving one or more results. These results are the further databases containing the searched words or keywords, and required to be read each and every document for determining the relevancy of the same. (Park et.al, 2014)

Example

The frequently found keywords in some sentence related to medical field of describing patient with 'pain', as the word 'pain'; in the given diagram, the total number of occurrence of the keyword is written in parenthesis.

Figure 4. Keyword mining result related to keyword: 'pain'

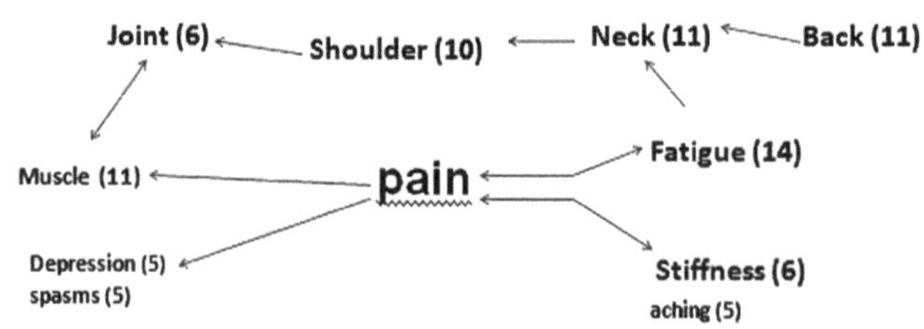

Machine Learning

Machine learning is the field which ideally refers to as the way machines does learning from the experiences acquired. The term "machine learning" is very much same as that of "artificial intelligence", provided that the learning phase is the main characteristic of an entity called intelligent elaborated in the broadest sense of the word. (Kavakiotis et.al, 2017)

The main purpose of machine learning methodology is constructing a system or a machine like computer system that can adapt and learn from its experiences. (Wilson et.al, MIT Press, 1999) An author named Mr. Mitchel, have given a more detailed and formal definition of machine learning as(Mitchell, 1997): A computer program is said to learn from experience E with respect to some class of tasks T and performance measure P, if its performance at tasks in T, as measured by P, improves with experience E.

Tasks of Machine Learning

The tasks of Machine learning tasks are broadly classified into three categories (Stuart and Norvig, 1995).

1. Supervised machine learning: in this, the system infers rules from given training data,
2. Un-Supervised machine learning: means the learning system infers the structure of unlabeled data,
3. Re-Inforcement machine learning: means the system interacts directly with a dynamic environment.

Neural Network

Neural networks are basically represents the modeling of human brain.(Esteban et.al, 2017) A human brain consists of neurons, also called the building blocks of brain. There are billions of neurons in a human brain, where each neuron having a connection point ranges between 1,000 and 100,000. In the human brain, information is stored in a distributed manner and human can does extraction of more than one piece of this information from memory in parallel whenever required.

In multi-layer artificial feed forward neural networks, neurons called units are placed just like as that in human brain.(Suman Rout et.al, 2020) Here each neuron/unit is connected to other neuron/unit with certain coefficients. During training or learning phase, the information is distributed on to these connection points so that the network performs learning.

Neural network consists of three layers:

1. Input layer
2. Intermediate layer/ Hidden layer
3. Output layer

Figure 5. Artificial Neural Network

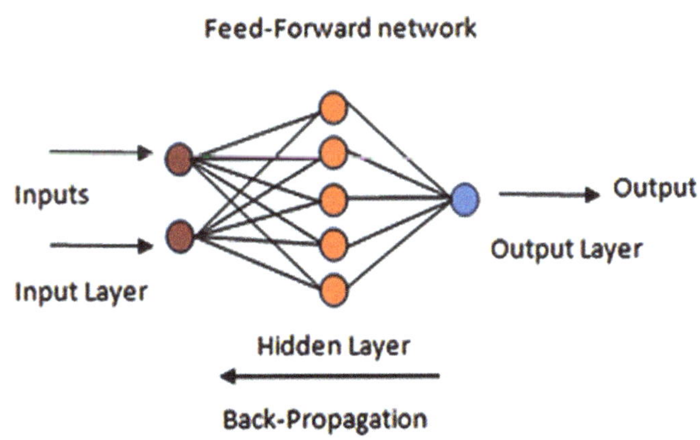

The training data set passed at the input layer. In the network, on the intermediate layer, each connection is assigned a weight. These weights are values which are learned from the events.

Support Vector Machines

A support vector machine (SVM) is also a machine learning algorithm which is used for classification and regression analysis. SVM follows the approach of supervised learning.(Kavakiotis et.al, 2017) This technique works by dividing data in to two categories. The outcome produced by SVM is in the form of graph with sorted data which are separated by margins between the two. SVM can be used in text categorization, image classification, handwriting recognition etc.

Figure 6. Support vector machine

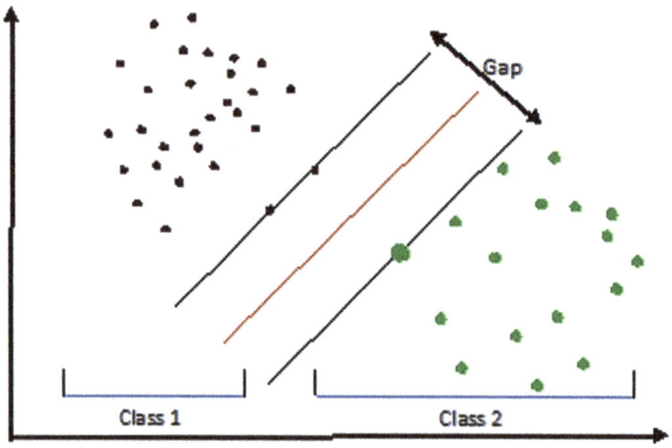

Apriori Algorithm

Apriori algorithm works by finding out most frequent item sets from large collection of data. The frequent item sets are discovered with the help of candidate generation (Kulkarni et.al, 2017). The algorithm is called Apriori just because the new item sets are generated on each stage by using prior knowledge. It follows the approach also called level-wise search where 'k' number of frequent item sets are used to find 'k+1' number of item sets.(Freeda and Florence, 2017)And for improving the efficiency of search, Apriori property is used for reducing the search space.

Apriori Property states that "All non-empty subsets of frequent item set must also be frequent".

The key concept of Apriori algorithm is its support measure factor.

Apriori algorithm follows bottom up approach, where frequent subsets are extended one item at a time.

K-Means Clustering

K-Means clustering technique is the most popular clustering algorithms in terms of its usage, its simplicity, ease of implementation along with its efficiency when considered the feature of complexity of algorithm. (Aggarwal and Aggarwal, 2012)

The grouping of k-means is based on proximity to each other according to the Euclidean distance. This algorithm works by partitioning 'n' number of objects from 'k' number of clusters. Here 'k' is an input parameter and partitioned a set of 'n' objects from 'k' cluster. The average value of the object is taken as the resemblance to the parameter to form the cluster. Cluster mean is being formed by selecting 'k' number of objects randomly. By comparing the similarities with other objects, the other objects are assigned clusters. For each data vector, the algorithm works by calculating the distance between the data vector and each centroid using the equation (Shah and Singh, 2012). The procedural steps of the K-means algorithm are shown through flow chart as given below:

Figure 7. Flow chart of working of k-means algorithm

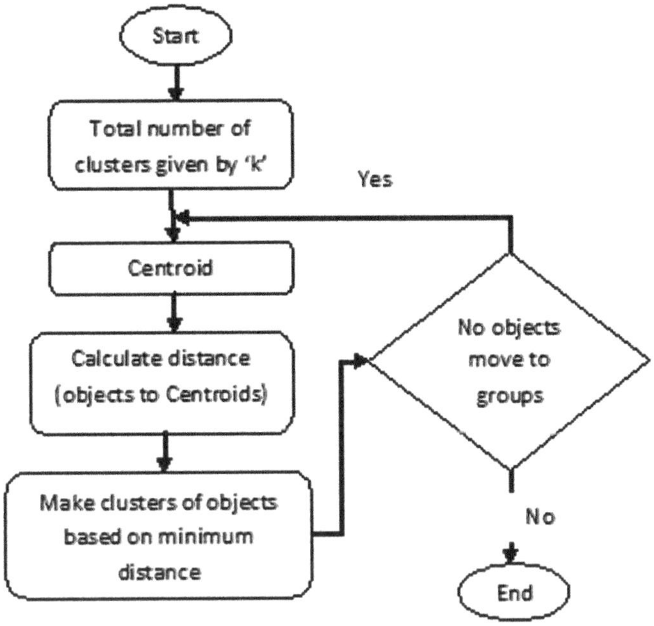

Natural Language Processing

Natural Language Processing (NLP) is used for enabling computers for understanding and processing human languages (Meystre et.al, 2008). As language is regarded as the way of communication by which one can speak, read and write. There arises a question that, can humans communicate with computers in their natural language? It becomes a challenge for developing NLP based applications because computers required structured data, and human speech is unstructured and ambiguous.

NLP research emphasizes on building computational models that can understand natural language. "Natural language" is language that is used to describe any language used by human beings, to differentiate it from programming languages and other data representation languages used by computers (Meystre et.al, 2008).

Technically, the main task of NLP is to make programmed computers for analyzing and processing huge amount of natural language data (Jindal and Sharma, 2018).

Phases in NLP: There are six phases in Natural language processing which are listed as below.

Phonetics

It deals with how the words get pronounced.

Morphological Analysis

In this phase individual words are analyzed and tokens such as punctuations are separated.

Syntactic Analysis

In this phase, linear sequencing of words is done to form structures showing relationship within words.

Semantic Analysis

In this phase, the structure that got created in earlier phase is assigned with meanings.

Discourse Integration

In this phase, dependencies among sentences are identified, which may lead to influencing the meaning of sentences.

Pragmatic Analysis

In this, the structure of sentence from above said phase is reinterpreted just to find out what it actually meant.

COMPARISON OF DIFFERENT DATA MINING TECHNIQUES

Below table gives the comparison based study of various data mining techniques along with their advantages and limitations.

LITERATURE REVIEW

For Literature review, approx.28 research articles related to mining of data or information in health care sector have been reviewed. The data given below explains the study of all these articles along with their description, journal info, author info, year of publication, datasets used, along with techniques used.

Text Based Mining Technique in Healthcare

Text mining can be used in healthcare industry, as the data in this industry is very much unstructured (Kavakiotis et.al, 2017). With the help of text mining implicit knowledge can be acquired that is hidden in the unstructured text. Information can be discovered from biomedical texts, such as identifying the reactions of any drug on patients, or in making prior decision about the symptoms drawn from patients.

Some of the research papers have been reviewed illustrating the use of text based mining in healthcare industry.

Figure 8. Natural language processing

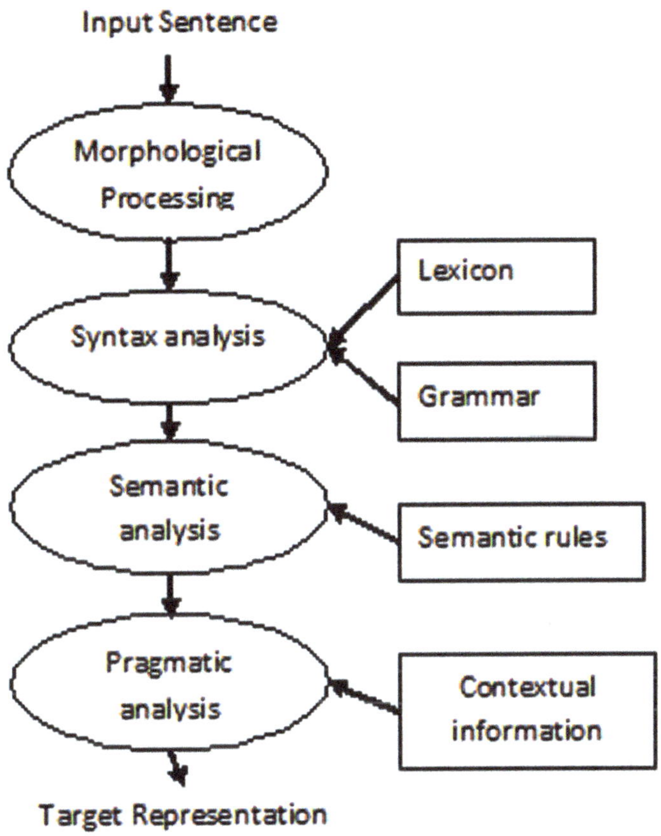

1. The researcher T. Katrien, et.al have come up with their article published in the year 2020, related to mining in healthcare data, had worked on text mining for extracting the information from healthcare data. The author uses the questionnaire for collecting the required information so that the data set can be generated for making decisions for betterment of health of patients. A total of 1661 patients analyzed from 2018 to 2019 to make questionnaire. The author uses the target domain as data related to smoking status in cardiovascular population. (Katrien et.al, 2020)
2. Another researcher Raja U,et.al have published an article based on text based mining in healthcare data in the year 2008, have elaborated the concept of text mining used in healthcare through the study. The author focuses on predictive modeling approach generated by text mining on Electronic clinical records. These models uses patients data or records and thus on its basis the errors in medical field are identified that results in deaths and significantly reducing these errors.(Raja U. et.al, 2008)
3. The researcher Frances B. Maguire et.al have come up with an idea of mining the data on the basis of text, where data considered was related to cancer registries, duly published in the year 2019, had also worked on text mining in healthcare by using the data set comprises of lung cancer data. The author uses flowchart for explanation. Author uses the technique of SAS along with text mining to find accurate and efficient lung cancer treatment text fields. (Maguire et.al, 2019)

Table 1. Comparison of different data mining techniques

S. No.	Techniques	Advantages	Limitations
1.	Text Based Mining	· Its predicting capability can benefit in finding best results. · Easy to implement. · Used widely in industries.	· Large number of large databases makes it slower to performance. · Requires large storage space. · Hard to handle with synonyms.
2.	Association Rule Based Mining	· Can relate many topics on the basis of associativity between them	· Large number of rule discovered. · Non-interesting rules are also discovered.
3.	Pattern Based Mining	· Used to generate compact and effective structures based on frequent patterns. · Similarity search can be achieved. · Provides high accuracy of results.	· Recognition of patterns is itself a tedious job. · Consumes time and space as new patterns needs to be stored.
4.	Keyword Based Mining	· Generates good precision and recall factors, and a large number of terms that are highly relevant yet non-obvious to the given input keyword.	· Faces problem with words having multiple meaning.
5.	Machine Learning	· Effective in generating predictive models	· Requires massive store of training data · Complexity level is high
6.	Neural Network	· Ability to work with incomplete data. · Used for predictive modeling. · Can be used for regression analysis and pattern recognition. · Fault tolerance · Self-learning results are drawn from experience within networks, deriving conclusions from a complex set of information.	· Consumes vast amount of memory, time and cost. · Hard to determine network structure. · Draws effective results but costly.
7.	Support Vector Machines	· Works well when margin of separation between classes is clear. · More effective in high dimensional spaces. · Effective in cases where number of dimensions is greater than the number of samples. · Memory efficient	· not suitable for large data sets. · Performance starts degrading when data set is noisy. · In cases where number of features for each data point exceeds the number of training data sample, the SVM performance starts lowering down.
8.	Apriori Algorithm	· Used for finding frequent item sets and association rules.	· High execution time · All subsets of frequent item sets has to be frequent too.
9.	K-Means Clustering	· Faster computation · Works well with similar clusters means same size and density.	· Does not work well if the clusters are of different sizes and different densities.
10.	Natural Language Processing	· Accuracy of result increases if relevant amount of information is provided. · Provides answers to questions in natural language.	· Does not have user interface. · can built for a single and specific task only · it is unable to adapt to new domains and problems because of limited functions.

4. Author Wencheng Sun et.al published their article based on mining the text in medical health records, in the year 2018, had worked on data processing and text mining on Electronic health records. Author uses text mining through named entity recognition(NER) and relation extraction(RE) approach, along with machine learning technique considering the fact that the data in medical fields is unstructured. (Kavakiotis et.al, 2017)
5. The researcher Revathi M. Nair et.al presented their survey paper on medical text mining, published in the year 2014, on text mining in healthcare explaining various text mining techniques that can be used in health care industry.(Revathi M. Nair and L. Sindh, 2019)

The table 2 given below will briefly explains the literature review of different research articles by different authors along with their working mode, advantages, datasets referred, and also the limitations of using the technique in healthcare system data.

Table 2. Brief literature review of text based mining technique in healthcare

Method	Related Work	Working Mode	Data Set	Advantages	Limitation
Text Based Mining	· Researcher T. Katrien, et.al · Raja U,et.al · Frances B. Maguire et.al · Wencheng Sun et.al · Revathi M. Nair et.al	· Use of Questionnaire. · Use of Predictive modelling approach · Combining technique of SAS with text mining · Use of NER & RE approach	· smoking status in cardiovascular population · Cancer registries	· Easy to implement on limited data of patients.	· Restricted to limited number of patients record. · Quality of evaluation is dependent on quality as well as completeness of input data.

Association Rule Based Mining in Healthcare

Lot of work has been done in this area of rule based mining in healthcare informatics. The Key amongst the uses is in matching patient's diagnosis with symptoms which correlates a lot with the use of knowledge based systems. Though, it is tough for inducing reliable rules in diagnostics from set of infinite number of permutations and combinations of symptoms because the resulting hypotheses can also have unsatisfactory prediction accuracy (Kulkarni et.al,2017). However, many researchers have come up with further enhancements and ideas in association rule generations for improving the prediction levels up to 90% along with (Park et.al, 2014) supervised learning methods.

Some of the research papers have been reviewed illustrating the use of association rule based mining in healthcare industry.(Kangethe et.al, 2014)

1. The researcher Chun An Chou, et. all(Chun An Chou et.al, 2020) with paper explaining rule based mining in health related data duly published in the year 2020, had worked on association rule based mining for extracting the information from healthcare data by discovering rules between patients data and diagnosis information etc.. This paper helps in identifying unplanned transfer to ICU from emergency department due to unexpected clinical deterioration is formulated as supervised learning problem. The target domain used was that of data set of unplanned ICU transferred patients record. This data set was collected between years 2007 and 2010. The author used rule based analytical methods for finding significant associations between risk factors with optimization and data mining. The author opted for this so as to improve critical care quality and also preventing mortality. 4 sub groups of patient were considered for making data set like:
    a. Infection,
    b. Cardiovascular/respiratory disease,
    c. Gastro-intestinal,
    d. Neurological disease

2. Another researcher Nikunj Domadia,et.al come up with their paper published in the year 2019, had worked on heart disease related data set of patients for generating association rules. The authors chose vertically partitioned data from healthcare data set.(Domadia et.al, 2019)
3. Researcher Akbar Telikani, et.al presented a survey paper on association rule mining duly published in year 2020 by describing the association rule mining in health care. The author reviewed the rules according to meta heuristic approach.(Telikani et.al, 2020)
4. The researcher Ashwini Rajendra Kulkarni, et. all have all published an article in the year 2017, based on association rule mining in healthcare. had worked on association rule mining along with apriori algorithm for finding frequent patterns, correlations, associations, casual structures among the sets of items or objects in transaction database, relational database. The data set used was based on Viral infective diseases.(Kulkarni et.al,2017)
5. Another researcher Stephen M. Kang'ethe, et.al with paper based on Extraction diagnosis patterns in electronic medical records using association rule mining published in the year 2014, had worked on Extraction of diagnosis patterns in electronic medical records using association rule mining with apriori algorithm. The target data set domain was Hypertension, depression, lipoids, diabeties mellitus data etc.(Kangethe et.al, 2014)
6. The researcher D.Sheilla Freeda, et.al have published an article on analysis of disease with the help of rule based mining in the year of 2017, The author also presented rule based mining methods of ARM along with SETM, AIS, Apriori algorithms. The data used for mining was comprise of diabetes data of patients used as target data domain. The claims SETM approach as the best method among other 3approach through study.(Freeda and Florence, 2017)
7. Another researcher M.Harahap, et.al published their article in the year 2017,mainly focusing on association rule based mining on disease population so that the medical needs for a patient can be recommended. The researcher used 10 dominant disease data set from patients prescriptions. These prescriptions then used for identifying the relationship between diseases and medicines and hence helps medical health professionals in curing disease and treating the patients. Disease and related medicines were used for recommendation of appropriate medicine. Prediction of disease is done through medicinal drugs given to patients. The author used rule mining approach along with k-means clustering and apriori algorithm.(Harahap et.al, 2017)
8. The author Lakshmi K.s.,et.al, also published their article in the year 2017, uses multicriteria for decision making by using association rule based mining.. This is the reviewed paper based study. The author considers the Correlation b/w diseases, diseases and symptoms, diseases and medicines. New methods for extraction of association rule from medical health records using NLP techniques were discussed. (Lakshmi K.s., G.Vadivu et.al, 2017)
9. The researcher Wasif Altaf, et.al come up with their survey paper on applications of rule based mining in medical health related data duly published in the year 2017 explaining how association rule mining is used in healthcare industry. (Altaf et.al, 2017)

The table given below will briefly explains the literature review of different research articles by different authors along with their working mode, advantages, datasets referred, and also the limitations of using the technique in healthcare system data.

Table 3. Brief literature review of association rule based mining in healthcare

Method	Related Work	Working Mode	Data Set	Advantages	Limitation
Association Rule Based Mining	· Researcher Chun An Chou, et.al · Nikunj Domadia,et.al · Akbar Telikani, et.al · Ashwini Rajendra Kulkarni, et.al · Stephen M. Kang'ethe, et.al · D.Sheilla Freeda, et.al · M.Harahap, et.al · Lakshmi K.s.,et. al · Wasif Altaf, et.al	· Use significant associations between risk factors with optimization and data mining. · Use of vertically partitioned data. · Identify relationships amongst a large set of variables in a given dataset. · Use of Meta heuristic approach · Use of Apriori algorithm · Prediction of disease through medicinal drugs.	· Unplanned ICU transfer patients record · Related to Heart disease · Related to Viral infective disease · Data related to diabetes mellitus data	· Helps in associating many topics. · Better prediction of diseases. · Amalgamation of different algorithms for finding association rules. · Training is faster.	· Large number of rules generated. · Non-interesting rules are also generated. · Different medicine names under same chemical structure. · Low algorithm performance

Pattern Based Mining in Healthcare

Pattern based mining can be used in healthcare industry for predicting the interesting patterns from time series data or patients detailed data from electronic health records. Some of the researchers are working in this area. Some research work done by various researchers have been reviewed and presented in this paper.

1. The researcher Jungsik Park, et.al with paper focusing mainly on fibromyalgia pain for identifying clinical distinctions duly published in the year 2014, had worked on fibromyalgia, a term in body pain. The author targeted the data set for doing research by collecting 399 memoires from FM data/ group website. The techniques used for fetching the required data was mainly pattern mining with keyword based text mining.(Park et.al 2014)
2. Another researcher O. Metsker, published their paper on pattern based mining in the year 2017, had worked on cardiology dataset for determining patterns based upon text mining done in healthcare. Data of patients treated from 2009 to 2016 in the cardiology ward in Almazov National Medical Research Centre was considered as target data set for performing research. (Metsker et.al, 2017)

The table given below will briefly explains the literature review of different research articles by different authors along with their working mode, advantages, datasets referred, and also the limitations of using the technique in healthcare system data.

Table 4. Brief literature review of pattern based mining in healthcare

Method	Related Work	Working Mode	Data Set	Advantages	Limitation
Pattern Based Mining	· Researcher Jungsik Park, et.al · O. Metsker	· Use of keyword based text mining. · Use of website for collecting information.	· Data related to fibromyalgia pain in patient · Data related to cardiology	· Easy to implement. · Use of pattern mining with keyword based text mining helps in extracting meaningful information from large set of input data.	· Extracted patterns are unstructured. · Required to structure the results.

Machine Learning in Healthcare

Machine learning in health care used for classification of patients with certain diseases and analyzing the data from large data store containing health related data or can say electronic health records from various healthcare departments.

Some research work has been done in this area and some of which is explained below through literature review.

1. The researcher named Hamed Majidi with his fellow researchers produced an article in the field of healthcare about predicting the likelihood of survival of patients suffering from cancer through machine learning technique. The author had worked on patients data related to cancer and patients suffering from chronic diseases as the target data set and builds the predicting models through machine learning method. The author had considered the data related to disease like: breast cancer, female genital cancers and prostate, and urinal cancer. The article was published in the year 2015 in the journal of Elsevier journal. (Majidi Zolbanin et.al, 2015)
2. The Researcher M. Maniruzzaman, et.al has come up with their research article based on machine learning. The author presented the article in the year 2017. The author used data set from health care data targeting diabetes related data of patients. The author had worked on classification of patients with diabetes from rest of the patients records with the help of machine learning technique. Data is analysed using cross validation approach. Total 768 patients records were taken of which 268 patients were having diabetes and 500 were controlled. (Maniruzzaman et.al, 2017)
3. Another author I.Kavakiotis, et.al come up with their research article on machine learning duly published in the year 2017. The author had worked on prediction and diagnosis of diabetes on patients. The target dataset used was of diabetic records of patients from healthcare related data. The technique of SVM along with learning algorithms and machine learning was used. (Kavakiotis et.al, 2017)
4. Another researcher Santiago Estaben and et.al have come up with their research article for developing and validating various different algorithms for classifying patient data from electronic health records data repository. The author uses the target data set consisting of data of patients suffering from diabetes from health records. The author have drawn 2 sample from year 2015 (n=800) and 2005 (n=1663) for derivation and validation where the inclusion criteria used was age= >=40 & <80 years of patient. The article was published in the year 2017. The machine learning technique along with neural network approach was used for fetching the required data and generating learning experiences. (Esteban et.al,2017)

The table given below will briefly explains the literature review of different research articles by different authors along with their working mode, advantages, datasets referred, and also the limitations of using the technique in healthcare system data.

Table 5. Brief literature review of machine learning in healthcare

Method	Related Work	Working Mode	Data Set	Advantages	Limitation
Machine Learning	· Researcher Hamed Majidi et.al · M. Maniruzzaman et.al · I.Kavakiotis, et.al · Santiago Estaben et.al	· Based on biological human brain system. · Use of predictive approach with supervised learning approach · Use of SVM for prediction of diseases · Uses neural network approach for developing and validating algorithm for classification of patient's record	· Data related to cancer · Data related to diabetes	· More accurate predictive models are built · Can helps in identifying relationships amongst dependent as well as independent variables. · More accurate results	· Hard to implement. · Hard to interpret. · High processing time if neural network is large. · Quality of evaluation is dependent on rules feed into the model for prediction.

Some more literature review is done in the field of data mining in healthcare related data. Some reviews are listed below:

1. The researchers Fatemeh et.al have published their survey based paper on discovering the knowledge from healthcare related data in 2019 year. The author focuses on knowledge data discovery in data mining in healthcare. The author surveyed research papers from past 10 years. The author concluded his survey by giving suggestions on making the strategy work on more data sets, and considering more database.(Soleimani Roozbahani et.al, 2019)
2. The Researcher Carlo et.al also has surveyed various papers from past years in the area of healthcare. The authors have discussed various researches and issues in the field of healthcare and also elaborated how AI can be used to enhance E-health. This survey paper was published in the year 2019.(Combi et.al, 2019)
3. The other author Estela S.Estape et.al have also done the survey based study on using data mining in healthcare for enhancing the care provided to patients and also thereby reducing the cost of it. This survey based paper has got published in the current year 2020.(Estape et.al, 2020)
4. Another author Subhash Chandra Pandey has published his review based paper on how one can improve the care provided to patients in terms of health. The author focuses on the impact data mining has on healthcare for enhancing the medical care and also reducing the cost of medical care. Also have discussed various techniques of data mining used in healthcare along with their pros and cons respectively. The author have concluded that, as the healthcare data is unstructured so collaborating more than one data mining techniques together for providing better results rather than using single technique. This review based paper was published in year 2016.(Subhash Chandra Pandey, 2016)
5. The researcher S. M. Meystre et. all have done their literature based review on finding patterns and then fetching out these patterns from medical based unstructured data. The author categorizes the medical text in to two categories: biomedical text and clinical text. The author uses NLP (Natural

Language Processing) technique for mining the information for further future predictions. This article has got published in the year 2008. (Freeda and Florence, 2017)

6. There was another review based study published in 2014 year by authors Mathew Herland et.al based on big data in healthcare informatics. The author proposes various levels of studying data in healthcare like molecural, tissues, patients and population based levels. Each level has certain level of questions for extracting the information so that care provided to patients can be enhanced. (Herlandet.al, 2014)
7. Another survey based paper was published by Wencheng Sun et.al in the year 2017, majerly focusing on the various different data mining techniques that can be used in health care data analysis along with their key features. (Wencheng Sun et.al, 2017)
8. Another review based paper by authors Ogundele I.O et.al published in the year 2018, comprises the review based study on techniques, tools, processes, and related works of data mining in the field of healthcare data analysis. The author concludes the article by explaining health analytics stages, data (source and transformation), and specific areas of application in data mining. This knowledge will then helps in reducing the cost spent and making accurate decisions from availability of voluminous and complex heath care data. (Ogundele I.O. et.al, 2018)

The data stated above briefly explains the literature review of different research articles by different authors along with their paper titles, author details, year of publication, journal details, data set referred, techniques used, a brief description of work done, along with limitations of using the technique in healthcare system data.

As data mining plays a vital role in health care analytics. In healthcare, the services provided to patients in order to cure the diseases they are suffering from, these medical practitioners can provide more effective and efficient services to patients only if the data extracted from medical data sources is knowledgeable and as per the requirements. This data extraction can be done in the form of patterns for making the right decision for solving the problem. All this is done to perform health analytics.

HEALTH ANALYTICS

The data extraction part from data mining in healthcare sector plays an important part in providing proper and sufficient care to patients.(A.Perer, 2012) These decisions can be made effective with the use of tools like, tools using statistics, tools based on computer, tools based on mathematical computation, tools using information technology etc. these tools helps medical practitioners, healthcare providers in making policies regarding better health care, also having improved working environments.

The health care related data are first collected from various health resources like hospitals, clinics, laboratories. After this, the collected data is then preprocessed. After this stage, the preprocessed data is then transformed. All this is done to perform health analytics.

There are four different ways in which health analytics can be performed and are mentioned below:

1. Descriptive analysis
2. Discovery analysis
3. Predictive analysis
4. Prescriptive analysis

Descriptive Analysis

In this analysis, the data is represented in the graphical form so that the medical practitioners or the health professionals can interpret the data easily for making the corrective diagnostic decisions. With this method, the patient details like, symptoms, diseases diagnosed, number of patients treated with diseases, procedure of diagnosis followed by doctors etc all these data details can be given for improving the conditions and health of patients. In short, descriptive analysis helps in giving the summarize details of the past (historical) data so that valid and valuable information can be further generated. Descriptive analysis can be done by individual (A.Perer, 2012) faculty of medical field since it is easy to use and the simplest method.

Discovery Analysis

In this method, the knowledge has been discovered through data mining process in healthcare sector in order to conduct new experiments in the medical field. For example, one can discover altogether new drugs for curing a disease from previously known drugs. Discovery analysis (A.Perer, 2012) also helps in discovering new treatment methods for curing the diseases also helps in discovering new finding about the disease and medications can be used for prevention of disease from past known discoveries.

Predictive Analysis

Predictive analysis mainly emphasizes on the information to be used. It gives the insight of what can happen in the near future. Thus it collects all the information and data from the past histories and then generates patterns from the datasets information extracted from history for predicting the future. As the healthcare related data is voluminous and very vast, so this feature makes predictive analysis techniques to be used in data mining. Several questions can be answered through this technique like: what are the medicinal drugs that can be used for treating the patients? What are the adverse effects of the disease on others? What are the signs and symptoms? How patients are reacting to a particular medicinal drug? Predicting (A.Perer, 2012) all these results of patients and then allocating resources properly. Predictive analysis also helps in identifying future probabilities and trends for predicting future occurrences.

Prescriptive Analysis

This analysis is applied when we have multiple options for solving a health related problem for giving the best prescriptive analysis. Several questions can be answered through this like: keeping in mind, how does someone respond to the potential future events, It helps in the field of healthcare in providing treatments and giving prescriptions (A.Perer, 2012) of medicinal drugs. Doctors can compare several medicinal drugs by comparing their positive effects and side effects before prescribing. Thus in this way, prescriptive analysis can be used in providing most accurate results from a problem.

DATA MINING APPLICATIONS

There are various areas in the field of healthcare where data mining can be used for better outcomes. Data mining plays a vital role in giving treatments to patients suffering from diseases, diagnosis of disease related decisions, preventive care, giving away prescriptions thus providing better care to patients by optimizing results. Since the health care related data is vast and unstructured and has information like patients record, personal information of patients, treatments provided, drugs prescribed, over all diagnosis status of patients and also the cost of diagnosis. All these data or information are needed for analyzing purposes and for extracting meaningful data and knowledge from healthcare related data.

Data mining applications in healthcare are listed below.

- Treatment effectiveness
- Healthcare management
- Fraud & abuse
- Hospital Infection Control
- Smarter Treatment Techniques

FUTURE RESEARCH OPPORTUNITIES

Here is the list of different research gaps found out during the literature review of various different research articles illustrating the implementation issues from previous work. The list given below also gives suggestions for future research opportunities.

- Research can be done to find out best correlations between condition of patient and reactions of drugs on them. This could help health professionals in giving treatments that may not be evident due to clinical research alone.
- As 90% of health data is unstructured, so research can be done to extract relevant information from unstructured data is itself is a challenge. So no single data mining techniques can give good results alone. And needs to do collaboration of more than one technique for better outcome also taking care of privacy of patient's data.
- There is a problem of process and method for organizing and classifying large amount of text. So research can be done on large amount of data.
- Can associate diseases together through support and confidence factor for finding out more specific causal relationship present within them for predicting more accurate diseases and then cure it with right medicine.
- More information about the co-morbid diseases can be further added to datasets for improving the effectiveness of prediction based models, and hence will result in lowering down the treatment costs.
- As different pharmaceutical companies uses different labels or names on medicines with same chemical composition. So research can be done in generating rules based on composition of medicines rather than names would considerably improve the prediction accuracy of system.

- As the quality of evaluation is dependent on quality as well as completeness of input data, and through algorithm for retrieving information for healthcare, the effect of time and clinical practice on the outcome and implicating misclassification needs to be taken into consideration.
- Data mining with machine learning in healthcare sector on big enriched datasets can be applied for prediction and diagnosis of diseases and can be used for identifying patterns for best results.
- As medical dictionary has medical terms in vast number hence needs standardization, as practioners uses different terms for diagnosis, issue of privacy of patient's personal data in EMR.
- Research can be done in health informatics by focusing on data from all levels to find correlations and connections between them by giving doctors more ways of diagnosis, treatments and helping their patients.
- Implementation of neural network approach can be done for accurate results.

CONCLUSION

As this is the review based paper, here in this paper previous work done in the field of data analysis in healthcare through data mining is reviewed. In this research article, the background, definition, and processes of data mining, techniques used in healthcare are discussed, benefits and drawback of those techniques is also mentioned. Also how these techniques were being used in prediction and providing better health care solutions to patients, and health practitioners as well. The descriptive, predictive, prescriptive and discovery health analytics were introduced. Sources and transformation of health data were discussed. Related works of previous research were reviewed in the literature review section, and specific application areas of data mining in healthcare were also mentioned. Along with it, the future research opportunities were discussed briefly in the end.

REFERENCES

Aggarwal, N., & Aggarwal, K. (2012). Comparative Analysis of kmeans and Enhanced Kmeans clustering algorithm for data mining. *International Journal of Scientific & Engineering Research.*

Altaf, Shahbaz, & Guergachi. (2017). Applications of association rule mining in health informatics, *AI Journal Under Springer, 47*, 313-340.

Chou, Cao, Weng, & Tsai. (2020). Mixed integer optimization approach to learning association rules for unplanned ICU transfer. *AI in Medicines Journal, 103.*

Combi & Pozzi. (2019). Clinical information systems and artificial intelligence: Recent research trends. *Yearbook of Medical Infirmatics Thieme Journal, 28*(1), 83-94.

Daliri. (2017). Data Mining for Health Care Industry: A Practical Machine Learning Tool. *Int. Res. J. Multidiscip. Stud., 3*(4).

Domadia, N., & Rao, U. P. (2019). Privacy preserving distributed association rule minning approach on vertically partitioned health care data. Procedia Computer Science, 148, 303-312.

Estape, Ortiz, Mays, & Laras. (2020). Data mining to transform clinical & translational research findings into precision health, AI in precision health under academic press. *Science Direct Journal*, 149-173.

Esteban, Tablado, Peper, Mahumud, & Ricci, Kopitowski, & Terrasa. (2017). Development and validation of various phenotyping algorithms for diabetes mellitus using data from EHR's. *Computer Method and Program in Bio-Medicine of Elsevier Journal, 152*, 53–70.

Garg, N., & Sharma, K. (2020). Sentiment Analysis of Events on Social Web. *International Journal of Innovative Technology and Exploring Engineering, 9*(6).

Han, J., Pei, J., & Kamber, M. (2011). *Data mining: concepts and techniques*. Elsevier.

Harahap, M., Husein, A. M., & Lubis, F. R. (2017). Mining association rule based on the disease population for recommendations of medical need. Journal of Physics, 1007.

Herland, Khoshgoftaar, & Wald. (2014). A review of data mining using big data in health informatics. *Journal of Big Data.*

Inbavalli. (2015). Efficient Analysis of Frequent item set Association Rule Mining Methods. *International Journal of Scientific & Engineering Research, 6*(4), 1-23. http://www.ijser.org/researchpaper%5cefficient-Analysis-of-Frequent-itemset-Association-Rule-Mining-Methods.pdf

Jain, D., Kumar, V., Khanduja, D., Sharma, K., & Bateja, R. (2019). A detailed study of big data in health care: case study of Brenda and IBM Watson. *International Journal of Recent Technology and Engineering, 7*(5).

Jindal & Sharma. (2018). A Review on Sentiment Classification: Natural Language Understanding. *Bentham Science Journal, Recent Patents on Engineering.*

Kangethe & Wagacha. (2014). Extracting diagnosis patterns in electronic medical records using association rule mining. *International Journal of Computer Applications, 108.*

Katrien, Groenhof, Koers, Blasse, de Groot, Grobbee, Bots, Asselbergs, Lely, & Haitjema. (2020). Data mining information from EHR producing high yield and accuracy for current smoking status. *Journal of Clinical Epidemiology, 118*, 100-106.

Kavakiotis, I. (2017). *Machine learning and data mining methods in diabetes research. Computational and Structural Biotechnology, 15.*

Kulkarni & Mundhe. (2017). Data mining technique: an implementation of association rule mining in healthcare. *IARJSET Journal, 4*(7).

Lakshmi, K. S., & Vadivu, G. (2017). Extracting association rule from medical health records using multi criteria decision analysis. Procedia Computer Science, 115, 290–295.

Maguire, Morris, Parikh-Patel, Cress, Keegan, Li, Lin, & Kizer. (2019). A text mining approach to obtain detailed treatment information from free text fields in population based cancer registries: a study of non-small cell lung cancer in California. *Plos One Journal, 14*(2).

Maniruzzaman, Kumar, Nishithkumar, Abedin, Islam, Suri, El-Baz, & Suri. (2017). Comparative approach for classification of diabetes mellitus data: machine learning paradigm. *Computer Method and Program in Biomedicine, 152*, 23-34.

Metsker, Bolgova, Yakovlev, Funkner, & Kovalchuk. (2017). Pattern based mining in E HR for complex clinical process analysis. Elsevier Journal, 119, 197-206.

Meystre, S. M., Savova, G. K., Kipper-Schuler, K. C., & Hurdle, J. F. (2008). *Extracting information from textual documents in E HR*. IMIA Yearbookof Medical Informatics.

Ogundele, I.O., Popoola, O.L., Oyesola, O.O., & Orija, K.T. (2018). A review on data mining in health care. *International Journal of Advanced Research in Computer Engineering & Technology, 7*(9).

Pandey. (2016). Data mining techniques for medical data: a review. *International Conference on Signal Pricessing, Comm., Power and Embedded Sys (SCOPES).*

Park, J., & Ryu, Y. U. (2014). FM: fibromyalgia: chronic pain: text mining to identify clinical distinctions and patient concerns. International Medical Journal of Experimental and Clinical Research.

Perer, A. (2012). Healthcare analytics for clinical and non-clinical settings. *Proceedings of CHI Conference.*

Raja, U., Mitchell, T., Day, T., & Hardin, J. M. (2008). Text mining in healthcare, applications and opportunities. *Journal of Healthcare Information Management, 22*(3), 52–56. PMID:19267032

Revathi, M. (2014). Survey on medical text mining. *International Journal of Computers and Applications.*

Rout, S. S., Verma, A., Choudhary, A. K., Sharma, K., & Chawla, P. (2020). Convolution Neural Networks for Plant Disease Identification. *International Journal of Engineering Research and Applications.* www.ijera.com

Russell, S., & Norvig, P. (2003). Artificial Intelligence: A Modern Approach (2nd ed.). Prentice Hall.

Shah, S., & Singh, M. (2012). Comparison of A Time Efficient Modified K-Mean Algorithm with K-Mean and K-Medoids algorithm. *International Conference on Communication Systems and Network Technologies.* 10.1109/CSNT.2012.100

Sharma, A., Sharma, R., Sharma, V. K., & Shrivatava, V. (2014). Application of Data Mining–A Survey Paper. *Int. J. Comput. Sci. Inf. Technol., 5*(2), 2023–2025.

Sheilla Freeda, D., & Lilly Florence, M. (2017). An overview of disease analysis using association rule mining. IJSER, 8(4).

Soleimani-Roozbahani, F., Ghatari, A. R., & Radfar, R. (2019). Knowledge discovery from a more than a decade studies on healthcare big data systems: a scientometrics study. Journal of Big Data, 6.

Sun, W., Cai, Z., Li, Y., Liu, F., Fang, S., & Wang, G. (2018). Data processing and text mining technologies on E-medical records. Hindawi Journal of Health Care Engineering.

Sun, W., Cai, Z., Liu, F., Fang, S., & Wang, G. (2017). A survey of data mining technology on electronic medical records. *IEEE: 19th International Conference on E-Health and Networking, Conference-19.*

Telikani, A., Gandomi, A. H., & Shahbahrami, A. (2020). A survey of evolutionary computation for association rule mining. Information Science Under Elsevier Journal, 524, 318-352.

Tomari, Razali, Zakaria, & Nurshazwani. (2015). *An empirical framework for automatic red blood cell morphology identification and counting.* Academic Press.

Varghese, D. P., & Tintu, P. B. (2015). A Survey on Health Data using Data Mining Techniques. *Int. Res. J. Eng. Technol.*, *2*(7), 56–2395.

Wilson & Keilthe. (1999). *MIT encyclopaedia of the cognitive sciences.* MIT Press.

Zolbanin, Delen, & Zadeh. (2015). Predicting overall survivability in comorbidity of cancers: a data mining approach. *Decision Support Systems, 74*, 150-161.

Chapter 2
Detection of Diabetic Retinopathy With Mobile Application Using Deep Learning

Sercan Demirci
https://orcid.org/0000-0001-6739-7653
Ondokuz Mayıs University, Turkey

Ali Murat Çevik
Ondokuz Mayıs University, Turkey

İrem Türkü Çınar
Ondokuz Mayıs University, Turkey

Ceyhun Tüzün
Ondokuz Mayıs University, Turkey

ABSTRACT

High glucose level disrupts the structure of the retinal layer in the eyes and causes diabetic retinopathy which is characterized with new pathologic blood vessels in the eyes. Although diabetic retinopathy is not clear at the beginning of the disease, it is the most common problem in people who have diabetes and causes blindness or cloudy vision if it is not diagnosed at the beginning of the disease. For early diagnosis of diabetic retinopathy, regular fundus controls and examination of the edema in the vessels of the retina are made periodically by ophthalmologists. With in the scope of this study, it is made possible to provide the early diagnosis and the level of diabetic retinopathy by using deep learning, image processing methods, and convolutional neural networks of the retina. In order to provide ease and rapid of diagnosis of the diabetic retinopathy in daily life, the diagnosis protocol has been turned into a mobile application. With the mobile application, both the diagnosis and more regular results of the diabetic retinopathy can be obtained easily and practically.

DOI: 10.4018/978-1-7998-6527-8.ch002

INTRODUCTION

Technology made our life easier by facilitating our work in most areas by bringing new innovations every day. Although it has been suggested that the advancement of every technological development brings along various damages, technology makes daily life easier for people and finalizes problems that cannot be solved or even partially solved by certain and existing methods. These advantages have increased the place and importance of technology for humanity and have brought a new dimension to the functioning of our age and human life.

Recently, in addition to the development of computer and communication technologies, the technology area called artificial intelligence is also receiving a lot of attention. Artificial intelligence is known as offering or exploring science field by using algorithmic solutions to problems based on the behavior of humans and living beings (Russell, 2016).

Increasing technological developments with acceleration have made it inevitable to be included in our life and seen and used math-based systems such as artificial intelligence, image processing, machine learning, and deep learning. Undoubtedly, the medical world comes first among them (Foster, 2014). Artificial intelligence and its fields provide the opportunity to obtain an early diagnosis and give faster results for the treatment of disease (Karaboğa, 2011). Studies on this area are increasing and developing day by day.

The fact that artificial intelligence in especially human health is used for the diagnosis of disease and produces good results and also gives good signs for the research of diabetic retinopathy and causes the studies on this subject to become widespread. Therefore, bringing to the literature new studies is very important.

There are almost 415 million diabetic patients in the world. It was reported that approximately 285 million of them have diabetic retinopathy, and the 40 to 45 million diabetic patients who have diabetic retinopathy are seriously threatening to see (Christian Nordqvist, 2017). Diabetic retinopathy is one of the leading causes of blindness in the world (Christian Nordqvist, 2017). Therefore, ophthalmologists suggested that diabetic patients need a more frequent eye test. With the early diagnosis of diabetic retinopathy; it is possible to prevent blindness as a result of diabetes and to improve the patient's vision. According to studies, it is predicted that patients with diabetic retinopathy will reach 370 million by 2030. Although these numbers are very serious and undeniable, to parallel the studies conducted with the development of technology aim to raise the awareness of the potentially risky patients, as well as the patients who have been diagnosed, and to reduce the number of patients.

Symptoms of diabetic retinopathy may be evident by the patient only at an advanced stage, but an ophthalmologist can detect the symptoms before reaching this stage. It is very important that diabetic patients have eye test at least twice in a year. In this way, the chances of early diagnosis and treatment of the diabetic retinopathy increase. Most commonly used methods detecting the diabetic retinopathy are expanded eye examination, fluorescein angiography (FA), and optical coherence tomography (OCT) (Clairhurts Eye Care, 2019).

Figure 1. Ophthalmoscope
(Clairhurts Eye Care, 2019)

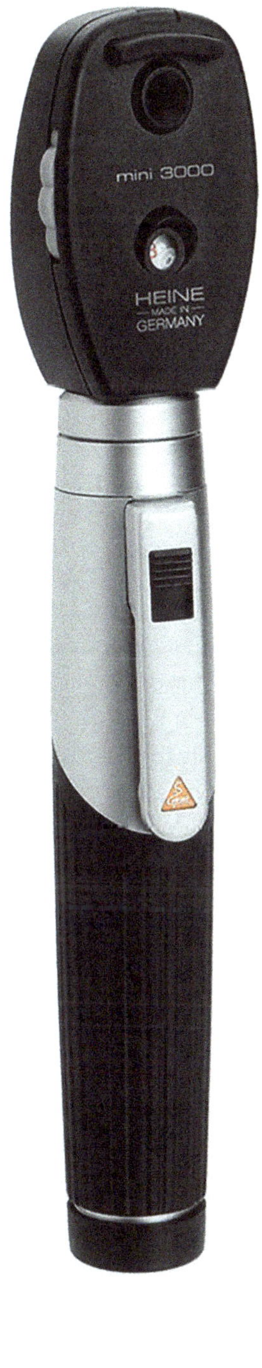

Technological systems such as artificial intelligence, image processing, deep learning, and machine learning are predicted to provide great assistance to medical professionals and students, the elderly, and people who are unfavorable in rural areas during the diagnosis and diagnosis stages of the disease. In this context, the methods used in the project and prepared the project benefited in a way that we can describe with a great degree in the stage of the project. In this study, the dataset was cleaned with the image processing method and made ready to use dataset. Data were prepared for the use of CNN technology during the deep learning phase.

Figure 2. Optical coherence tomography (OCT)
(Eye Care, 2019)

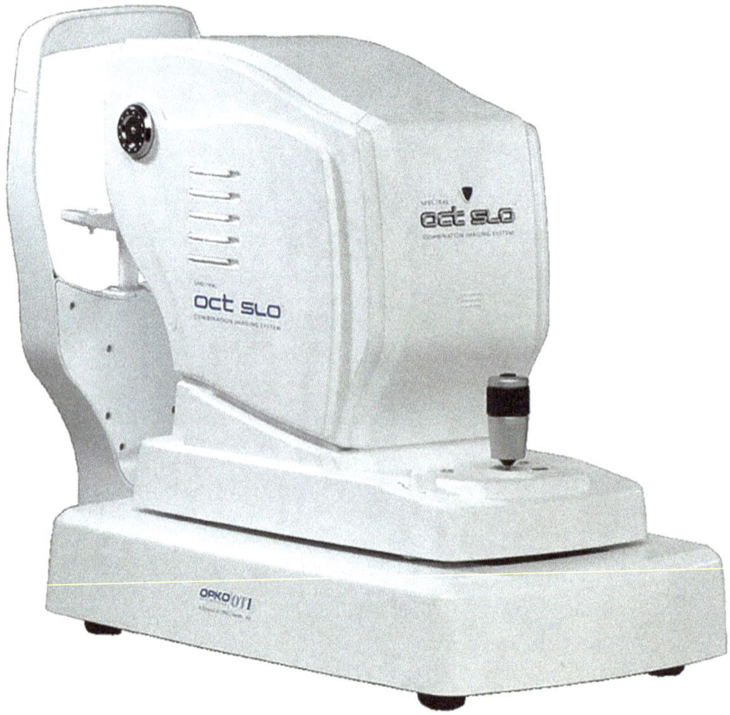

Figure 3. Image of healthy retina photo
(IEEE DataPort, 2019)

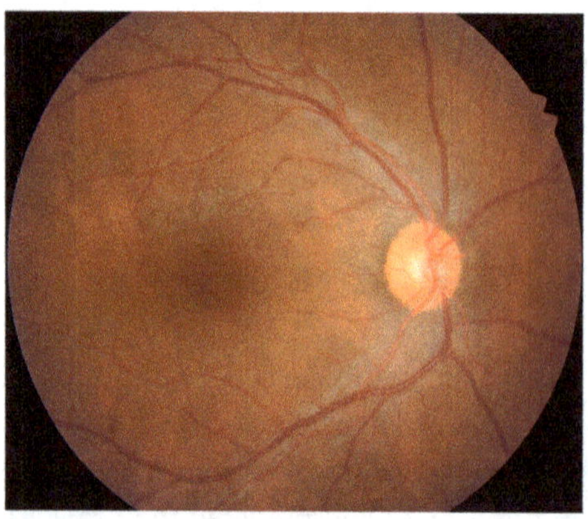

Figure 4. Image of retinal disease
(IEEE DataPort, 2019)

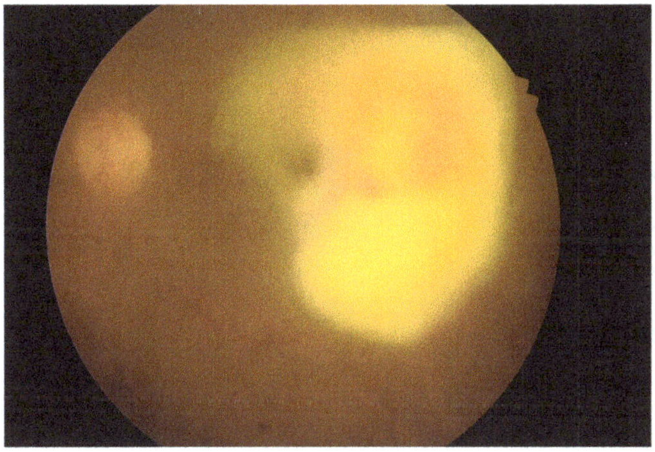

Convolutional Neural Networks (CNN) is preferred for use in this project because it has a high success rate in image processing-based subjects. Training and prediction processes of the artificial neural network have been completed and included in the mobile application (Hubel, 1968). In mobile application development, both Android and iOS operating systems showed high performance in the application. Dart programming language is preferred by using Flutter SDK. The mobile application was tested on both tablets and smartphones. In this artificial intelligence and mobile application-based study, it is aimed to contribute to an early and easier diagnosis of diabetic retinopathy.

Figure 5. Image of retinal disease
(IEEE DataPort, 2019)

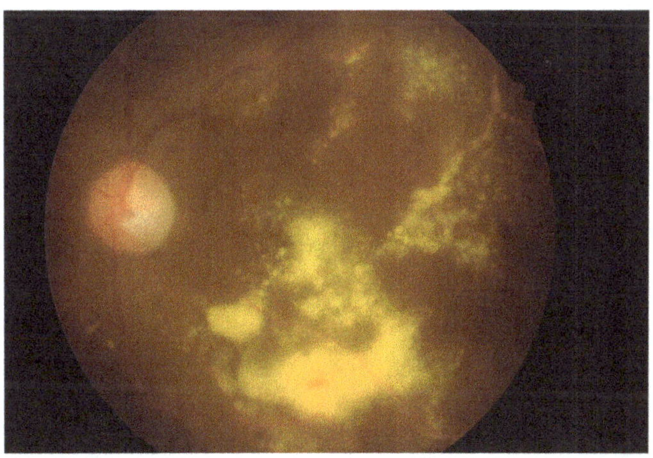

Figure 6. Light NPDR
(IEEE DataPort, 2019)

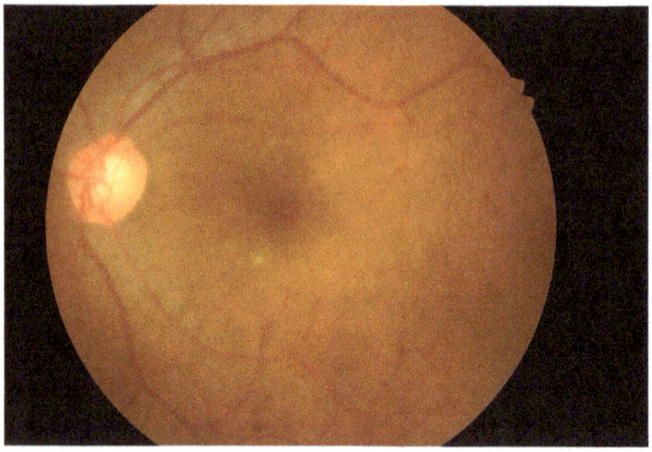

BACKGROUND

In this section, it is mentioned that studies in the literature related to diabetic retinopathy about the removal of retinal vessels. Literature reflected these studies in the two separate classes. The retinal vascular removal methods are classified into two groups; rule and supervised based. The algorithm in rule based methods, which is used to extract and successfully model the vessel using methods such as vessel tracking, mathematical form, adaptive thresholding, can distinguish bifurcation points and intersection points of the vessels. In supervised based methods, the retina vessels, called pixel processing or pixel classification, are also removed with the help of a classifier. Most of the current studies have been done mostly with supervised based methods. In this project, supervised based methods were used.

Figure 7. ModerateNPDR
(IEEE DataPort, 2019)

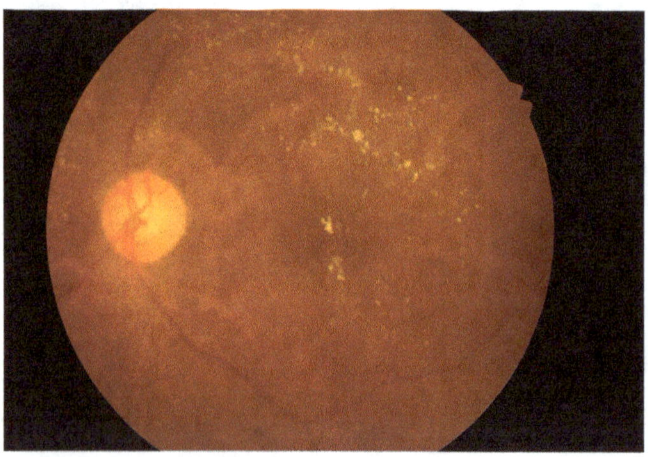

Figure 8. Severe NPDR
(IEEE DataPort, 2019)

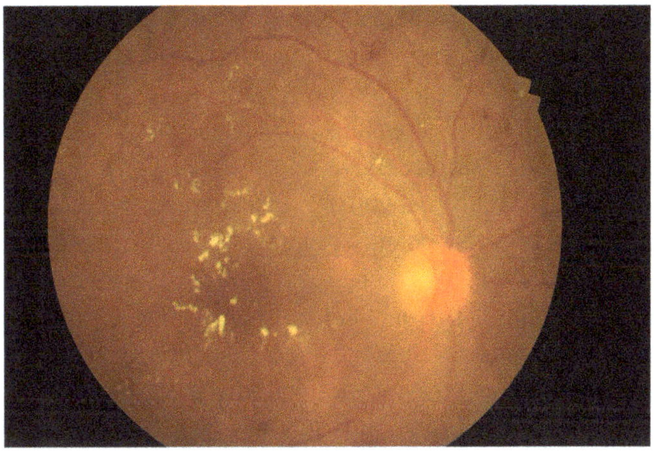

Figure 9. PDR
(IEEE DataPort, 2019)

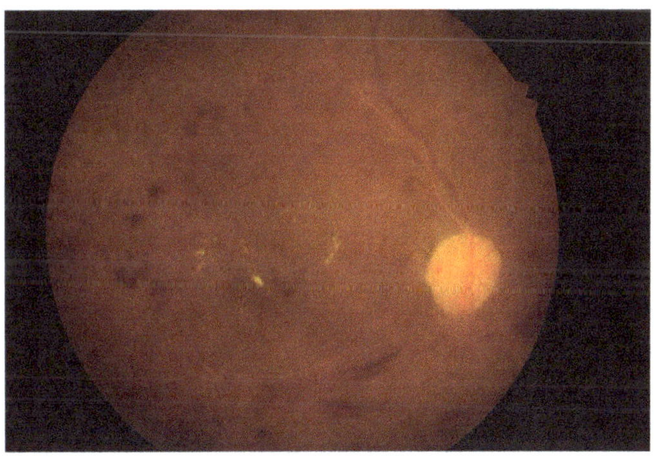

RULE BASED OR MODEL BASED METHODS

In rule based vascular monitoring method, retinal vascular structure is obtained by following the vascular center lines. This process carried out from a starting point. The starting point can be selected manually or automatically. In published the first study used rule based method it was mentioned that extracted the vascular points manually used the features of veins such as the vein width of the veins, the beginning and endpoints of the veins, the direction and neighborhoods of the veins with the help of a matching filter (Chaudhuri S, 1989). Adaptive tracking algorithm consisting of recursive three stages to extract the retina network structure was preferred as an idea (Liu I, 1993). Following this study, it is determined only bifurcation point and intersection point of vein by removing the manual data entry with the width, orientation and neighborhood information of the veins (Zhou, 1994). The algorithm of fuzzy clustering is presented to determine areas with veins or without veins (Tolias Y. A., 1998). Then, studies have been put forward to extract automatically determining the vascular points instead of manually determining the vascular points. In this study, the determination of the starting point is taken as reference according to the points where the contrast and saturation values are the least in the divided grid method of the images. Neighboring veins, which were encountered throughout the reference point, were determined according to their number and angle (Liu, 1993).

After these studies to extract the retina network structure, a math-based method has been proposed. After contrast operation, top-line transformation, a numerical method, was used and the retinal network structure was mapped (Walter T, 2001). By the beginning of 2001, a four-step method was developed to obtain the retinal network structure. This method consists of four steps consisting of remove noise, vessel pattern extraction, cross curvature evaluation, linear filtering stages, respectively (Gang L., 2002). Another method for the retina network structure extraction was the vessel images model through the Gauss function in 2002. Numerical based vessel structures are modeled with the help of Gauss functions. After modeling, vessel measurements were made using Gauss's filter (Jiang X., 2003). For the first time, retinal vascular network was obtained using the local thresholding method (Mendonca A.M, 2011).

Following this, vascular intersections were determined. Genetic algorithm approach was proposed in the studies carried out to optimize the sensitivity of a matched-filtering (Al-Rawi M., 2007). The hybrid method idea was created by using the matched-filtering and ant colony algorithms together to extract the retina network structure and this idea was the first in this sense as a way of approach (Cinsdikici M.G., 2009).

SUPERVISED BASED METHODS

Supervised Based Methods, categorized as second class, are based on pixel classification or pixel processing methods. Pixels are examined in two different classes as vein and not vein. It is tried to train the classifiers with the help of data or values on the images selected manually or automatically. The first supervised based approach in the literature is the use of the proposed backpropagation multilayer artificial neural network for determining the retinal vascular network. The image obtained from histogram synchronization, smoothing, and edge detection operations is divided into a square of 20x20 and the input vector of the artificial neural network is created. Then, it was classified and categorized as either a vein or not a vein as a central output value (Gardner G.G., 1996).

In another study, a multilayer perceptron neural network was created to determine the retinal vascular network. After recording the first principal component to classify each pixel on the retina image, the artificial neural network was fed with an input vector of 10x10 (Sinthanayothin C., 1999). As a result of image processing, optic disc region was determined by using saturation values in the data and vascular extractions from fundus images were performed using artificial neural networks (Sinthanayothin, 1999). Then, Hipwell developed an automated technique rather than a manual technique for the diagnosis of diabetic retinopathy in digital red-free fundus images as a result of training 102 fundus images (Hipwell, 2000). A classifier idea, using the closest neighbor algorithm to extract the retinal vascular network, has been proposed. In this approach, 31 component feature vectors are used (Niemeijer M., 2004).

The vessel structure was detected by using color fundus images via support vector machines (Zhang X, 2005). Thanks to regression processes, damaged vessels were evaluated (Lupascu, 2008). Classification of the attributes was made by using feed-forward neural networks, and the vessel structures were determined. In this study, the classification process was made based on the analysis of 124 retinal images (Yun., 2008). Thanks to the global thresholding method, the optical disc region has been identified, and classification algorithms have been tested using image processing and histogram techniques (Lu, 2010).

Since supervised based methods are based on image processing and fundus images, studies have progressed in this direction. Then, it was detected microaneurysms with the help of mathematical morphology and 'Naive Bayes' classifier (Sopharak, 2013). As a result of Mookiah studies, it was prepared an automatic screening system for non-proliferative diabetic retinopathy (NPDR) and DR detection (Mookiah, 2013). The idea of a system for detecting damaged vessels in the images has been proposed. This system was created by using different algorithms such as k-means algorithm and support vector machine (Naqvi, 2015). In the retina images processed in 2015, multi-layer sensor neural networks were used for the detection of the disease. In the analysis of the studies, statistic methods such as standard deviation, mean, and entropy were used (Bhatkar,2015).

PROPOSED APPROACH

In 2018, Chetoui suggested detecting diabetic retinopathy by using tissue features. Thanks to this idea, in this study, local energy-based and local triple patterned shape histograms were used. Classification of the project has been completed by using support vector machines (Chetoui, 2018).

In this section, detailed information about the content of the methods, which is used in this project and mobile application, is given. In this project, the valuable studies and their methods that took place in the literature were analyzed, and we focused the idea about this question "How can we make this project better?".

As it is mentioned in the introduction section, Convolutional Neural Networks was used during the deep learning phase in this project. Among the most important reasons for using the Convolutional Neural Networks are its "up to date", used in artificial intelligence studies in medicine, and its success rate in model training and prediction. Convolutional Neural Network algorithms are applied in many different areas such as natural language processing (NLP), biomedical, especially in the field of image and sound processing. This project has been the preference of the best results, especially in the field of image processing.

The project was started with the pre-processing phase and then a mobile application was developed synchronously. While the deep learning part of the project is being carried out, front-end user interface development has been made in the mobile application and the draft has been prepared. In pre-processing, image processing has been done for five thousand datasets that we have. The steps are as follows just like Figure 10:

- All images are cropped and resized using the resize script and pre-processing script.
- Images without retinopathy were projected using the rotation script; Images with retinopathy were reflected and rotated 90, 120, 180 and 270 degrees.
- After rotating and reflecting with and without retinopathy, the class imbalance has been resolved and detected several thousand images have retinopathy.
- In total, there are 5000 images processed by the neural network.

- All images were converted to NumPy Arrays using the conversion script. NumPy Arrays combined images and tags in an array and send the images to CNN.
- The model was created by using the TensorFlow and Keras libraries. For CNN, encoding was done by using anaconda as IDE and Jupyter Notepad within anaconda.
- The pictures are tagged and parsed the pictures used to train them in two different sequences according to the labeling.
- The pictures were then brought to a fixed size (255*255) by grayscale method.
- The images are then passed through CNN and are called learning.
- The trained model can be saved and then tested with pictures.

Figure 10. Steps of the proposed approach

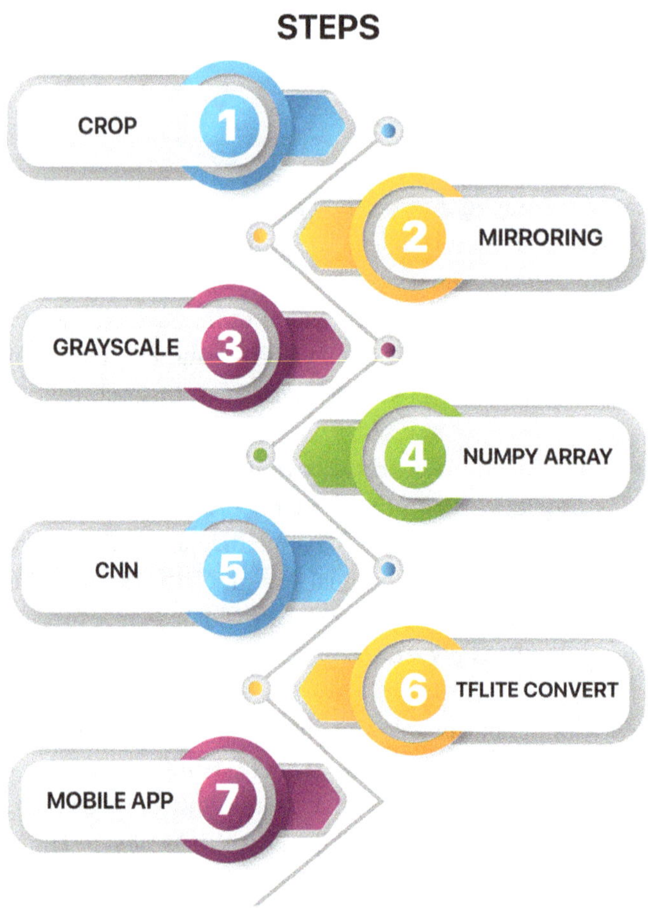
STEPS
CROP
1
2
MIRRORING
GRAYSCALE
3
4
NUMPY ARRAY
CNN
5
6
TFLITE CONVERT
MOBILE APP
7

As a result, 2 double values were obtained. We understood that the image is tested with these values, is closer to which cluster. For example [0.8966925 0.10330744] according to this result, 89% of the images belong to the first cluster. The success rate is higher than 0.7.

EyeNet uses three convolutional layers, each with a depth of 32. EyeNet is easy to use as it does not require an internet connection. Additionally on the model the local device can classify. No internet connection is required for the application to work. When deep learning is completed with the Convolutional Neural Networks, the integrated operation of the developed mobile application was provided. The flowcharts are as follows just like Figure 11.

Figure 11. Flowchart of the mobile application

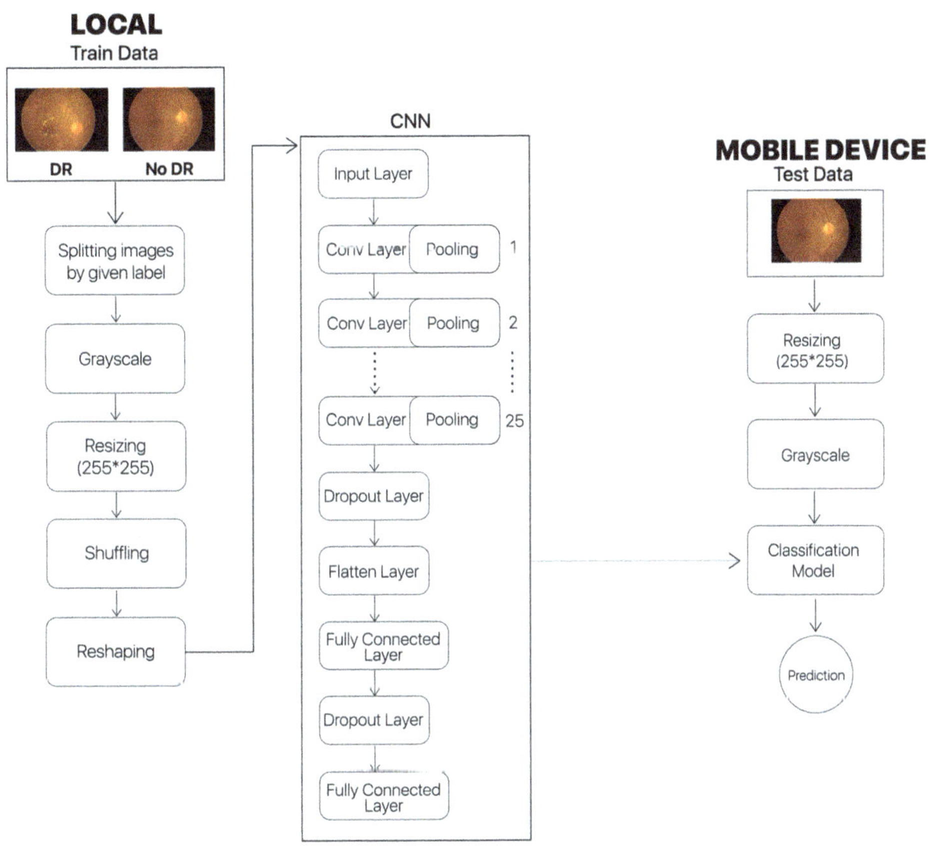

Next, information is given to have an idea about Flutter SDK and Dart language before moving on to exchange information about the mobile application. While flutter allows you to easily create a user interface, quickly add attributes, and fix bugs, it is also a cross framework that is on the agenda with its work on mobile devices with IOS and Android operating systems (Flutter, 2018).

Flutter SDK offers native application development environment, widgets include all critical platform differences such as scrolling, navigation, icons, and fonts to provide native performance on both iOS and Android (Flutter, 2018). Worldwide organizations have been developing applications with Flutter. Being open-source can be assumed as one of the most important advantages for us. Because Flutter is a flexible SDK, it can be used in Windows, Linux, or Mac environments. No experience needed in mobile application field to develop mobile applications with Flutter. The mobile application and application prototypes can be developed by learning Flutter, which uses the darts programming language, with little or no coding knowledge. Applications that reflect brand identity can be designed with Flutter, based on 2D mobile applications development on Android and iOS platform. It is also possible to develop mobile applications that require camera, location data, internet, storage and other 3rd Party SDKs using Flutter, just like on Native platforms (Maraci, 2017). While mention of the dart language above, of course, I think it is useful to explain it a little bit.

The Dart programming language published by Google in 2011 is used to develop mobile applications using the Flutter SDK. It has been standardized by Ecma. Its an open-source language is one of the best features that will work for us. Dart language is similar to the code sequence of the C programming language which is class-based and object-based. It can be translated into the JavaScript language or native language on the system it is running on. Interfaces support abstracts, generic type, and optional types (Medium, 2018). It should be remembered that mobile applications and web servers, web applications, and IoT improvements can be made together by using mobile and Flutter SDK. Detailed information about the mobile application will be found in the next subtitle.

ABOUT MOBILE APPLICATION

Nowadays, although people are more conscious compared to the past and medicine is developing rapidly, chronic diseases and epidemics are rapidly spreading in this century. In fact, "Covid-19", which is a global problem and has been declared a pandemic, can be shown as the most recent example of this. There are approximately 415 million diabetic patients all over the world (Christian Nordqvist, 2017).

Although this number is the highest in the last 100 years and expected to be close to 629 million in the next 25 years (Medicine, 2019). The fact that the numbers are so high and create a great risk throughout the world played a role in the diagnosis process and the treatment methods for these diseases. Of course, the importance of computer technologies, machine learning systems, and artificial intelligence is an undeniable fact. Recently, many diseases can be diagnosed with machine learning techniques using artificial intelligence, and in this manner, the treatment process of diseases is accelerated, for example, cancer, etc. Therefore, considerable progress has been observed in computer-aided solutions in medical applications. However, an important point is that any disease cannot be diagnosed and treated with simple medical findings and different imaging and analysis are even required, for the diagnosis processes.

The main aim of this study is to solve the problem of medical diagnosis via artificial intelligence and make it a mobile application that has not been used in previous studies. In this mobile application, it is provided to diagnose the disease both by pulling the processed data from the image processing thanks to the image processing and by using the simultaneous eye photo with the help of the internal camera of the mobile device and 20 Dioptric Lens integrated with the apparatus to the mobile device. In this study, an image processing (IP) and deep learning focused system has been designed for the diagnosis of diabetic retinopathy (DR) disease. The system in question produces a classification oriented solution that capable of dealing with the data that requires a lot of analysis and that requires precision and that is a kind of machine learning sub-field that includes convolutional neural networks in deep learning. Thus, supervised based methods have been used in this study. In order to increase the diagnostic performance of the convolutional neural networks technique, two different IP (Image Processing) techniques were included in the pre-processing process, and even intelligent optimization was used in order to achieve the success of these techniques at the optimum level.

Table 1a. Dataset tag created by Javathunderman

Tag Number	Tag Number
0	Patient
1	Healthy

(Arjun, 2017)

Table 1b. Dataset tags of IDrid

Tag Number	Other
0	No Disease
1	Mild NPDR
2	Moderate NDPR
3	Serious NDPR
4	NDPR

(IEEE DataPort, 2019)

When the literature was considered and the MESSIDOR dataset in the literature was taken into account for the diagnosis of disease studies within the scope of this study, a total of 1200 retina images were performed. One of the data sets planned to be used in our study is a small data set created by GitHub user "javathunderman" from DR definition data set in Kaggle (Arjun, 2017). The data set consists of 2079 various retina images, which are taken at high resolution. In this study, 90% of these images were planned for model training, and the rest of them is planned to be used for testing and it was made as planned. The disease rating in the images was made in two ways.

The first of these is "healthy" with a label value of 0, and the second is "patient" with a label value of 1. These values are obtained from data set tag created by the user with the Github username "Javathunderman" like Table 1a.

Figure 12a. Interest over time
(Google, 2019)

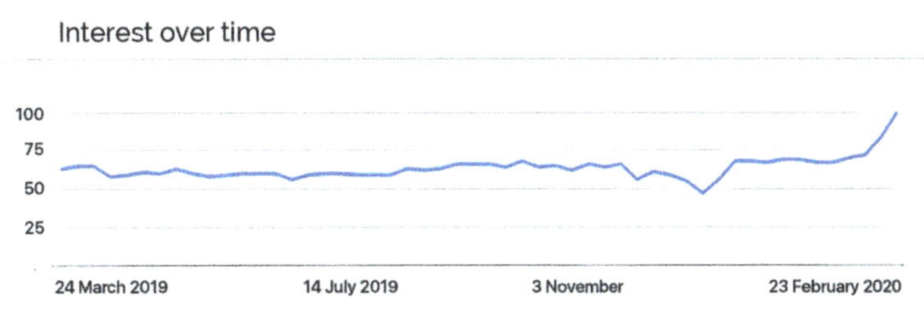

Another data set is the IDRid database which has been planned to be used as in Table 1b. This data set was taken by retina specialists at an eye clinic in Nanded, Maharashta, using the Kowq VX-10 digital fundus camera. There are 516 retina photos in total with 4288x2848 pixels. This data set is classified into 5 categories by experts. These categories are "No Disease, mild NPDR, moderate NPDR, severe NPDR, and PDR" values separated by 0, 1, 2, 3, 4 labels, respectively just like Figure 3, Figure 4, Figure 5, Figure 6, Figure 7, Figure 8 and Figure 9.

Figure 12b. Interest by region
(Google, 2019)

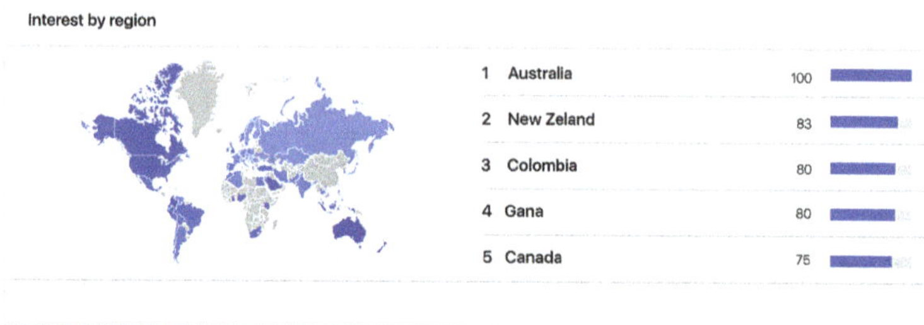

In the 21st century, we research almost everything that stuck in our minds thanks to mobile devices along with us and the internet which can give us instant information. Unfortunately, although all the information we obtain from the internet is not correct, it can give wrong information and cause people to be panic. According to the Global Web Index [Figures 12a,b,c] data, people, between the ages of 16-64 around the world, using smartphone and social media approximately takes 2 hours and 54 minutes per person in a day! In countries such as the Philippines and Nigeria, this rate rises to 4 hours. The United States ranks 8th in this order with 1 hour 57 minutes. In the most searched categories in over the world in the Google search engine related to "health" [Figure: 12a] increased by 1400%.

When comparing people according to apply to health institutions and to research their complaints on Google, it is clearly seen that internet searches are preferred. The information related to "Diabetic Retinopathy" supports these results. Puerto Rico, Malaysia, Nepal, Ghana, and the UK are ranked top about doing research Diabetic Retinopathy on Google.

Figure 12c. Countries
(Google, 2019)

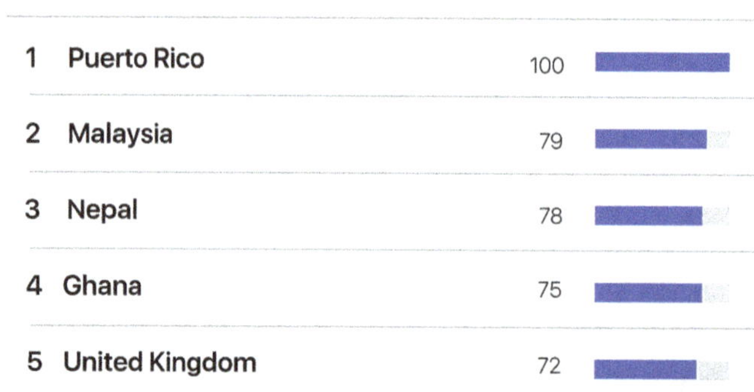
1 Puerto Rico
100
2 Malaysia
79
3 Nepal
78
4 Ghana
75
5 United Kingdom
72

Figure 13. Information Schema About Mobile Application

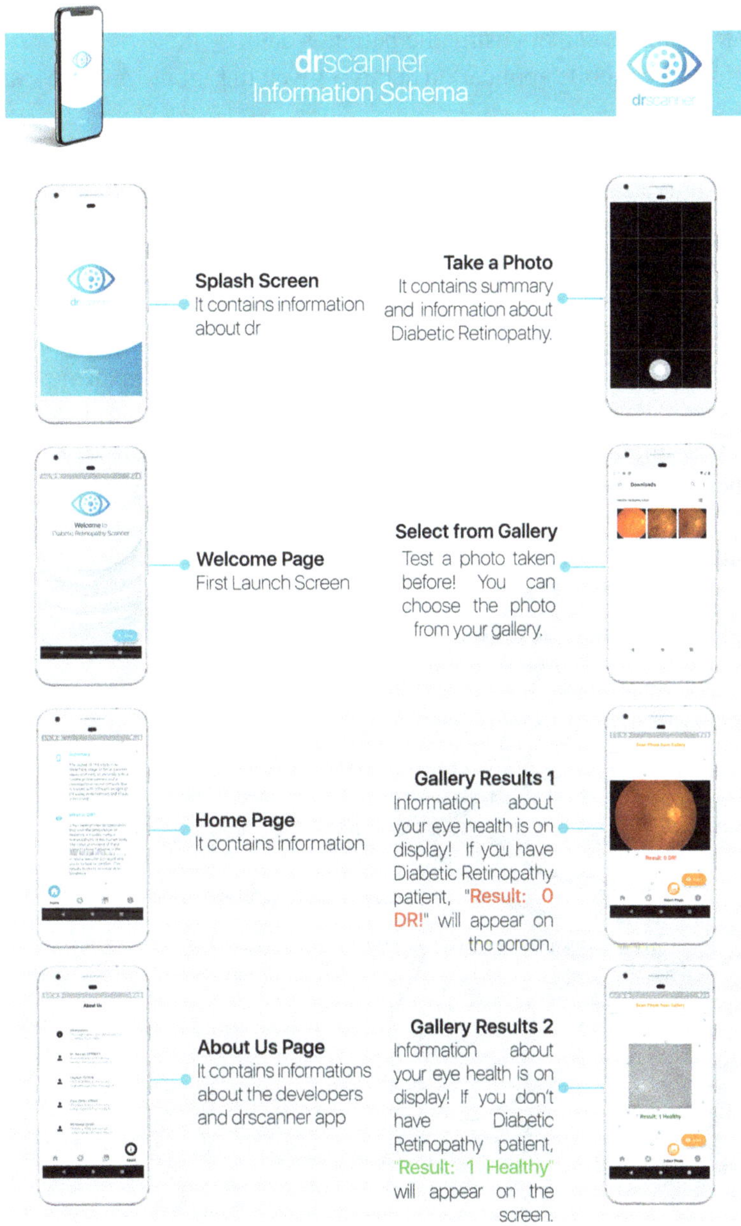

Diabetic Retinopathy can cause blindness, this risk makes it very important. In this context, the project "Mobile Application Development for Diagnosis of Diabetic Retinopathy" has been inevitable. In addition to facilitating daily life while making this application; It is aimed to reach and help the doctors, medical students, patients and the suspicious masses.

In this project, an artificial intelligence-supported mobile application was developed for iOS and Android mobile devices by using Flutter SDK, an up-to-date and useful mobile application development environment, to speed up the diagnosis of diabetic retinopathy disease and to bring the computer science and medicine a little closer. In this mobile application, which is compatible with every mobile device, the degree of the disease is automatically determined in seconds by taking fundus photographs through the 20D lens integrated into the camera using the patient's data.

The usage scenario of the mobile application detail is given in Figure 14. If we examine this scenario in detail;

Screening results are given in 2 groups as "Result: 0 Healthy", "Result: 1 Diabetic Retinopathy". With the principle of "universal colour seriousness experience"; green in case of normal level (Figure 13.), red in case of more serious (Figure 13.) were used.

If a healthy eye is tested with a mobile application, as seen in the scenario; the interface gives us the "Healthy" result. This green color indicates that the eye is healthy and there is no problem according to user experience.

The red alert tone gives the user a hazard warning that serious visual impairments and symptoms that may lead to blindness may develop in the future. The user receiving this warning should seek help from a specialist by not neglecting the symptoms of the disease as soon as possible. This information should be remembered because this situation can cause vision loss. For this reason, in the in-app notifications, the warning "it is recommended to get support from a health institution" is stated.

USAGE OF MOBILE APPLICATION

Figure 14. Diagnosis of diabetic retinopathy

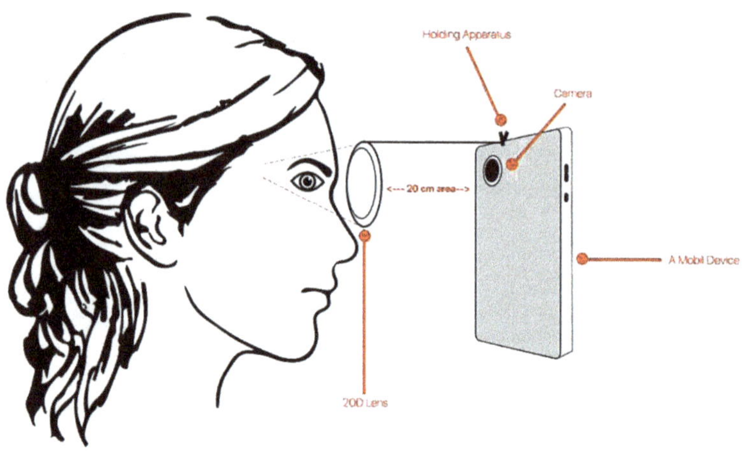

The interface designed specifically for all users of all ages to operate easily is as shown in Figure 13. Simplicity is preferred in UI design in order to facilitate usage and provide practicality in the interface that minimal perspective kept the foreground. The usage scenario of the mobile application with 20D lens, detailed is given in Figure 14.

SOLUTIONS AND RECOMMENDATIONS

Mobile application was run in this section. The content of the application is provided. The pages of the mobile application are displayed in the content. The results are given in a separate section.

Figure 15a. Splash screen

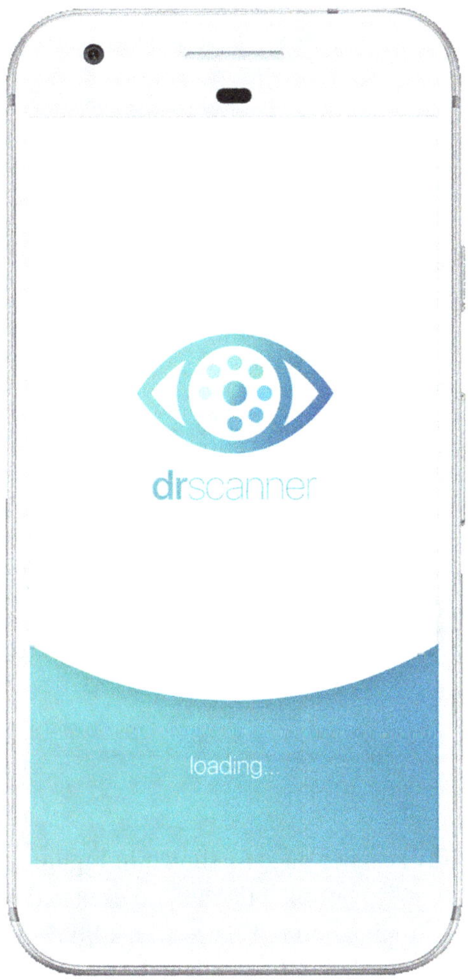

When first opening the application, the splash screen (figure 15a) is shown. When most mobile application opens, there will be a screen that shows the logo and the name of the application for a few seconds before going away. This screen is called the splash screen. This screen can be thought like a losing screen. After splash screen, welcome page of the application will open.

Figure 15b. Welcome To diabetic retinopathy

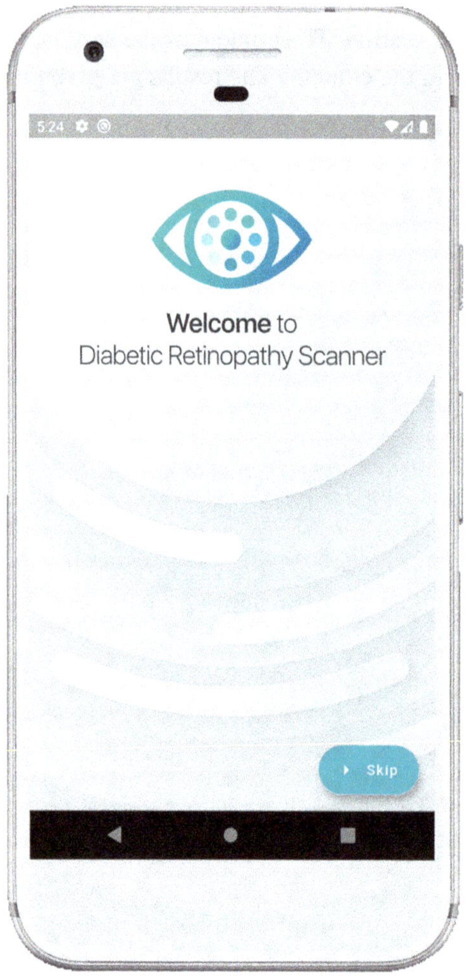

Welcome to diabetic retinopathy scanner page as shown in Figure 15b, is designed to welcome the user to the application. Clicking the skip button will lead the user to the main page.

In the home page of the mobile application in Figure 15c, a little summary of how to use the application and information about diabetic retinopathy is given. In the main page as well as the other pages menu section, navigation of other pages can be made.

As soon as clicking the "Select Photo" button in Figure 15d, the desired photo from the retina images, which is taken via the 20D lens or previously saved in the gallery, is selected and uploaded to the application. Selected retina photos will be displayed in the Downloads section.

As shown in Figure 15e, the photo taken from the gallery is shown and the result of the model is written accordingly. If the retina is healthy it writes healthy otherwise it diabetic retinopathy is written to the page.

In the camera page in Figure 15f, with the help of a 20d lens, the retina image is taken and uploaded to the application and processed through tflite model. With the result that the model gives, according page will open up.

Figure 15c. Home page

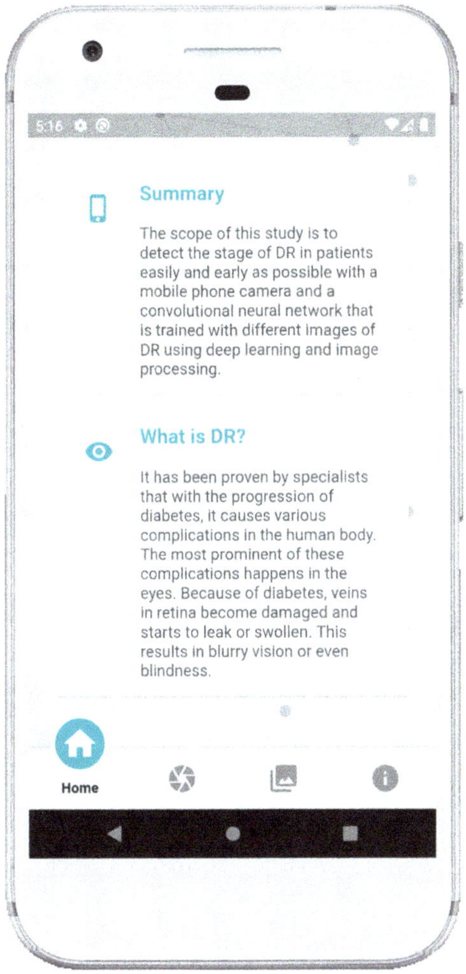

The about us page, as shown in Figure 15g, contains information about the developers of the application. These pieces of information are name, surname, university, and email addresses.

In this section, the success rate of the trained model and outputs of the application are given. By using the tflite file that is converted from trained Keras model in the application, the patient's diabetic retinopathy status can be determined with 0.78 success rate. The screenshots obtained from the mobile application named "Diabetic Retinopathy Scanner" that is developed under the "Development of a mobile application for detection of diabetic retinopathy" project are shown in Figure 16a, Figure 16b, Figure 16c, Figure 16d and Figure 16e, respectively.

Figure 15d. Select photo

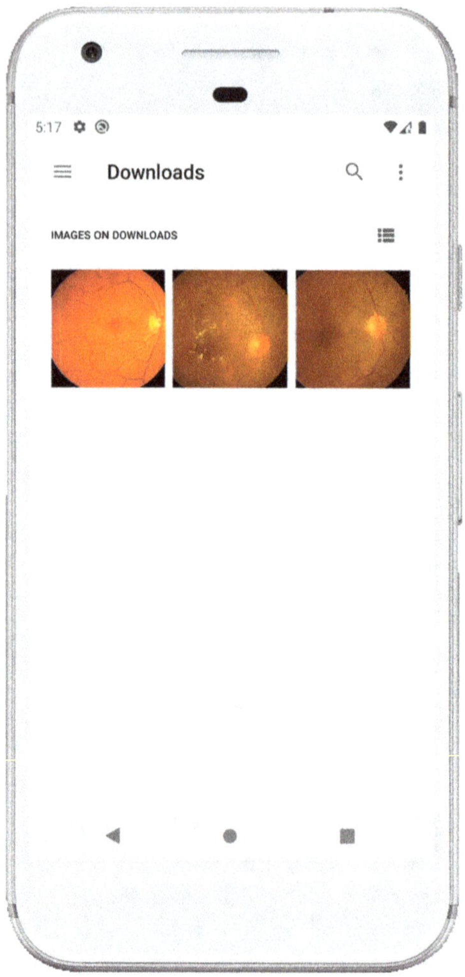

FUTURE RESEARCH DIRECTIONS

In the future of this project, it's planned to increase the data size and improve the model score. It is also planned that with better labeling and classifying, to see not only if the patient has diabetic retinopathy but also with a grade of retinopathy the patient has.

Figure 15e. Scan from gallery

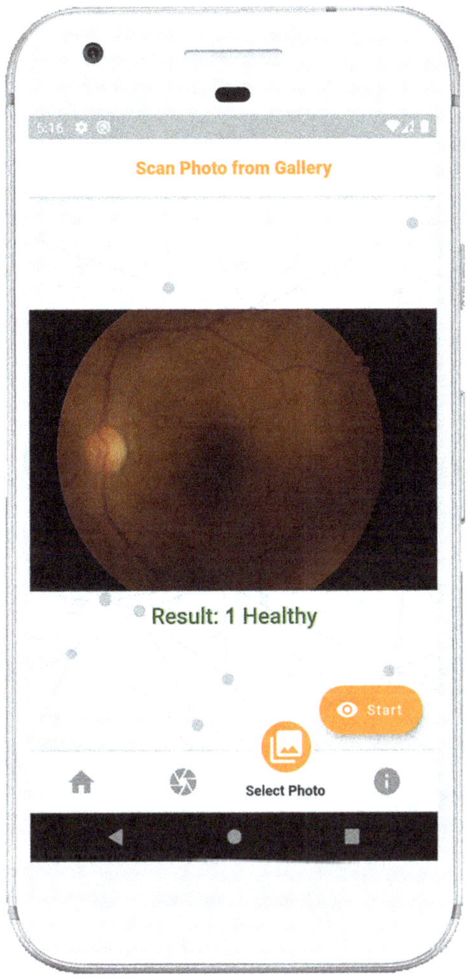

CONCLUSION

According to the data that was released in 2015 by the International Diabetes Federation, one out of every eleven has diabetes. Also half of the patients do not know that they have diabetes. For this reason, people do not realize that they have diabetic retinopathy. There are comprehensive studies being made today for analyzing medical images. In this chapter, diabetic retinopathy (DR) was tried to be detected by using colored retina images. With the help of deep learning this problem was solved using two methods: preprocessing and classification. In general, variables and methods used in this work are going to ease the work done for the detection of DR in diabetes research and treatment centers.

Figure 15f. Scan from gallery

Figure 15g. About us

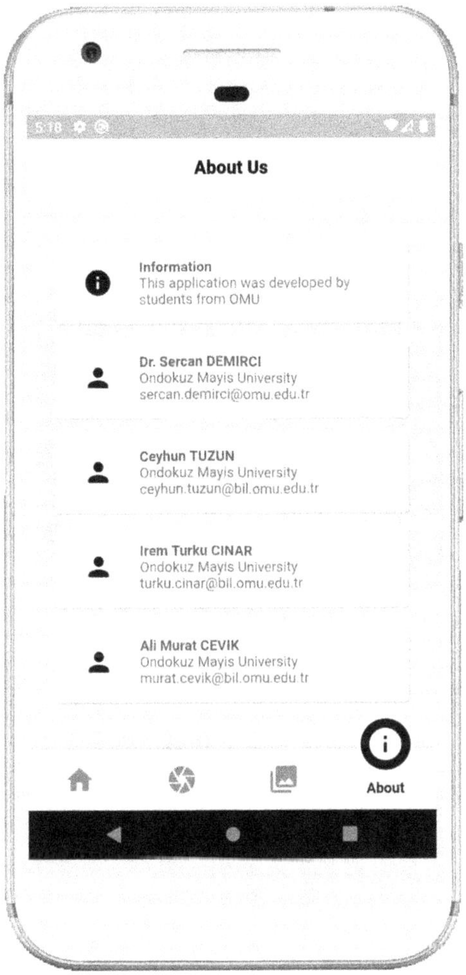

Figure 16a. Result: 0 DR!

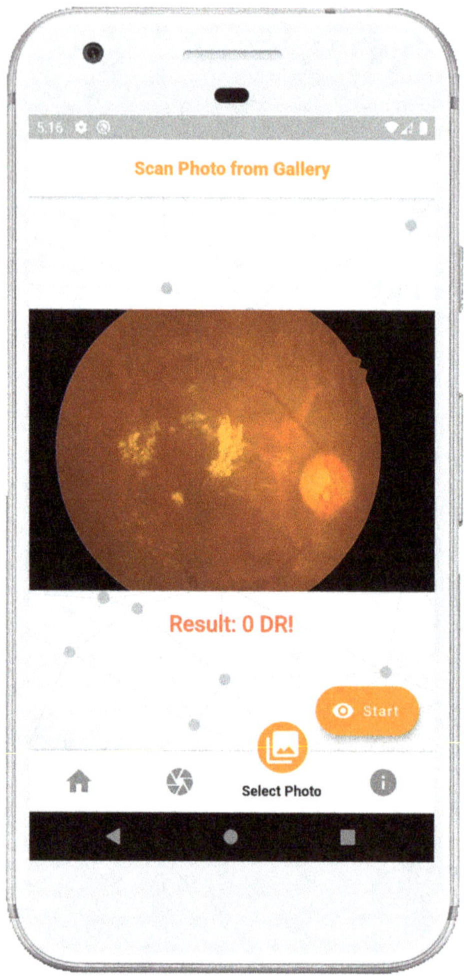

Figure 16b. Result: 1 Healthty

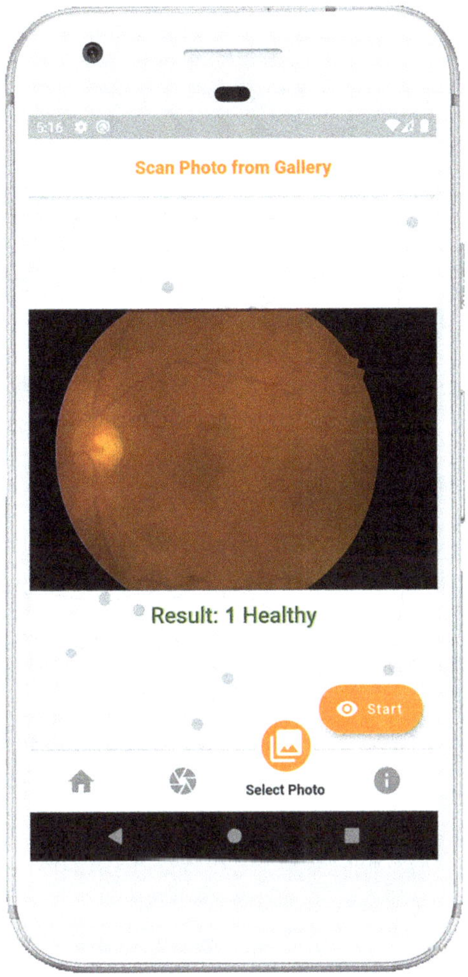

Figure 16c. Result: 0 DR!

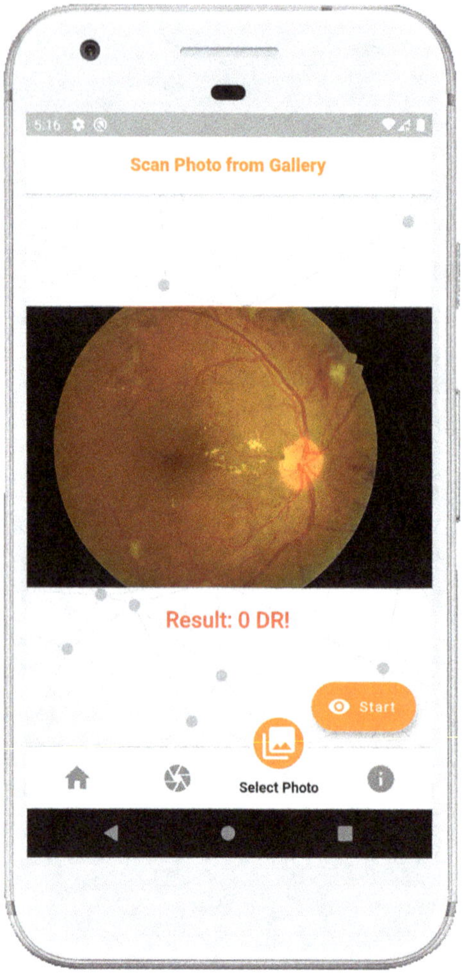

Figure 16d. Result: 1 Healthty

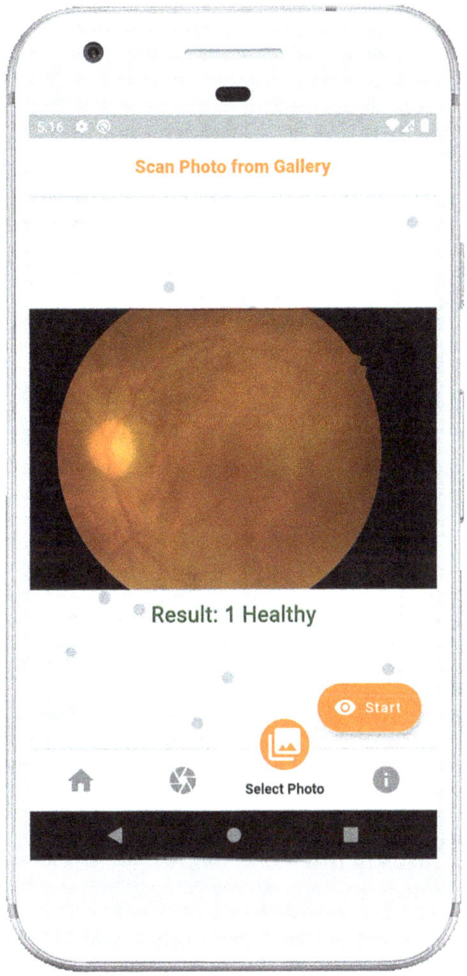

Figure 16e. Result: 0 DR!

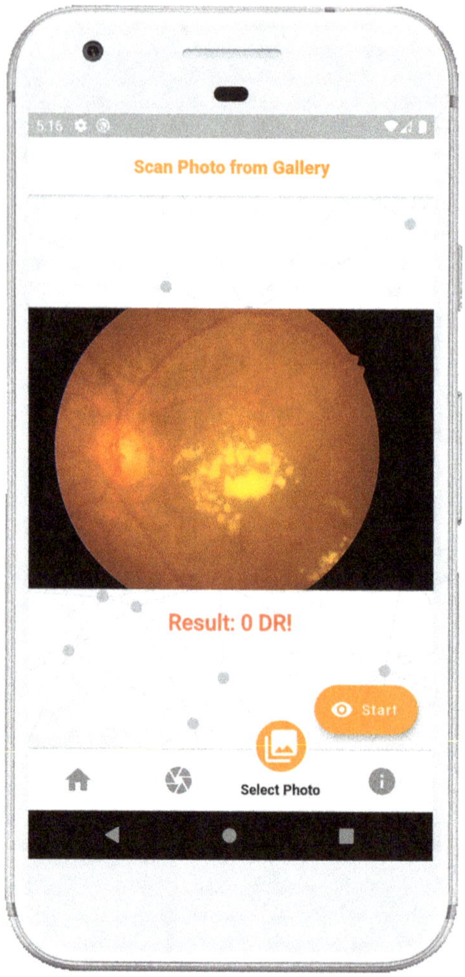

REFERENCES

Al-Rawi, M., & Karajeh, H. (2007). Genetic algorithm matched filter optimization for automated detection of blood vessels from digital retinal images. Comput. Methods Programs Biomed., 87, 248–253.

Arjun. (2017). *Retinopathy Dataset*. Retrieved from https://github.com/javathunderman/retinopathy-dataset

Bhatkar, A. P., & Kharat, G.U. (2015). Detection of Diabetic Retinopathy in Retinal Images using MLP Classifier. *2015 IEEE International Symposium on Nanoelectronic and Information Systems*, 331-335. 10.1109/iNIS.2015.30

Chaudhuri, S., Chatterjee, S., Katz, N., Nelson, M., & Goldbaum, M. (1989). Detection of blood vessels in retinal images using two-dimensional matched filters. IEEE Trans. Med. Imag., 8(3), 263–269.

Chetoui, M., Akhloufi, M. A., & Kardouchi, M. (2018). Diabetic Retinopathy Detection Using Machine Learning and Texture Features. *2018 IEEE Canadian Conference on Electrical & Computer Engineering (CCECE)*. 10.1109/CCECE.2018.8447809

Christian Nordqvist. (2017). *What to know about diabetic retinopathy*. Retrieved from https://www.medicalnewstoday.com/articles/183417.php

Cinsdikici, M. G., & Aydin, D. (2009). Detection of blood vessels in ophthalmoscope images using MF/ant (matched filter/ant colony) algorithm. Comput. Methods Programs Biomed., 96, 85–95.

Eye Care. (2019). *OCT Göz Cihazı*. Retrieved from http://www.clairhursteyecare.com/retinal-digital-imaging

Flutter. (2019). *Flutter*. Retrieved from https://flutter.dev/

Gang, L., Chutatape, O., & Krishnan, S. M. (2002). Detection and measurement of retinal vessels in fundus images using amplitude modified second-order Gaussian filter. IEEE Trans. Biomed. Eng., 49, 168–172.

Gardner, G. G., Keating, D., Williamson, T. H., & Elliott, A. T. (1996). Automatic detection of diabetic retinopathy using an artificial neural network: A screening tool. Br. J. Ophthalmol., 80, 940–944.

Global Web Index Data. (2020). Retrieved from https://www.cybermagonline.com/turkiye-internette-vakit-gecirmede-dunya-dorduncusu

Google. (2019). *Googletrends*. Retrieved from https://www.googletrends.com

Hipwell, J. H., Strachan, F., Olson, J. A., McHardy, K. C., Sharp, P. F., & Forrester, J. V. (2000). Automated Detection of Microaneurysms in Digital Red-free Photographs: A Diabetic Retinopathy Screening Tool. *Diabetic Medicine*, *17*(8), 588–594. doi:10.1046/j.1464-5491.2000.00338.x PMID:11073180

Hubel, D. H., & Wiesel, T. N. (1968). Receptive Fields and Functional Architecture of Monkey Striate Cortex. *The Journal of Physiology*, *195*(1), 215–243. doi:10.1113/jphysiol.1968.sp008455 PMID:4966457

IEEE DataPort. (2019). *Indian diabetic retinopathy image dataset (IDRID)*. Retrieved from https://ieee-dataport.org/open-access/indian-diabetic-retinopathy-image-dataset-idrid

Jiang, X., & Mojon, D. (2003), Adaptive local thresholding by verificationbased multithreshold probing with application to vessel detection in retinal images. IEEE Trans. Pattern Anal. Mach. Intell., 25(1), 131–137.

Karaboğa, D. (2011). *Yapay Zeka Optimizasyon Algoritmaları*. Nobel Yayın Dağıtım.

Koprowski, R., & Skufca, J. D. (2014). Machine learning, medical diagnosis, and biomedical engineering research-commentary. *Biomedical Engineering Online*, *13*(1), 94. doi:10.1186/1475-925X-13-94 PMID:24998888

Liu I. & Sun Y. (1993). Recursive tracking of vascular networks in angiograms based on the detection-deletion scheme. *IEEE Trans. Med. Imag., 12*(2), 334–341.

Lu, S., & Lim, J. H. (2010). Automatic Optic Disc Detection Through Background Estimation. *17th IEEE International Conference on Image Processing*, 833-836. 10.1109/ICIP.2010.5653473

Lupascu, C. A., Tegolo, D., & Rosa, L. D. (2008). Automated Detection of Optic Disc Location in Retinal Images. *21st IEEE International Symposium on Computer Based Medical Systems*, 17-22. 10.1109/CBMS.2008.15

Maraci. (2017). *Flutter*. Retrieved from https://wmaraci.com/nedir/flutter

Medicine. (2019). *Dünyada Diyabet Hastasi.* Retrieved from https://www.aa.com.tr/tr/saglik/dunyada-diyabet-hastasi-sayisi-2045te-629-milyona-ulasacak/1643626

Medium. (2018) *Flutter*. Retrieved from https://medium.com/@halilozel1903/dart-programlama-dili-eeafb64ad300

Mendonca, A. M., & Campilho, A. (2011). Segmentation of retinal blood vessels by combining the detection of centerlines and morphological reconstruction. *IEEE Transactions on Medical Imaging*, *25*(9), 1200–1213p. doi:10.1109/TMI.2006.879955 PMID:16967805

Mookiah, M. R. K., Rajendra-Acharya, U., Martis, R. J., Chua, K. C., Lim, C. M., Ng, E. Y. K., & Laude, A. (2013). Evolutionary Algorithm Based Classifier Parameter Tuning for Automatic Diabetic Retinopathy Grading: A Hybrid Feature Extraction Approach. *Knowledge-Based Systems*, *39*, 9–22. doi:10.1016/j.knosys.2012.09.008

Naqvi, S. A., Zafar, M. F., & Haq, I. U. (2015). Referral System for Hard Exudates in Eye Fundus. *Computers in Biology and Medicine*, *64*, 217–235. doi:10.1016/j.compbiomed.2015.07.003 PMID:26231313

Niemeijer, M., Staal, J., Ginneken, B. v., Loog, M., Abramoff, M. D., Fitzpatrick, J., & Sonka, M. (2004). Comparative study of retinal vessel segmentation methods on a new publicly available database. SPIE Med. Imag., 5370, 648–656.

Russell, S. J., & Norvig, P. (2016). *Artificial Intelligence: A Modern Approach*. Pearson Education Limited.

Sesan. (2019). *Oftalmoskop Vitalitaet VM-P110*. Retrieved from https://www.denizlermedikal.com/oti-oct-goz-cihazi/Foster

Sinthanayothin, C., Boyce, J. F., Cook, H. L., & Williamson, T. H. (1999). Automated localisation of the optic disc, fovea and retinal blood vessels from digital colour fundus images. Br. J. Ophtalmol., 83, 902–910.

Sinthanayothin, C., Boyce, J. F., Cook, H. L., & Williamson, T. H. (1999). Automated location of the optic disc, fovea, and retinal blood vessels from digital color fundus images. *The British Journal of Ophthalmology*, *83*(8), 902–910. doi:10.1136/bjo.83.8.902 PMID:10413690

Sopharak, A., Uyyanonvara, B., & Barman, S. (2013). Simple Hybrid Method for Fine Microaneurysm Detection from Non-dilated Diabetic Retinopathy Retinal Images. *Computerized Medical Imaging and Graphics*, *37*(5), 394–402. doi:10.1016/j.compmedimag.2013.05.005 PMID:23777979

Tolias, Y. A., & Panas, S. M. (1998). A fuzzy vessel tracking algorithm for retinal images based on fuzzy clustering. IEEE Trans. Med. Imag., 17(2), 263–273.

University of Iowa Carver College of Medicine. (2019). *Diabetic Retinopathy: From One Medical Student to Another.* https://webeye.ophth.uiowa.edu/eyeforum/tutorials/Diabetic-Retinopathy-Med-Students/Classification.htm

Walter, T., & Klein, J. C. (2001). Segmentation of color fundus images of the human retina: Detection of the optic disc and the vascular tree using morphological techniques. Lecture Notes in Computer Science, 282–287.

Yun, W. L., Rajendra Acharya, U., Venkatesh, Y. V., Chee, C., Min, L. C., & Ng, E. Y. K. (2008). Identification of Different Stages of Diabetic Retinopathy Using Retinal Optical Images. *Information Sciences*, *178*(1), 106–121. doi:10.1016/j.ins.2007.07.020

Zhang, X., & Chutatape, O. (2005). Top-down and Bottom-up Strategies in Lesion Detection of Background Diabetic Retinopathy. *IEEE Computer Society Conference on Computer Vision and Pattern Recognition (CVPR'05)*, *2*, 422-428.

Zhou, L., Rzeszotarski, M. S., Singerman, J., & Chokreff, J. M. (1994). The detection and quantification of retinopathy using digital angiograms. *IEEE Transactions on Medical Imaging*, *13*(4), 619–626p. doi:10.1109/42.363106 PMID:18218540

ADDITIONAL READING

Gonzales, R. C., & Woods, R. E. (2002). *Digital image processing*. Pearson.

Ketkar, N. (2017). Introduction to keras. In *Deep learning with Python* (pp. 97–111). Apress. doi:10.1007/978-1-4842-2766-4_7

Okur, E., & Turkan, M. (2018). A survey on automated melanoma detection. *Engineering Applications of Artificial Intelligence*, *73*, 50–67. doi:10.1016/j.engappai.2018.04.028

Yun, W. L., Rajendra Acharya, U., Venkatesh, Y. V., Chee, C., Min, L. C., & Ng, E. Y. K. (2008). Identification of Different Stages of Diabetic Retinopathy Using Retinal Optical Images. *Information Sciences*, *178*(1), 106–121. doi:10.1016/j.ins.2007.07.020

KEY TERMS AND DEFINITIONS

Convolutional Neural Network: It is a class of deep neural networks, most commonly applied to analyzing visual imagery.

Deep Learning: It is a machine learning method using multiple layers of nonlinear processing units to extract features from data.

Diabetic Retinopathy: It is a diabetes complication that affects eyes. It's caused by damage to the blood vessels of the light-sensitive tissue at the back of the eye.

Image Processing: It is a method to perform some operations on an image, in order to get an enhanced image or to extract some useful information from it.

Machine Learning: Machine learning is an application of artificial intelligence that provides systems the ability to automatically learn and improve from experience without being explicitly programmed.

Mobile Application: A mobile application, most commonly referred to as an app, is a type of application software designed to run on a mobile device, such as a smartphone or tablet computer.

Retinal Fundus: The interior lining of the eyeball, including the retina, optic disc, and the macula.

Chapter 3
Android-Based Skin Cancer Recognition System Using Convolutional Neural Network

Sercan Demirci
https://orcid.org/0000-0001-6739-7653
Ondokuz Mayıs University, Turkey

Durmuş Özkan Şahin
https://orcid.org/0000-0002-0831-7825
Ondokuz Mayıs University, Turkey

Ibrahim Halil Toprak
Ondokuz Mayıs University, Turkey

ABSTRACT

Skin cancer, which is one of the most common types of cancer in the world, is a malignant growth seen on the skin due to various reasons. There was an increase in the number of the cases of skin cancer nearly 200% between 2004-2009. Since the ozone layer is depleting, harmful rays reflected from the sun cannot be filtered. In this case, the likelihood of skin cancer will increase over the years and pose more risks for human beings. Early diagnosis is very significant as in all types of cancers. In this study, a mobile application is developed in order to detect whether the skin spots photographed by using the machine learning technique for early diagnosis have a suspicion of skin cancer. Thus, an auxiliary decision support system is developed that can be used both by the clinicians and individuals. For cases that are predicted to have a risk higher than a certain rate by the machine learning algorithm, early diagnosis could be initiated for the patients by consulting a physician when the case is considered to have a higher risk by machine learning algorithm.

DOI: 10.4018/978-1-7998-6527-8.ch003

INTRODUCTION

The cancer is defined as the emergence of malignant tumors when the division of cells or tissues are seen aberrantly and multiply. The uncontrolled growth of cancer cells in the body of an individual is the main reason of cancer including distinct illnesses (Lancaster Cancer Center, 2020). Despite the wide variety of cancer types, these distinct diseases are seen as the result of abnormal cell growth. When a treatment is not provided for the disease, it can cause severe health problems and loss of lives. One of these types is skin cancer (Medical News Today, 2020). Skin cancer is usually divided into two groups. These are non-melanoma and melanoma types (Armstrong and Kricker, 1995). According to the report of the World Health Organization (WHO), a range between 2 and 3 mil. people experience non-melanoma type skin cancer every year, while more than 100000 people have melanoma type skin cancer (WHO Report-1, 2020). Although melanoma is not seen very commonly, the disease is the deadliest of skin cancer types (Kasap et al., 2015).

According to another report of the WHO, it has been predicted more than 9 mil. individuals died from cancer in 2018 (WHO Report-2, 2020). Skin cancer is commonly encountered as a cancer causing death. According to the data obtained from the report, the most common cancers are given in Figure 1. When Figure 1 is examined, skin cancer cases are seen very much over the world. As with any cancer case, skin cancer is likely to cause death. Considering this situation, skin cancer is one of the serious problems that need to be addressed.

Figure 1. Globally highly seen cancer types

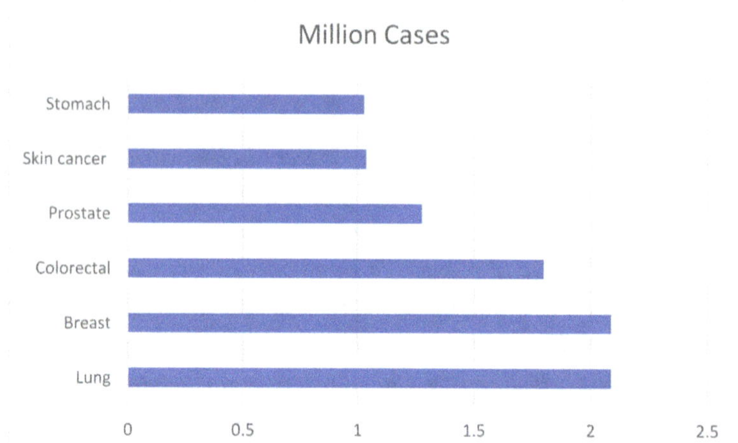

Skin cancer occurs when an error (mutation) is seen in the cells' DNA in the skin. Such mutations are the reason of growing uncontrollably and create a huge amount of cancerous cells (Narayanan et al., 2010). Much of the DNA damage in skin cells comes from ultraviolet (UV-ultraviolet light) radiation found in sunlight and the lights used in solariums. Besides, some factors will increase the risk of skin cancer (Saladi and Persaud, 2005). These include light skin color, sunburn history, excessive sun exposure, sunny or high-altitude climates, skin moles, precancerous skin lesions, family skin cancer history, personal skin cancer history, weakened immune system, and radiation exposure.

Motivation and Contribution

Dermatologists make the diagnosis of skin cancer mainly by visual evaluation of pathological skin. However, since this is a subjective assessment, it is mostly based on the experience of the dermatologist. With the advances in technology, computer-aided systems have started to be used in the determination of skin cancer as in many diseases. Especially with the development of image processing technologies, the detection of skin cancer can be performed more easily and accurately compared to painful and costly methods such as biopsy. In the literature, for the detection of skin cancer many methods based on image processing and application of computer algorithms have been preferred. However, mobile application-based diagnostic systems are limited and mobile applications are needed. In this study, a skin cancer detection system working on a mobile application system based on deep learning was developed. In this way, the skin cancer detection system, which can work directly on Android devices, is developed and contributed to the literature. When compared to other studies in the literature, the main contribution of this study can be summarized as follows:

- The most important advantage of the proposed diagnostic system is that can work on tablets and phones with Android operating system. The fact that the Android operating system is the most used mobile operation in the world will enable many patients or doctors to access the system.
- As patients and doctors are active on the developed system, early diagnosis will be provided. Thus, patients who are likely to have skin cancer detected by the system will be encouraged to apply to the nearest health institution. Thereby, the number of people who die from a dangerous disease, skin cancer, will be reduced.
- Skin cancer diagnosis system specific to the proposed Android operating system is enriched with CNN, one of the deep learning techniques. Since there is CNN in the infrastructure of the system, there is no direct feature extraction step based on image processing techniques. Because the feature extraction phase is automatically done by CNN.
- This study sheds light on how readers can design such a system and how to construct its infrastructure.

Organization

The chapters of the book are given as: literature review has been performed via background section in the second chapter. In section 3, a convolutional neural network from deep learning techniques will be explained. The infrastructure of the mobile application-based skin cancer diagnosis system developed in section 4 will be discussed. In section 5, the results obtained in the study will be given. Finally, information about the conclusions and future works will be given for the researchers who want to work in this field in section 6 and 7.

BACKGROUND

There are many ways to treat skin cancer (Mogensen and Jemec, 2007). Generally, two steps are followed by doctors to diagnose skin cancer. These are physical examination and biopsy steps. In the first step, the color, shape and shape changes in the skin are examined by the expert by hand and eye. Then the biopsy step is started. In this step, a piece is taken from where it is possible to have cancer. This piece is examined by a pathologist under a microscope and then diagnosed. If the disease is diagnosed, the treatment process is started. In the treatment of skin cancer, it can change depending on many factors such as the location of tumor, patient's age, progression degree, margins and dimensions, and the stage of the disease (Martinez and Otley, 2001). Generally, surgical intervention, regional treatments, radiotherapy and chemotherapy methods are applied to cure cancer cells (Neville et al., 2007).

Cancer disease covers a challenging process from diagnosis to recovery. In each of these challenging processes, there are doctors specialized in various fields and assistant health professionals. Besides, much medical equipment is used. Recently, due to the advancements in information technologies as computer software and hardware, many studies based on the computer have been developed to help physicians diagnose cancer (Kourou et al., 2015; Hu et al., 2018). Some of these studies are as follows:

- Brain tumor recognition (Manogaran et al., 2018)
- Breast cancer recognition (Azar and El-Said, 2014)
- Skin cancer recognition (Nahata and Singh, 2020)
- Lymph cancer recognition (Varol and İşeri, 2019)
- Thyroid cancer recognition (Anand and Koundal, 2020)
- Prostate cancer recognition (Puech et al., 2007)
- Lung cancer recognition (Polat and Güneş, 2008)
- Colorectal cancer recognition (Ito et al., 2019)
- Bladder cancer recognition (Liao et al., 2011)
- Pancreatic cancer recognition (Zhang et al., 2010)

Most of these studies are used retrieving data, computer algorithms, and image processing. Data mining could be stated as a branch in the field of artificial intelligence. Data mining can also be explained as the method for accessing and mining information among large-scale data (Han et al., 2011). In other words, it is the realization of the relations with computer programs that provide predictions from big data stacks. Automatic computer learning is the system modeling making estimations via mathematical and statistical operations over data (Alpaydın, 2020). There are many algorithms in machine learning. The structures and ways of working of these algorithms are different from each other. With these algorithms estimation, clustering and classification processes are performed. Image processing is the technique of obtaining useful information on digital images (Gonzales and Woods, 2002). There are many studies on skin cancer with the use of these three techniques together or separately (Hameed et al., 2016; Okur and Turkan, 2018). These studies are summarized as follows:

For the skin cancer diagnosis clinically, some techniques are found in the literature. These include ABCD rule (Stolz 1994), 7-point checklist (Argenziano et al., 1998) and Menzies method (Menzies et al., 1996). The most widely implemented method among these methods is the ABCD rule. In the ABCD method, A corresponds to the asymmetry, B to the border, C to the color, and D to the diameter. With the creation of this information, some conclusions can be made about the bulk by obtaining the ABCD score. Each of the ABCD values can be given as an input to machine learning algorithms as a feature. There are many studies in the literature using this approach (Kasmi and Mokrani, 2016; Ozkan and Koklu, 2017)

Segmentation could be noted as a technique used for the disease (Oliveira et al., 2016). Ilkin et al. (2018) finds the area of melanoma via dermatological images using the Mean Shift algorithm, which is also among the clustering methods. In the study, firstly, RGB color channel values are obtained from tested images. After the color channel values are obtained, the image is flattened. After this step, the core bandwidth is obtained, which determines the size of the window to be moved over the image to access the data points in the image matrix. After the window size is determined, the Mean Shift algorithm is run on the image to segment the melanoma areas. Researchers are tested using a data set of 70 different dermatological melanoma images. A comparison is made between the performance of the system and the improved Canny edge detector algorithm. According to the results of the, it is observed that the segmentation performed with the Mean Shift algorithm yielded more successful results than the segmentation carried out via improved Canny edge detector algorithm.

Ilkin et al. (2020) uses the K-means clustering algorithm in terms of segmenting melanoma lesions on skin images. The results obtained by choosing 2 different center values in the K-means algorithm are compared with Mean Shift and Canny edge detection algorithms. The center values used are 2 and 4. To measure the success of the developed system, 70 macroscopic melanoma skin cancer images taken from the MED-NODE system are used. According to the findings of the study, it is noted that the lesion segmentation process on macroscopic melanoma skin images observed more successful results when the K-means clustering algorithm has been used for the basic segmenting algorithm in lesion segmentation procedures. The most successful result is obtained when the center value is 4. In addition to these studies, some of the popular clustering algorithms and statistical technique are also used in skin cancer segmentation. For example (Datar et al., 2008) use self-organization mapping, (Abbas et al., 2013) use Otsu's thresholding, and (Silveira et al., 2009) use expectation-maximization.

In recent years, deep learning models have been preferred instead of classical machine learning and image processing techniques. The high success regarding machine learning models by neural networks in image classification (Krizhevsky et al., 2012) encourages researchers to use deep learning in computer-aided diagnostic systems (Litjens et al., 2017). Deep learning studies are also implemented on skin cancer (Do et al., 2018; Zhang et al., 2019; Barata and Marques, 2019). Large data sets are needed for deep learning models to be successful. Also, the deep learning network has an overfitting problem. To cope with these problems, as much data as possible should be used in a balanced way. However, it is not always possible to have balanced and big data. For the solution of this problem, Ayan and Ünver (2018) recommend the data augmentation technique for skin lesions by making use of the deep learning technique.

Sahin and Alpaslan (2020) propose a SegNet architecture-based system for the segmentation of lesions on the skin. Besides, researchers are examining the effects of preprocessing steps on skin segmentation performance, such as data magnification, color consistency, and hair removal on skin lesions. DullRazor (Lee et al., 1997) method is used for hair removal. Shades of the gray algorithm are used for Color Constancy. ISBI2016 dataset is used in the study. The dataset contains a total of 900 images. In the study, 0.907 performance is obtained according to the Accuracy metric without the preprocessing step. With the usage of the preprocessing step, the performance is improved to 0.935.

Akyel and Arici (2020) propose a new approach to hair removal and lesion segmentation based on UNET and image processing algorithms. Masks obtained by deep learning are optimized with image processing algorithms and it is aimed to predict lesion masks more accurately. ISIC 2018 data set is used in the study. 80% of the data is devoted to training and 20% to be a test set. When the results are examined, it is observed that success is 92% in lesion hair cleaning, and success is 94% in lesion segmentation.

Ünver and Ayan (2019) propose a hybrid model for lesion segmentation. In the study, the model based on a deep convolutional neural network called You Only Look Once (YOLO) is combined with the GrabCut algorithm. For the level of performance of the hybrid model, two important datasets have been benefitted. These are PH2 and ISBI 2017 datasets. 94% performance is obtained from the PH2 dataset according to the accuracy metric. Besides, the success is achieved by 96.4% in ISBI 2017 data set. Apart from the accuracy metric, performance is compared with specificity, Dice coefficient and Jaccard index metrics. To illustrate, 90% sensitivity was obtained for the recommended hybrid model in the ISBI 2017 dataset. The proposed model gives more successful results compared to other deep learning models. It gives close results compared to the models available in the literature.

Yıldız (2019) aims to diagnose a computer-aided melanoma. In the study, more than one deep learning model and classical machine learning algorithms are used. Deep learning models are AlexNet, GoogLeNet, ResNet and VGGNet models. Besides these methods, traditional artificial intelligence methods such as machine learning, nearest neighbor algorithm and support vector machine (SVM) are also tried. The name of the deep learning model proposed in the study is C4Net. 3920 dermoscopy images are used from the ISIC dataset. When the results of the study are examined, it is emphasized that the C4Net deep neural network model, which has a 96.94% accuracy, has higher classification performance than other methods. The most successful of the classical machine learning algorithms is the support vector machine. This result is 93.72% according to the accuracy metric.

Tan et al. (2019) suggest a hybrid lesion segmentation architecture. Particle swarm optimization, one of the heuristic algorithms, is combined with the deep learning model. Convolutional neural networks (CNN) from deep learning techniques are applied. Researchers add some search algorithms to the particle swarm algorithm. In this way, derivatives of the algorithm are created. Some added search algorithms are simulated annealing, levy flight, helix behavior, and differential evolution. Besides these methods, fuzzy C-Means clustering algorithm, one of the clustering techniques, is used. Particle swarm optimization and its variants are preferred for the optimization of the CNN parameters and the centroids of the Fuzzy C-Means clustering algorithm. In the study, 3 different data sets are used. These are PH2, ISIC 2017, and Dermofit Image Library. It is emphasized that the proposed methods give better results in all 3 datasets than the existing methods in the literature.

Albahar (2019) has suggested a novel classification model classifying skin lesions as either malign or benignant lesions in accordance with a new regularization method. CNN, one of the deep learning methods, is used as the classification technique. According to the comparison of the technique recommended with the previous relevant research in the literature, it could be noted that the best result has been obtained so far.

CONVOLUTIONAL NEURAL NETWORK

Information about convolutional neural network will be given in this section. Deep learning enables computational models consisting of more than one processing layers to obtain the representations of data with multi-level abstraction. These techniques are used in many other areas such as speech recognition (Noda et al., 2015), object recognition (Cao et al., 2015), drug discovery (Chen et al., 2018), and processing of genomic data (Zou et al., 2019). The complicated structures in big datasets are discovered by deep learning. These datasets use the back propagation algorithm for the indication of changed internal parameters by a machine. Such parameters are preferred to obtain data on the representation of each layer. Convolutional neural network is also included in the category of deep learning. Significant achievements in image, video, speech and sound processing are achieved with CNN (Khan et al., 2019).

A convolutional neural network consists of Both input and output layers are found in a CNN. There are also a multi-hidden ones. In these layers, convolutional neural network processes the image. These layers are convolutional layer, activation layer, pooling layer in other words down sampling, flattening layer, and fully connected layer. Figure 2 shows a representative CNN network.

Figure 2. An example of CNN architecture

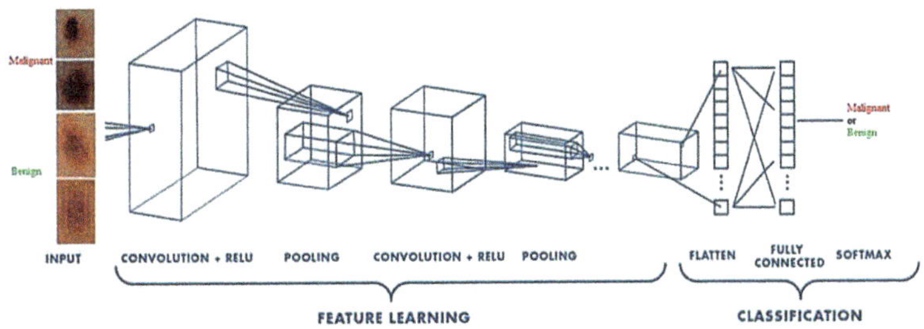

The convolutional layer is used to determine properties. It is used in an activation layer system to promote nonlinear features. In order to decrease the number of weights and to check suitability, the pooling layer is preferred. The flattening layer prepares the data for the classical artificial neural network. The completely attached layer is the classic artificial neural network using classification. CNN uses the classic artificial neural network to solve the classification problem while using other layers to identify and use features.

According to classical machine learning algorithms, there is usually a feature extraction step on the raw data. There is no general method in the feature extraction phase. There is a different feature extraction in image processing, and different feature extraction in natural language processing. Feature extraction with hierarchical transformations is performed in conventional neural networks or other deep learning algorithms. With convolutional layers, features are extracted and produced. This layer is a simple filtering process that is used for many processes in image processing.

The activation layer usually comes after the convolutional layers. In this layer, one of the activation functions is preferred. Nonlinear functions such as sigmoid and tahn are used in classical artificial neural networks. However, in CNN studies, Rectifier (ReLu) function is generally preferred. The representation of ReLu is given in Equation 1.

$$\mathrm{ReLu}(Z) = \max(0, Z) \tag{1}$$

Pooling is performed after using convolutional and activation layer. Reducing the number of features is the main role of the layer. Thus, incompatibility in the network will be checked. Various pooling operations are available. The most prominent one could be stated as max pooling. Average pooling as well as L2-norm pooling working with the same mentality are available.

Preparing the data for the input of the recent and the most significant layer is the responsibly of the flattening layer, completely attached one. Artificial neural networks receive input data from a one-dimensional array. Therefore, it needs that the matrices received from the convolutional and pooling layers have been converted into a one-dimensional array. Otherwise, the input cannot be given to the completely attached layer and the classification process cannot be performed. After the data is converted to a single dimension, it is given to a completely attached layer. Finally, the classification process has been carried out.

ARCHITECTURE OF THE DEVELOPED APPLICATION

In this section, the techniques used during the development of the application will be mentioned. 2140 images are used to train the CNN network. The images used are taken from the ISIC dataset. Half of these pictures are malignant skin cancer samples, while the remaining half are non-cancer pictures. The architecture of the recommended skin cancer detector has been given in Figure 3.

Within the scope of the project, the most commonly used tools and methods are used for skin cancer detection. The Python programming language is preferred to create the image classification model. This is because it offers easy and flexible software development and a large number of libraries. The application uses the Tensorflow library (Abadi et al., 2016). Tensorflow is an open-source library created by Google for end-to-end machine learning. Besides, OpenCV library (Bradski and Kaehler, 2008) is used during the pre-processing of the images.

When Figure 3 is examined, firstly the pictures are separated according to their labels. Then, the photos are converted to gray level through the **cv2.IMREAD GRAYSCALE** function in the OpenCV library. When the pictures are colorful, the pictures have 3 different layers. In this case, the computation cost will increase. However, if grayscale images are used, each cell of the images can be expressed as a number between 0 and 255. In this case, fewer computation costs will occur. For this reason, in many model image classification studies, instead of using colored images, grayscale images are used. At the last stage of the pre-processing step, the pictures are converted to 128x128 dimensions. In this way, a more efficient CNN model will be created. After the grayscale and scaling process, the stage of training of the CNN is started. The duration of the training phase varies according to the data set used.

For pictures to be passed through a convolutional layer the reshaping step is implemented. After this step, pictures are given to the input layer. There are 3 convolutional layers in total in the designed model. The properties of the convolutional layers used in the model are Conv2D(), filter = 32, Conv2D(), filter = 64 and Conv2D(), filter = 128, respectively. Convolutional layers are used with the ReLu activation feature. Max pooling has been performed after each convolutional layers. The max-pooling operation used is MaxPool2D().

Dropout layer is added to avoid overfitting of the model. In creating this, **Dropout()** function is used. Flatten layer is added to give input to fully connected layer. The **Flatten()** function is used to create the flatten layer. The final step is the preparation of the resulting model. For this, fully connected layer must be used. Two completely attached layers are used. The first one is created by **Dense(1024)** function, while the second one is created by **Dense(2)** function. In the first completely attached layer, various operations are done about what the result of the model will be. The second completely attached layer is the output of the model. Since it is a two-class problem, there are two outputs. After all these steps are applied in order, a model that distinguishes between malignant cancer and benign cancer images is created. For the classification process to be performed on the mobile device, the model obtained must be kept on a remote server. Therefore, the model obtained is saved in **h5 (.hdf)** format and kept on a remote server. After this stage, the model is ready to classify the given pictures and can be used as desired.

Figure 3. Architecture of the developed application

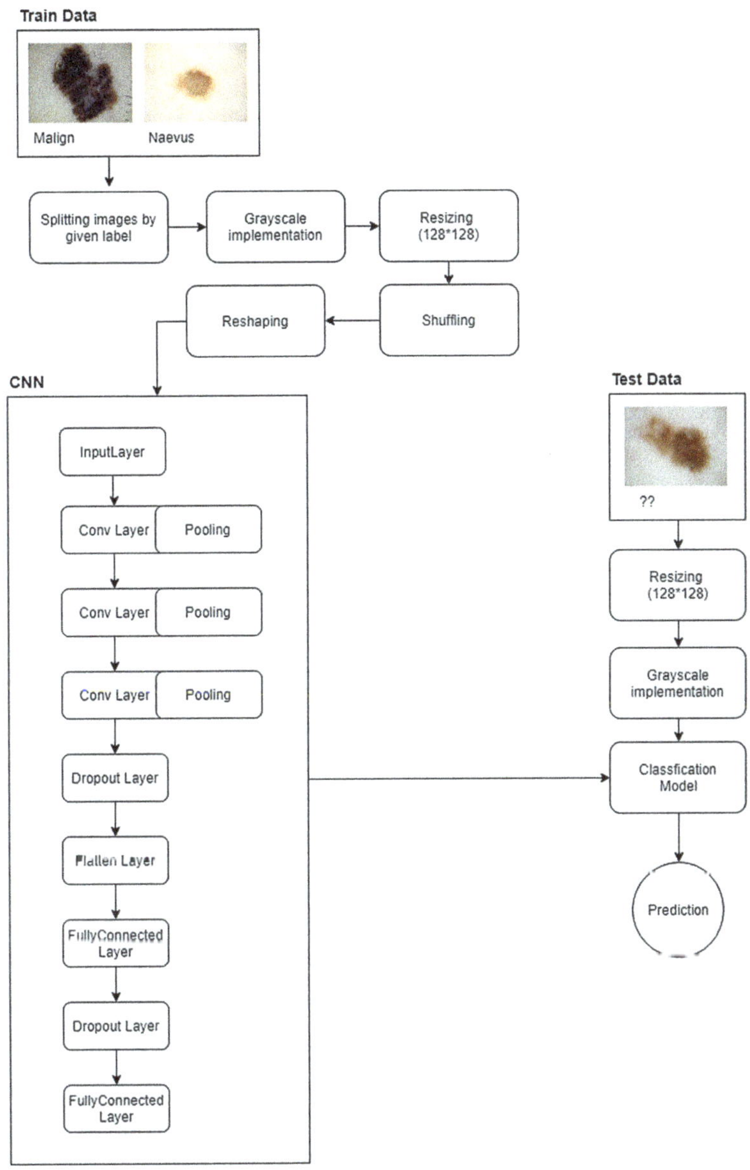

In the project, the Firebase (Firebase, 2020) solution offered by Google is used for the server solution. Firebase offers solutions such as real-time database, notification, and ML Kit. It is a service that is used in many different areas today. The model saved in the **h5** format is uploaded to the server using the **Custom Model** feature listed under the **ML Kit** package offered by Firebase. This system works as follows: The model created according to Tensor Flow Lite standards is uploaded to Firebase. This model is downloaded from the related applications and the picture to be tested is examined on this model. At the last stage, the test result is calculated. In order to use this feature, the model created must have a **.tflite** extension. The **TFLiteConverter** tool in the Tensorflow library is used for this conversion process.

Figure 4a. Registration screen

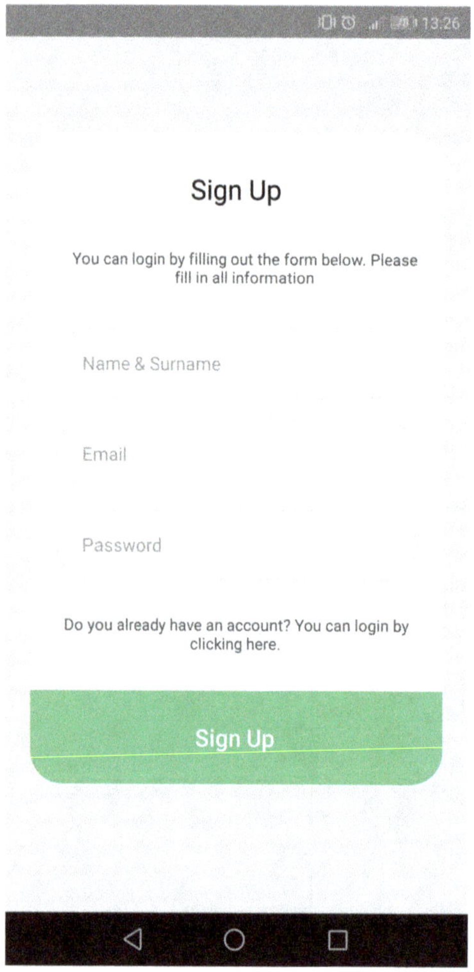

The mobile application developed within the scope of the project is developed in the Android Studio environment using the Java programming language to operate on smartphones with the Android operating system. Firebase framework is used during mobile application development. These are the **Firestore** offered by Firebase as the database, **Cloud Messaging Service** to send notifications, **Firebase Functions** to catch database changes, and **ML Kit** to accommodate the classification model. Upon completion of these steps, the mobile application is available for use.

SOLUTIONS AND RECOMMENDATIONS

In this section, the outputs obtained by running the application will be given and interpreted. When the application is run for the first time, the login screen is displayed. The reason is that certain user data are collected and the permanence of the data is ensured. In addition notifications are sent to the users. Users who have never registered before can register for the system. In addition, registered users can log in to the system via e-mail and the password they have specified. The recording screen has been presented in Figure 4a and the login screen is presented in Figure 4b.

Figure 4b. Login screen

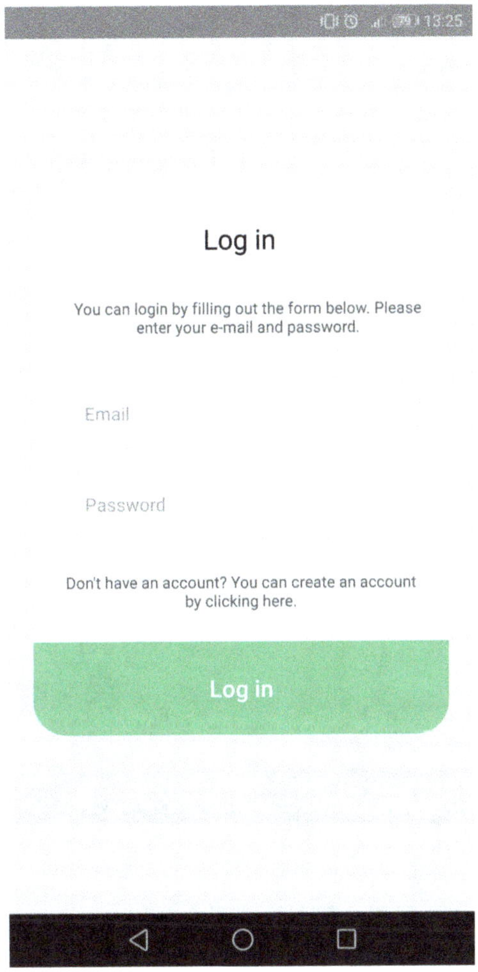

If the user has not created a record yet, an information message is displayed stating that a record has not been created before. By clicking the button on the bottom right of the page, users can upload to system the lesions on their bodies by taking photos. This situation is given in Figure 5.

Figure 5. Home screen

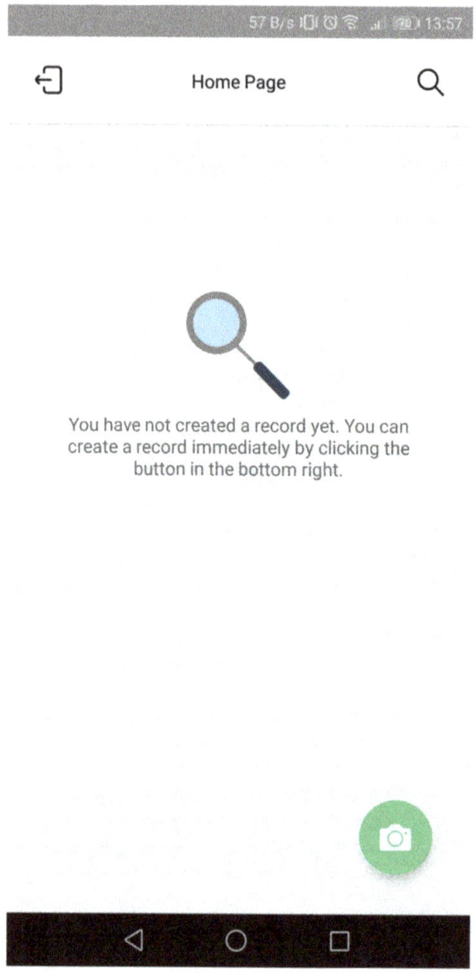

After clicking the button given in Figure 5 and opening the camera application, the picture is directed to the next page, the cropping page, for the user to crop. Following the changes made on this page, the picture is prepared for testing and passed through the model existing on the server. The result of the model is reported to the user and a record of this lesion is created on the user's homepage. The relevant page is given in Figure 6.

Figure 6. Operating the camera and cropping screen

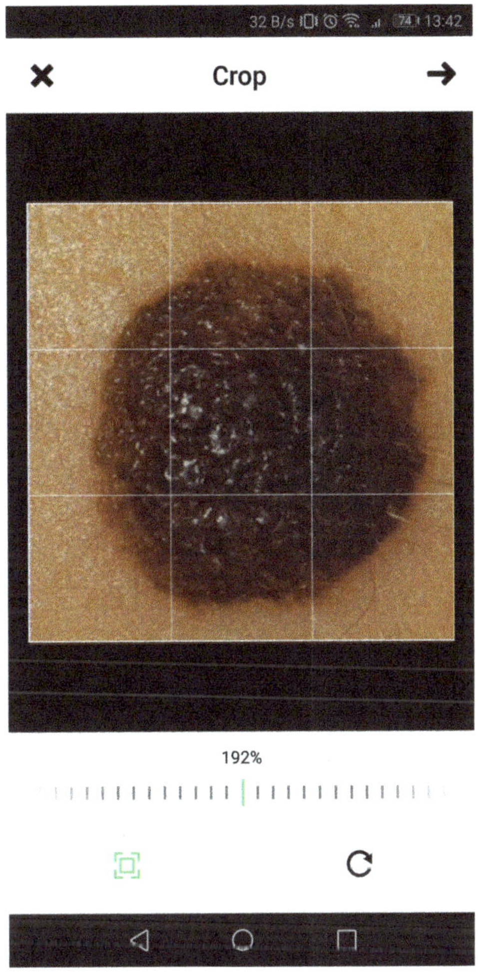

There are four hazard levels defined in the system. These are green, yellow, orange and red, respectively. These colors are determined according to the probability values given by the CNN model. The green level has been determined as risk free. In other words, it is a non-cancer lesion. The danger levels of lesions with this level are less than 0.25. The yellow level is not as strong as green, but it is determined as risk-free. The hazard levels of this level of lesions estimated by the model are less than 0.5. The next level, the orange level, was identified as risky. The hazard levels of the lesions with this level are higher than 0.5 by the model. The last level, red, is determined to be quite dangerous. The hazard levels of this level of lesions detected by the model are higher than 0.75. In Figure 7(a) and Figure 7(b), the evaluation of the lesions loaded by users and the results of this evaluation are shown.

The risk levels of the lesions and whether they are risky or not can be seen from the list on the homepage. There is an explanation of the color risk level of the circle around the lesion pictures in the list elements on the home page, and the explanation in whether the related lesion is risky or not. If the record was examined by a doctor, the information that the related record was examined by the doctor is shown on the list. On the screen that opens after clicking on the list element, the user can see the full picture of the lesion, the detailed description, and the comment made by the doctor, if any. The list and detail page have been presented in Figure 7a and Figure 7b.

Figure 7a. Patient 1's results

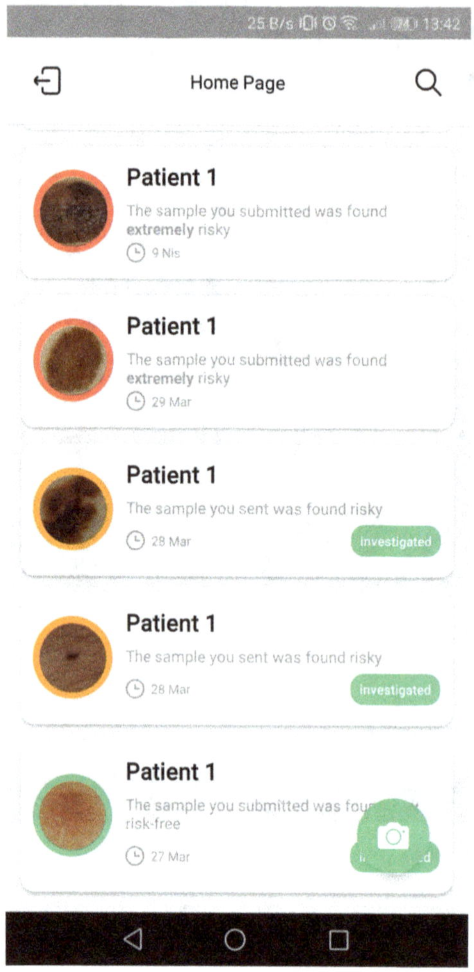

When Figure 7a is examined, Patient 1 loads 5 lesions into the system. According to the model evaluation, 2 of the loaded lesions are marked red, 2 are yellow and 1 is green. When Figure 7b is examined, Patient 2 loads 5 lesions into the system. According to the model evaluation, all lesions loaded are marked in red. Some lesions in Figure 7a and Figure 7b write "examined" in the green form on the right side. This is an important part of the developed application. This information indicates that related lesions are examined by a doctor registered in the system. While the system is being designed, a doctor's control is added in order to pass the predictions made through a secondary control. This feature is mostly designed for countries and regions where access to health services is limited. The biggest problem in such places is the insufficient number of doctors. It is aimed to bring an urgent patient with the doctor through this system.

Figure 7b. Patient 2's results

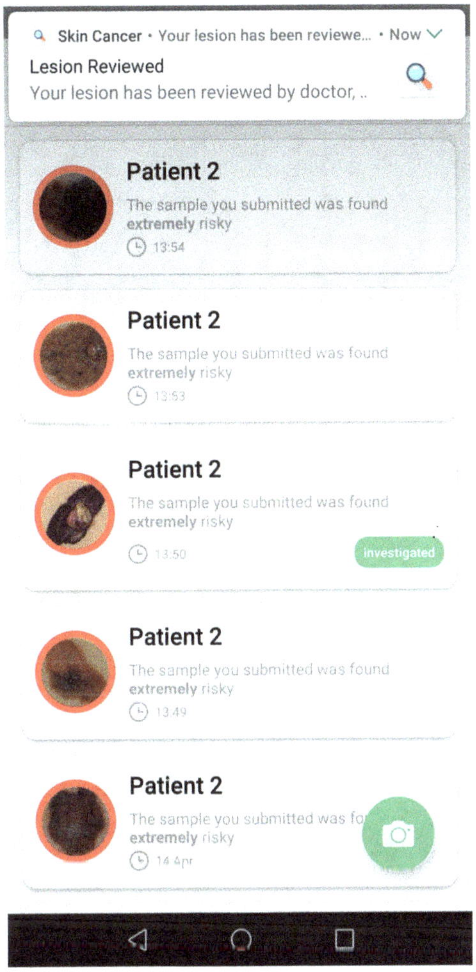

The entry of doctors into the system is like normal users. Doctors are marked as doctors in the system by a flag variable in the database. Doctors have the authority to access an extra page that normal users cannot see. If they are marked as a doctor, users can access this page via the search button in the upper right. This page is a list screen listing the lesions entered into the system. This list can be filtered by the doctor based on their level and whether they have been examined. When this list is clicked on, the doctor can see the control result made by the system and can send the examinations about the lesion to the user by using the input elements at the end of the page. Related pages are given in Figure 8a and Figure 8b.

Figure 8a. doctor lesion list screen

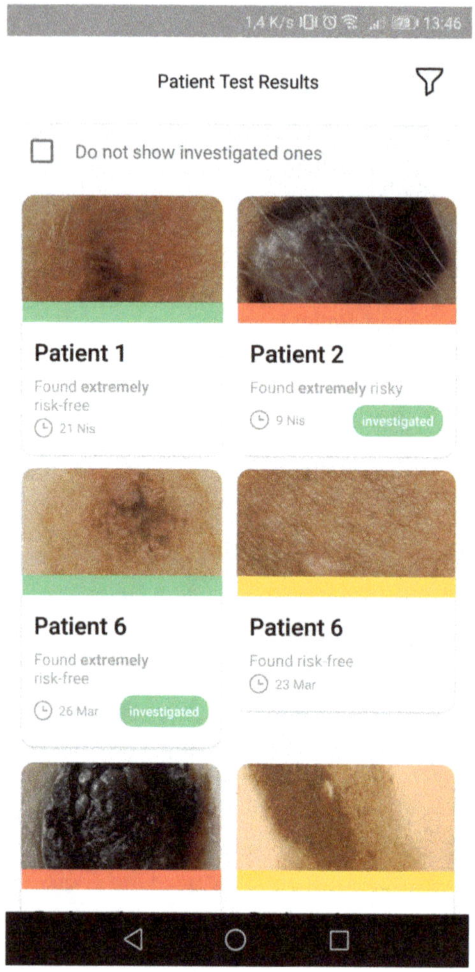

It is possible to send notifications to all users in the system via the administration panel. In addition, 2 automatic notification sending status has been added to the system. The first is to notify doctors when a red level lesion falls on the system. Another is to send a notification to the lesion owner when a doctor examines a lesion. When a new lesion assessed in red is loaded on the system, the notification appears as shown in Figure 9.

When the screen of the patient is examined, a lesion not evaluated by the doctor is seen as in Figure 10a. However, if the patient's lesion has been examined, it appears as in Figure 10b. With the application, patients are given detailed information both by the doctor and by the deep learning model. In this way, the patient will access information about the lesion. The main purpose of the study is to raise awareness for people who may be skin cancer. Besides, early diagnosis will be provided by obtaining information about lesions with the application.

Six different images that are not used in the training phase are given to the CNN model to evaluate the overall success of the system. While four of these six photos are non-disease images, the rest are images with skin cancer. The images in Figure 11 are the non-diseased images given to the model.

Figure 8b. Doctor lesion detail screen

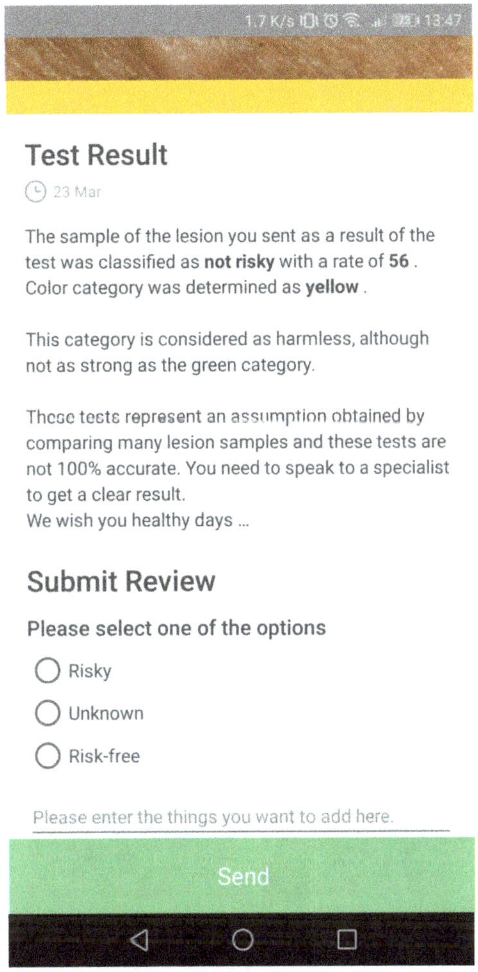

Let the images given in Figure 11 be given the names Naevus-1, Naevus-2, Naevus-3 and Naevus-4 respectively. The estimation results of the CNN model for each image are as given in Table 1.

According to Table 1, the image named Naevus-1 is estimated as harmless, that is, non-diseased cancer type with a probability of 96%. A similar situation is achieved in other non-diseased images. Achievements from other image samples are 99%, 99% and 98%, respectively. Considering Table 1, when the performance of the system is evaluated, the system can reach high performance rates. The diseased images given to the CNN model are given in Figure 12.

Let the images given in Figure 12 be given the names Malign-1 and Malign -2 respectively. The estimation results of the CNN model for each image are as given in Table 2.

According to Table 2, the image named Malign-1 is estimated as skin cancer with 99% probability. A similar situation is obtained from the image named Malign-2. The probability of the image named Malign-2 to be a diseased image is 97% according to CNN model. Considering Table 2, when the performance of the system is evaluated, the system can reach high performance rates. In general, when the results are examined, the skin cancer detection rate of the system is at a remarkable level.

Figure 9. Loading of the lesion evaluated as red

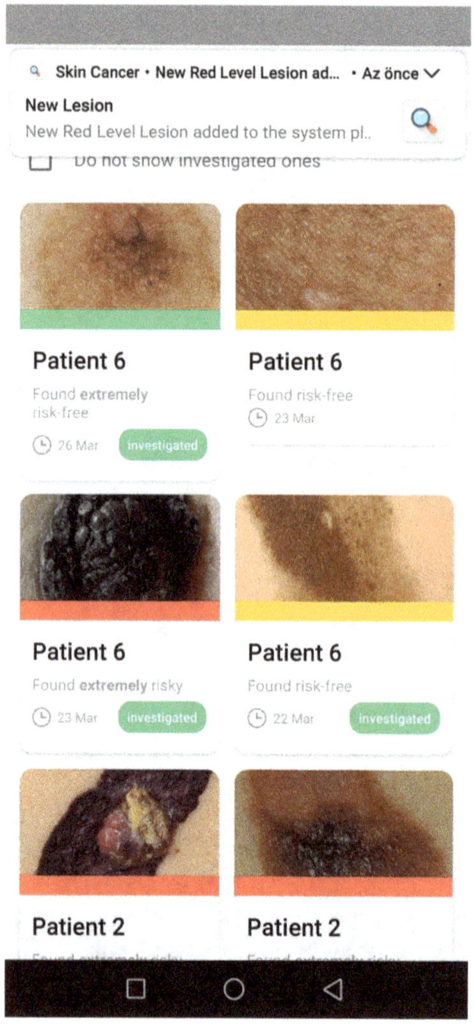

FUTURE RESEARCH DIRECTIONS

With the development and cheapness of computer hardware, the computation is getting easier. One of the best examples of this is machine learning algorithms using neural networks. These types of algorithms are operating with the data of previous years. But they were not popular due to the lack of computer hardware to run these networks. With the developments in the field of hardware in recent years, deep learning algorithms can be operated easily. Therefore, deep learning networks have been replacing classical machine learning algorithms in recent years. The biggest deficiency of deep learning algorithms is that it requires a lot of data during the training phase. For this reason, sufficient data sets are needed to conduct effective studies on deep learning. After obtaining a sufficient data set, classification performance can be increased with deep learning models. The convolutional neural network (CNN) was preferred in the research. There are many deep learning algorithms. Studies on skin cancer diagnosis can be done using other deep learning models. Also, hybrid structures can be created by combining these models. In this way, the classification performance can be increased. A significant challenge of skin cancer detection systems operating through artificial intelligence is lesion cleansing. This issue is one of the open problems. Many researchers continue to work on this. To solve this problem, efficient segmentation algorithms are needed. Classification performance will undoubtedly increase if a remarkable preprocessing step is made before machine learning or deep learning techniques. Detector systems for skin cancer operating on server-client architecture is recommended in the present paper. Deep learning steps are carried out on the server-side. On the mobile application side, the image to be tested is pre-processed and sent to the server-side. Considering the limited memory and processor capacity of the mobile device, it is quite difficult to operate the deep learning network on the mobile device. For these reasons, the server-client architecture is inevitable. The transfer learning model, one of the popular methods in recent years, can be used instead of the server-client architecture. If such a model is added directly on the mobile device, the picture will be tested directly on the mobile device.

Figure 10a. Lesion detail for patient without investigation

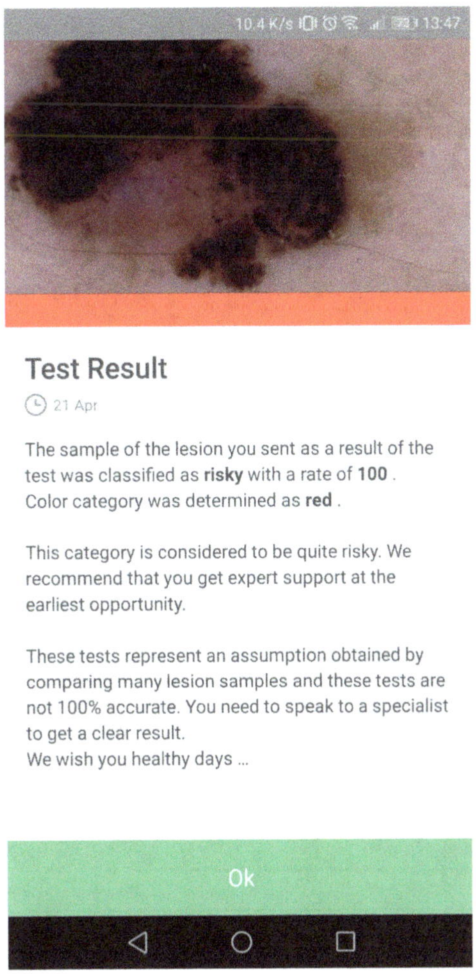

Figure 10b. Lesion detail for patient with investigation

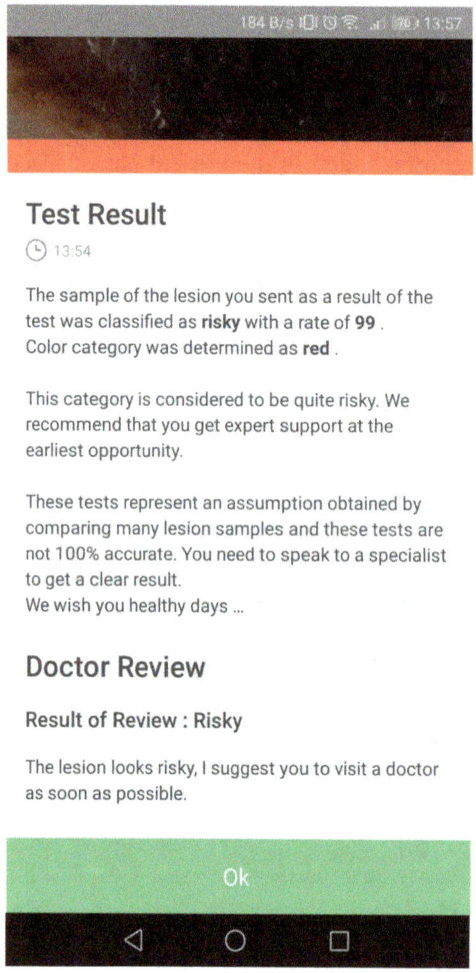

Figure 11. Naevus images given to the CNN model

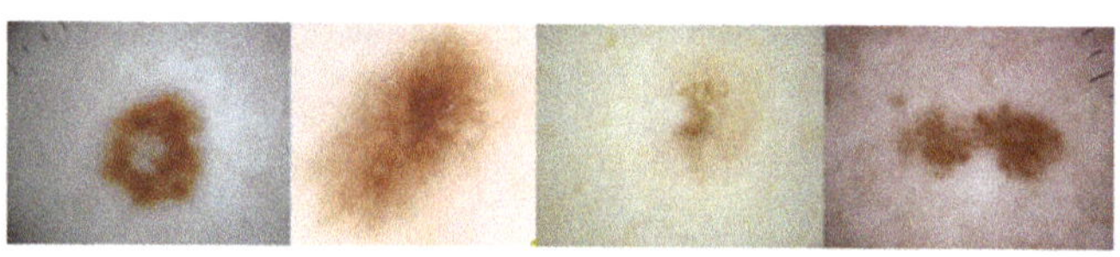

Table 1. Prediction results of naevus images given to the CNN model

Image Name	Prediction Results
Naevus-1	0.96
Naevus-2	0.99
Naevus-3	0.99
Naevus-4	0.98

Figure 12. Malign images given to the CNN model

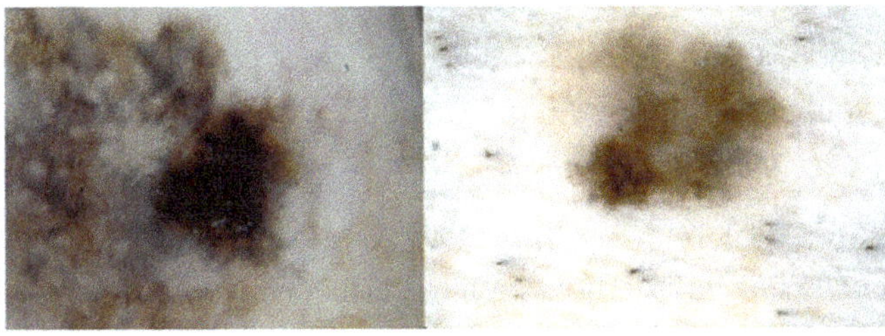

Table 2. Prediction results of malign images given to the CNN model

Image Name	Prediction Results
Malign-1	0.99
Malign-2	0.97

CONCLUSION

Skin cancer is malignant growth seen as the result of abnormal spread of the skin cells for many reasons. Skin cancer, like all other types of cancer, is a disease in which early diagnosis is extremely critical. In the detection of the disease, experts diagnose with 2-step verification. These stages are both difficult to apply and painful for patients. The first of these stages is the visual examination of the lesion. At this stage, experts examine in the lesion according to a rule called ABCD rule. At this stage, if the case is considered to be risky, the biopsy stage, which is the second stage, is passed. As a result of this stage, a definitive determination is made. When the first stage is examined, the visual examination of the experts can be carried out with some algorithms. In this study, it has been shown that the first stage can work on computers thanks to the increase in the processing power of computers and the good predictions of machine learning and deep learning algorithms. In this study, an image classification model was created by using deep learning and sufficient data sets. This model is operated in a server environment. It is estimated whether the pictures sent to the server over the mobile application are at risk of cancer. With this application, patients upload their photos to the system and see the results. At the same time, the doctors in the system give information about the patient's result. Early diagnosis of the disease is very important. For this reason, before the patients go to the doctor, the patients undergo the control of the doctor by uploading the photos of the wounds on their skin. In this way, time will be saved for the patients and early diagnosis will be made. Patients in critical situations will be admitted to the hospital in a short time. In future studies, it is aimed to use the system by large masses with the support of mobile applications. In addition, it will be emphasized to elevate the correctness of the estimations with data obtained from the users over time.

REFERENCES

Abadi, M., Barham, P., Chen, J., Chen, Z., Davis, A., Dean, J., & Kudlur, M. (2016). Tensorflow: A system for large-scale machine learning. In *12th {USENIX} Symposium on Operating Systems Design and Implementation ({OSDI} 16)* (pp. 265-283). USENIX.

Abbas, Q., Garcia, I. F., Emre Celebi, M., Ahmad, W., & Mushtaq, Q. (2013). A perceptually oriented method for contrast enhancement and segmentation of dermoscopy images. *Skin Research and Technology*, *19*(1), e490–e497. doi:10.1111/j.1600-0846.2012.00670.x PMID:22882675

Akyel, C., & Arici, N. (2020). *Cilt Kanserinde Kıl Temizliği ve Lezyon Bölütlemesinde Yeni Bir Yaklaşım. Politeknik Dergisi*. Early Access.

Albahar, M. A. (2019). Skin lesion classification using convolutional neural network with novel regularizer. *IEEE Access: Practical Innovations, Open Solutions*, *7*, 38306–38313. doi:10.1109/ACCESS.2019.2906241

Alpaydın, E. (2020). *Introduction to machine learning*. MIT Press.

Anand, V., & Koundal, D. (2020). Computer-Assisted Diagnosis of Thyroid Cancer Using Medical Images: A Survey. In *Proceedings of ICRIC 2019* (pp. 543-559). Springer. 10.1007/978-3-030-29407-6_39

Argenziano, G., Fabbrocini, G., Carli, P., De Giorgi, V., Sammarco, E., & Delfino, M. (1998). Epiluminescence microscopy for the diagnosis of doubtful melanocytic skin lesions: Comparison of the ABCD rule of dermatoscopy and a new 7-point checklist based on pattern analysis. *Archives of Dermatology*, *134*(12), 1563–1570. doi:10.1001/archderm.134.12.1563 PMID:9875194

Armstrong, B. K., & Kricker, A. (1995). Skin cancer. *Dermatologic Clinics*, *13*(3), 583–594. doi:10.1016/S0733-8635(18)30064-0 PMID:7554506

Ayan, E., & Ünver, H. M. (2018). *Data augmentation importance for classification of skin lesions via deep learning. In Electric Electronics, Computer Science, Biomedical Engineerings' Meeting (EBBT)*. IEEE.

Azar, A. T., & El-Said, S. A. (2014). Performance analysis of support vector machines classifiers in breast cancer mammography recognition. *Neural Computing & Applications*, *24*(5), 1163–1177. doi:10.100700521-012-1324-4

Barata, C., & Marques, J. S. (2019). Deep Learning For Skin Cancer Diagnosis With Hierarchical Architectures. In *IEEE 16th International Symposium on Biomedical Imaging (ISBI 2019)* (pp. 841-845). IEEE.

Bradski, G., & Kaehler, A. (2008). *Learning OpenCV: Computer vision with the OpenCV library*. O'Reilly Media, Inc.

Cao, Y., Chen, Y., & Khosla, D. (2015). Spiking deep convolutional neural networks for energy-efficient object recognition. *International Journal of Computer Vision*, *113*(1), 54–66. doi:10.100711263-014-0788-3

Chen, H., Engkvist, O., Wang, Y., Olivecrona, M., & Blaschke, T. (2018). The rise of deep learning in drug discovery. *Drug Discovery Today*, *23*(6), 1241–1250. doi:10.1016/j.drudis.2018.01.039 PMID:29366762

Datar, M., Padfield, D., & Cline, H. (2008). Color and texture based segmentation of molecular pathology images using HSOMs. In *5th IEEE International Symposium on Biomedical Imaging: From Nano to Macro* (pp. 292-295). IEEE. 10.1109/ISBI.2008.4540990

Do, T. T., Hoang, T., Pomponiu, V., Zhou, Y., Chen, Z., Cheung, N. M., Koh, D., Tan, A., & Tan, S. H. (2018). Accessible melanoma detection using smartphones and mobile image analysis. *IEEE Transactions on Multimedia, 20*(10), 2849–2864. doi:10.1109/TMM.2018.2814346

Firebase. (2020). *Firebase is Google's mobile platform that helps you quickly develop high-quality apps and grow your business.* Retrieved from https://firebase.google.com/

Gonzales, R. C., & Woods, R. E. (2002). *Digital image processing*. Pearson.

Hameed, N., Ruskin, A., Hassan, K. A., & Hossain, M. A. (2016). A comprehensive survey on image-based computer aided diagnosis systems for skin cancer. In *10th International Conference on Software, Knowledge, Information Management & Applications (SKIMA)* (pp. 205-214). IEEE. 10.1109/SKIMA.2016.7916221

Han, J., Pei, J., & Kamber, M. (2011). *Data mining: concepts and techniques*. Elsevier.

Hu, Z., Tang, J., Wang, Z., Zhang, K., Zhang, L., & Sun, Q. (2018). Deep learning for image-based cancer detection and diagnosis– a survey. *Pattern Recognition, 83*, 134–149. doi:10.1016/j.patcog.2018.05.014

Ilkin, S., Aytar, O., Gençtürk, T. H., & Şahin, S. (2020). Dermoskopik Görüntülerde Lezyon Bölütleme İşlemlerinde K-ortalama Kümeleme Algoritmasının Kullanımı. *Gazi Üniversitesi Fen Bilimleri Dergisi Part C: Tasarım ve Teknoloji, 8*(1), 182–191. doi:10.29109/gujsc.625378

Ilkin, S., Tayfur, T., & Şahin, S. (2018). Ortalama Kayma Algoritması Kullanılarak Dermatolojik Görüntüler Üzerindeki Melanomlu Alanların Tespiti. *IMASCON Uluslararası Marmara Fen ve Sosyal Bilimler Kongresi*, 780-787.

Ito, N., Kawahira, H., Nakashima, H., Uesato, M., Miyauchi, H., & Matsubara, H. (2019). Endoscopic diagnostic support system for ct1b colorectal cancer using deep learning. *Oncology, 96*(1), 44–50. doi:10.1159/000491636 PMID:30130758

Kasap, S., Pektaş, M. L., Dere, Y., & Altıparmak, M. (2015). Retrospective Evaluation of Skin Cancer Patients in Muğla. *Muğla Sıtkı Koçman Üniversitesi Tıp Dergisi, 2*(3), 34-7. Retrieved from https://dergipark.org.tr/tr/download/article-file/409758

Kasmi, R., & Mokrani, K. (2016). Classification of malignant melanoma and benign skin lesions: Implementation of automatic ABCD rule. *IET Image Processing, 10*(6), 448–455. doi:10.1049/iet-ipr.2015.0385

Khan, A., Sohail, A., Zahoora, U., & Qureshi, A. S. (2019). *A survey of the recent architectures of deep convolutional neural networks.* arXiv preprint arXiv:1901.06032.

Kourou, K., Exarchos, T. P., Exarchos, K. P., Karamouzis, M. V., & Fotiadis, D. I. (2015). Machine learning applications in cancer prognosis and prediction. *Computational and Structural Biotechnology Journal, 13*, 8–17. doi:10.1016/j.csbj.2014.11.005 PMID:25750696

Krizhevsky, A., Sutskever, I., & Hinton, G. E. (2012). Imagenet classification with deep convolutional neural networks. *Advances in Neural Information Processing Systems*, 1097–1105.

Lancaster Cancer Center. (2020). *Review Types of Cancer.* Retrieved from http://www.lancastercancer-center.com/disease-drug-information/review-types-of-cancer/

Lee, T., Ng, V., Gallagher, R., Coldman, A., & McLean, D. (1997). Dullrazor®: A software approach to hair removal from images. *Computers in Biology and Medicine*, *27*(6), 533–543. doi:10.1016/S0010-4825(97)00020-6 PMID:9437554

Liao, T. W. (2011). Diagnosis of bladder cancers with small sample size via feature selection. *Expert Systems with Applications*, *38*(4), 4649–4654. doi:10.1016/j.eswa.2010.09.135

Litjens, G., Kooi, T., Bejnordi, B. E., Setio, A. A. A., Ciompi, F., Ghafoorian, M., & Sánchez, C. I. (2017). A survey on deep learning in medical image analysis. *Medical Image Analysis*, *42*, 60–88. doi:10.1016/j.media.2017.07.005 PMID:28778026

Manogaran, G., Shakeel, P. M., Hassanein, A. S., Kumar, P. M., & Babu, G. C. (2018). Machine Learning Approach-Based Gamma Distribution for Brain Tumor Detection and Data Sample Imbalance Analysis. *IEEE Access: Practical Innovations, Open Solutions*, *7*, 12–19. doi:10.1109/ACCESS.2018.2878276

Martinez, J. C., & Otley, C. C. (2001). The management of melanoma and nonmelanoma skin cancer: A review for the primary care physician. *Mayo Clinic Proceedings*, *76*(12), 1253–1265. doi:10.4065/76.12.1253 PMID:11761506

Medical News Today. (2020). *What to know about cancer.* Retrieved from https://www.medicalnews-today.com/articles/323648

Menzies, S. W., Ingvar, C., Crotty, K. A., & McCarthy, W. H. (1996). Frequency and morphologic characteristics of invasive melanomas lacking specific surface microscopic features. *Archives of Dermatology*, *132*(10), 1178–1182. doi:10.1001/archderm.1996.03890340038007 PMID:8859028

Mogensen, M., & Jemec, G. B. (2007). Diagnosis of nonmelanoma skin cancer/keratinocyte carcinoma: A review of diagnostic accuracy of nonmelanoma skin cancer diagnostic tests and technologies. *Dermatologic Surgery*, *33*(10), 1158–1174. doi:10.1097/00042728-200710000-00003 PMID:17903149

Nahata, H., & Singh, S. P. (2020). Deep Learning Solutions for Skin Cancer Detection and Diagnosis. In *Machine Learning with Health Care Perspective* (pp. 159–182). Springer. doi:10.1007/978-3-030-40850-3_8

Narayanan, D. L., Saladi, R. N., & Fox, J. L. (2010). Ultraviolet radiation and skin cancer. *International Journal of Dermatology*, *49*(9), 978–986. doi:10.1111/j.1365-4632.2010.04474.x PMID:20883261

Neville, J. A., Welch, E., & Leffell, D. J. (2007). Management of nonmelanoma skin cancer in 2007. *Nature Clinical Practice. Oncology*, *4*(8), 462–469. doi:10.1038/ncponc0883 PMID:17657251

Noda, K., Yamaguchi, Y., Nakadai, K., Okuno, H. G., & Ogata, T. (2015). Audio-visual speech recognition using deep learning. *Applied Intelligence*, *42*(4), 722–737. doi:10.100710489-014-0629-7

Okur, E., & Turkan, M. (2018). A survey on automated melanoma detection. *Engineering Applications of Artificial Intelligence*, *73*, 50–67. doi:10.1016/j.engappai.2018.04.028

Oliveira, R. B., Mercedes Filho, E., Ma, Z., Papa, J. P., Pereira, A. S., & Tavares, J. M. R. (2016). Computational methods for the image segmentation of pigmented skin lesions: A review. *Computer Methods and Programs in Biomedicine*, *131*, 127–141. doi:10.1016/j.cmpb.2016.03.032 PMID:27265054

Ozkan, I. A., & Koklu, M. (2017). Skin Lesion Classification using Machine Learning Algorithms. *International Journal of Intelligent Systems and Applications in Engineering*, *5*(4), 285–289. doi:10.18201/ijisae.2017534420

Polat, K., & Güneş, S. (2008). Principles component analysis, fuzzy weighting pre-processing and artificial immune recognition system based diagnostic system for diagnosis of lung cancer. *Expert Systems with Applications*, *34*(1), 214–221. doi:10.1016/j.eswa.2006.09.001

Puech, P., Betrouni, N., Viard, R., Villers, A., & Leroy, X. (2007). Prostate cancer computer-assisted diagnosis software using dynamic contrast-enhanced MRI. In *29th Annual International Conference of the IEEE Engineering in Medicine and Biology Society* (pp. 5567-5570). IEEE. 10.1109/IEMBS.2007.4353608

Sahin, N., & Alpaslan, N. (2020). SegNet Mimarisi Kullanılarak Cilt Lezyon Bölütleme Performansının İyileştirilmesi. *Avrupa Bilim ve Teknoloji Dergisi*, 40-45.

Saladi, R. N., & Persaud, A. N. (2005). The causes of skin cancer: A comprehensive review. *Drugs of Today (Barcelona, Spain)*, *41*(1), 37–54. doi:10.1358/dot.2005.41.1.875777 PMID:15753968

Silveira, M., Nascimento, J. C., Marques, J. S., Marçal, A. R., Mendonça, T., Yamauchi, S., Maeda, J., & Rozeira, J. (2009). Comparison of segmentation methods for melanoma diagnosis in dermoscopy images. *IEEE Journal of Selected Topics in Signal Processing*, *3*(1), 35–45. doi:10.1109/JSTSP.2008.2011119

Stolz, W. (1994). ABCD rule of dermatoscopy: A new practical method for early recognition of malignant melanoma. *European Journal of Dermatology*, *4*, 521–527.

Tan, T. Y., Zhang, L., Lim, C. P., Fielding, B., Yu, Y., & Anderson, E. (2019). Evolving ensemble models for image segmentation using enhanced particle swarm optimization. *IEEE Access: Practical Innovations, Open Solutions*, *7*, 34004–34019. doi:10.1109/ACCESS.2019.2903015

Ünver, H. M., & Ayan, E. (2019). Skin lesion segmentation in dermoscopic images with combination of YOLO and grabcut algorithm. *Diagnostics (Basel)*, *9*(3), 72. doi:10.3390/diagnostics9030072 PMID:31295856

Varol, A. B., & İşeri, İ. (2019). Lenf Kanserine İlişkin Patoloji Görüntülerinin Makine Öğrenimi Yöntemleri ile Sınıflandırılması. *Avrupa Bilim ve Teknoloji Dergisi*, 404-410.

World Health Organization Report. (2020a). *How common is skin cancer?* Retrieved from https://www.who.int/uv/faq/skincancer/en/index1.html

World Health Organization Report. (2020b). *Canser*. Retrieved from https://www.who.int/news-room/fact-sheets/detail/cancer

Yıldız, O. (2019). Melanoma detection from dermoscopy images with deep learning methods: A comprehensive study. *Journal of the Faculty of Engineering and Architecture of Gazi University*, *34*(4), 2241–2260.

Zhang, G., Shen, X., Chen, S., Liang, L., Luo, Y., Yu, J., & Lu, J. (2019). DSM: A Deep Supervised Multi-Scale Network Learning for Skin Cancer Segmentation. *IEEE Access: Practical Innovations, Open Solutions*, *7*, 140936–140945. doi:10.1109/ACCESS.2019.2943628

Zhang, M. M., Yang, H., Jin, Z. D., Yu, J. G., Cai, Z. Y., & Li, Z. S. (2010). Differential diagnosis of pancreatic cancer from normal tissue with digital imaging processing and pattern recognition based on a support vector machine of EUS images. *Gastrointestinal Endoscopy*, *72*(5), 978–985. doi:10.1016/j.gie.2010.06.042 PMID:20855062

Zou, J., Huss, M., Abid, A., Mohammadi, P., Torkamani, A., & Telenti, A. (2019). A primer on deep learning in genomics. *Nature Genetics*, *51*(1), 12–18. doi:10.103841588-018-0295-5 PMID:30478442

ADDITIONAL READING

Albahar, M. A. (2019). Skin lesion classification using convolutional neural network with novel regularizer. *IEEE Access: Practical Innovations, Open Solutions*, *7*, 38306–38313. doi:10.1109/ACCESS.2019.2906241

Deng, L., & Yu, D. (2014). Deep learning: methods and applications. Foundations and trends in signal processing, 7(3–4), 197-387.

Esteva, A., Kuprel, B., Novoa, R. A., Ko, J., Swetter, S. M., Blau, H. M., & Thrun, S. (2017). Dermatologist-level classification of skin cancer with deep neural networks. *Nature*, *542*(7639), 115–118. doi:10.1038/nature21056 PMID:28117445

Gonzales, R. C., & Woods, R. E. (2002). *Digital image processing*. Pearson.

Ketkar, N. (2017). Introduction to keras. In *Deep learning with Python* (pp. 97–111). Apress. doi:10.1007/978-1-4842-2766-4_7

Okur, E., & Turkan, M. (2018). A survey on automated melanoma detection. *Engineering Applications of Artificial Intelligence*, *73*, 50–67. doi:10.1016/j.engappai.2018.04.028

Oliveira, R. B., Mercedes Filho, E., Ma, Z., Papa, J. P., Pereira, A. S., & Tavares, J. M. R. (2016). Computational methods for the image segmentation of pigmented skin lesions: A review. *Computer Methods and Programs in Biomedicine*, *131*, 127–141. doi:10.1016/j.cmpb.2016.03.032 PMID:27265054

KEY TERMS AND DEFINITIONS

Deep Learning: It is an advanced version of artificial neural networks from machine learning techniques.

Expert System: It is computer software used to solve problems in an information field. The logic of these software; when information is stored in databases and then problems are encountered, it is tried to reach results with inferences made on these databases.

Image Processing: It is a method that can identify with different techniques to obtain useful information based on digitized images according to the relevant need.

Lesion: It is the general name given to any abnormal tissue in the organism that is often destroyed by disease or trauma.

Machine Learning: It is the modeling of systems that make predictions by using mathematical and statistical processes on data.

Melanoma: It is a skin cancer that begins in cells called melanocytes, which give the skin its color.

Segmentation: It is usually the first stage of image analysis. Image segmentation can be described as dividing an image into meaningful regions in which different features are held.

Chapter 4
mHealth:
A Resolution in Improving Global Health

Ritu Punhani
Department of Information Technology, Noida, India

Sonia Saini
Amity Institute of Information and Technology, Amity University, India

Nimriti Varun
Amity University, India

Rahul Rustagi
Amity University, India

ABSTRACT

mHealth or mobile healthcare has become an increasingly important issue in several disciplines such as health communication, public health, and health promotion. This enables the users to use portable devices such as smartphones, smart bands, or tablets for health monitoring. The users have the ability to utilize software applications to interact with mobile devices and store relevant data for further classification and diagnosis. The apps then process the gathered data using the given algorithms and provide the user with personalized diagnosis, and further recommendations for treatment and even suggestive measures to improve general health and fitness. Another benefit of mobile technology is that the data and health statistics of a single patient can be compared with large data sets to facilitate treatment and proper guidance. Doctors, nurses, and other health professionals use mobile devices to access patient information, databases, and resources. Help in today's world is just a click away.

DOI: 10.4018/978-1-7998-6527-8.ch004

INTRODUCTION

mHealth is the use of mobile and wireless technologies to promote the accomplishment of health objectives. The growing use of cell phones is one reason why this trend is making rapid progress. The chapter offers an introduction to this new area and an outline of best practices for the creation of mHealth solutions.

mHealth is short for mobile health, medical practice and health care on mobile devices, phones, PDAs and computers. Being an industry, the field of mHealth has faced an unprecedented growth in recent years, due to growing adoption in developed countries and increasingly available mobile devices. Many people are familiar with eHealth, the healthcare industry that uses smartphones, phones, satellite networks and displays. mHealth Technology conducts related functions, such as tracking vital signs, delivering reports to physicians and facilitating remote assessment, tablets, smart phones and other handheld devices.

mHealth focuses on collecting information quickly to identify diseases, monitor diseases and provide timely information to the public in developing countries. Mobile health (mHealth) is especially relevant in remote regions where doctors and nurses may not be accessible to provide services. Healthcare workers employed in these remote areas rely on mHealth for timely updates on the handling of diseases and can also acquire implementable health information to be passed on to those in their vicinity. This mobile health system also speeds up training and education on health conditions for medical students and interns operating in remote communities.

BACKGROUND

mHealth (mobile health) is the general term used in medical care for the use of cell phones and other wireless technology. mHealth's most popular use is the use of mobile apps to inform patients about preventive health care services. Nevertheless, mHealth is also used for disease control, care assistance, tracking epidemic outbreaks and management of chronic conditions. mHealth started to came into bigger picture with the use of the most basic mobile technology, that is through the SMS alerts – which certainly has demonstrated ability to affect behaviours in a way that is superior to radio and TV campaigns. Then came the smartphones and smart devices, that completely upgraded the whole scenario. As a result of these technical developments, at the point of need the potential for increased access to information and two-way communication became more accessible. Advances in mobile software and hardware combined with expanded availability of connected devices have contributed to rapid growth in the demand for health apps. Latest reports indicate that more than 259,000 mHealth applications are available today in app stores and account for about 3.2 billion downloads per year (Singh & Landman, 2017). The clinical evidence supporting the use of applications independently of other treatments is still very small, and this has contributed to scepticism among huge healthcare organizations about the part applications could fulfil in healthcare. The mHealth industry is seeing a significant increase in wearable devices due to the growing demand of the consumers to keep track of their personal health. Originally developed to keep consumer usability in mind, these apps, equipped with the latest technologies, are now in the constant update and growth process to introduce newer industry developments The best result amongst the wearables is undoubtedly, the smartwatches. These smartwatches are attached to the app, mostly on mobile phones, which is installed in smart devices. One of the major factors that drive wearable device demand is the proliferation of mHealth technology by healthcare professionals, hospitals, insurers, software development companies, and so on. In essence, healthcare apps now are becoming a substantial part of the integrated health IT functions. Nonetheless, apps tend to displace older innovations in many areas, such as replacing specialized messaging systems for people with autism, and replacing wearable bands with mobile recognition built in smartphone lock screens (Singh & Landman, 2017). Obstacles like privacy issues and lack of incorporation into the electronic medical record have restricted the influence of apps, but mHealth has tremendous potential to reshape the delivery of healthcare in the future. Ethical consideration from the early development stages of such systems should be involved in maximizing the potential of mHealth to the fullest and applying it in an ethically sound way (Singh & Landman, 2017).

HISTORY

mHealth originally began in the area of biomedical engineering and it then started focusing at wireless and sensor technologies and how these technologies could be integrated to track people's health at a distance. And then, what we saw in the very early days were stuff like remote cardiac monitors that developed to continue looking at things like glucose control/diabetes monitoring and other types of sensor technologies. At the same time, particularly in developing countries, this newly discovered access to mobile communications infrastructure(s) and simple handsets allowed people in parts of the world who never really had access to fixed-line telephones to have access to a communication and information source.

So many of the early, mHealth initiatives actually came out of research in developed countries out of requirement because they didn't historically had access to very basic communication or information resources or networks in remote areas, so now people are able to access emergency medical transportation services, they are now likely to reach their health care providers with concerns, and healthcare providers have been able to organize their practice even more efficiently by leveraging mobile technology.

And a lot of that work started mostly in the early 2000, what we saw then over time was a more systemic trend in the mHealth room to start creating mobile health apps for cell phones, and then what we ended up with was stuff like Frontline SMS, which was essentially an SMS based service, a very broad based service that can be used for something that is routinely applicable to health or some of the early work of the UNICEF Innovations Team, from which came Rapid SMS, which offered a platform for interacting and SMS-based structured communications and data collection and messaging. So, some of these early projects were utilized to provide training mechanisms for health professionals to handle their customer base more efficiently and how to use them for issues like supply chain management, and one of UNICEF's early implementations was the procurement monitoring of Plumpy'Nut, which is basically a dietary supplement for children suffering from extreme malnutrition, and since then topics such as Frontline SMS or Rapid SMS have been used to tackle a wide variety of health problems, including early newborn detection for HIV, to promote the prevention of mother-to-child transmission, to birth registration, to provide rapid diagnostic support services for community health staff as well as standardized clinical monitoring (Mechael, 2012).

NEED FOR MHEALTH

The need for mHealth in the world has never been higher than in the recent years. The rapid improvements in the technological sector and the drastic relationship that has been formed between the fields of medical endeavours and bio-technology synchronisation has fuelled the desire in hearts of the patients and even people with just genuine concern for their health now want to make sure that the ability of self-diagnosis and fact checked customised knowledge is in their hands all the time.

As per the company of Accenture, patients are now more comfortable with a blend of realistic and digital approach. A move in the patients' perspectives and the preparation to utilize mHealth devices to deal with their wellbeing has been shown in a research. Around 66% of patients are willing to integrate mHealth and creativity into their recovery strategy. Accommodation is the main catalyst and impetus behind such acceptance of virtual medical services (Anonymous, 2017).

Figure 1. Views on the use of mHealth
Source: Healthcare Intelligence Network

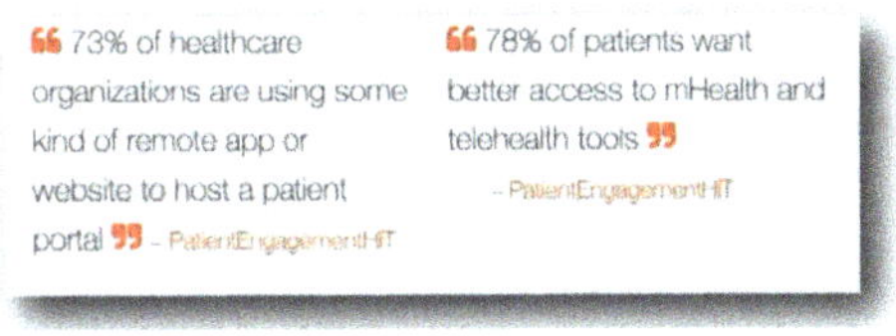

The dawn of virtual medical care culminated in the formation of mHealth as the platform for improving patient involvement. Patient involvement is accomplished as health care providers and patients join together to collaborate for better clinical treatment and outcomes. New initiatives in mHealth improve patient involvement and contentment levels by balancing the needs of patients with the skills of doctors and helping them find a middle ground for an optimal overall solution, increasing access to treatment and facilities, and further offering customised assistance and support through these networks (Anonymous, 2017).

STATISTICS

- Around 93% of the physicians believe that the mobile health apps can help in improving a patient's health outcome.
- Around 60% of physicians believe that half of their patients would like a mobile app that reminds them about their appointments.
- Nearly 67% physicians believe that the commitment to medication is a major health issue in which a mHealth app further linked to EHR could make a long lasting positive impact.
- Research shows that more online patient involvement at providers like Palo Alto Medical Foundation result in a 90% satisfaction rate among both patients and physicians.
- 97% of American healthcare providers still offer no branded patient engagement mobile apps to their patients. (Boston Technology Corporation, n.d.).

Patient care and engagement have improved drastically since the inception of the apps that constitute mhealth, along with eliminating the incidence of curable diseases. The content and connectivity provided to patients via the mHealth apps is guided, meaningful and offers assistance at various levels of care.

This preparation and customization outcomes in greater patient involvement, improved health satisfaction and lower readmission rates.

DEVICES AND SOFTWARE

The introduction of mobile devices has changed the healthcare narrative to a very large extent. Mobile devices are now considered an integral part in health care settings, prompting fast development in the improvement of medical programming (applications) for these stages. Various applications are presently accessible to help Health Care Personnel (HCP) with a huge number of significant assignments, for example, data and time the executives; health record support and the access; interchanges and counselling; reference and data gathering; persistent administration and observing; clinical dynamic; and medical instruction and preparing (Ventola, 2014).

The number of benefits and advancements that HCPs could garner using this technology is unparalleled, maybe most essentially broader accessibility of such devices, which has been appeared to help better clinical dynamic and improved patient outcomes. However, some HCPs stay hesitant to receive their use (Ventola, 2014). Despite the advantages they offer, better benchmarks and approval works on with respect to mobile medical applications should be set up to guarantee the best possible use and combination of these undeniably refined apparatuses into medical practice. These measures will raise the boundary for section into the medical application advertise, expanding the quality and wellbeing of the applications as of now accessible for use by HCPs (Misra, 2013).

Healthcare experts utilize medical devices and applications for various reasons, the greater part of which can be assembled under five general classifications: organization, health record support and access, interchanges and counselling, reference and data social occasion, and healthcare training. The numerous utilizations for mobile devices and sorts of medical applications that fall under these classifications are talked about in the accompanying segment (Ventola, 2014).

Mobile Devices and Applications

The inception of mobile digital devices has extraordinarily affected various aspects of life, including medication. Health care experts can now maximize the use of mobile phones or laptop PCs with the features they used to require a cell phone, pager or a computer to operate. Tablets and smartphones integrate communication and networking into a single unit that could be kept in hand or just be put in a handbag, making it simple to reach and be used for caring purposes (Mosa et al., 2012). Expanding to audio and video, new mobile gadget models deliver better evolved highlights, like web-looking, frameworks locating worldwide (GPS), excellent cameras, and sound recorders. Mobile phones have essentially turned into handheld PCs with these highlights, such as amazing processors and working systems, massive recollections, and high-res displays (Ventola, 2014).

Figure 2. Generation of Mobile Phones
Source: Sumnerone, 2018

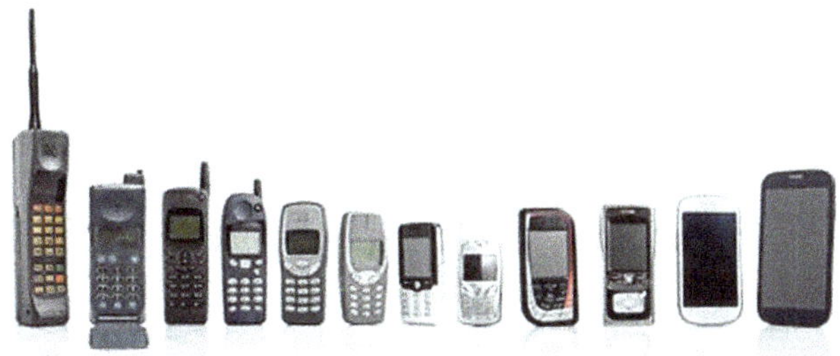

Medication is one of the many areas that were significantly affected by mobile app accessibility. It is evident in various HCP reports that show a high rate of ownership of these apparatuses used by health care workers in several medical practices and training. Mobile phones and tablets have succeeded workflow architectures as the main tools for processing work done by health care professionals.

One core motive driving the far-reaching appropriation of mobile devices by medical professionals has always been the need for preferable transparency and also dataset formation for the utility of medical care. Optimally, HCPs expect exposure to a wide variety of assets in a clinical environment, which include:

1. **Correspondence Capacities:** Video conferencing, voice calls, emails and other content (Mosa et al., 2012).
2. **Educational Assets:** Course readings, rules, medical writing, medicate references (Mosa et al., 2012).
3. **Clinical Programming Applications:** Ailment conclusion helps, medical mini-computers (Mosa et al., 2012).

Prior to the coming of age of mobile devices, these used to be the assets which were mostly given by desktop computers, which doesn't satisfy the concern for portability in health care technology. When attempting to resolve that concern, some health care institutions set up concise, remote mobile data stations, for instance, Computers on Wheels (COWs) or Workstations on Wheels (WOWs) (Mosa et al., 2012). Through the use of mobile apps, doctors are increasingly entering a pool of freely accessible data through their smartphones and tablets.

Large part, the accelerated adoption of mobile devices in medical field has been motivated by the availability and functionality of medicinal software applications or "apps." (Aungst, 2013). Apps are pieces of software designed to work on a computer or mobile device to achieve a specific goal. Speedier processors, better memory, compact batteries and highly powerful open-source software executing complex functions have paved the way for the production of a flood of technical and personal clinical mobile device software (Ozdalga et al., 2012).

Figure 3. Importance of Healthcare Apps
Source: Redbytes, 2017

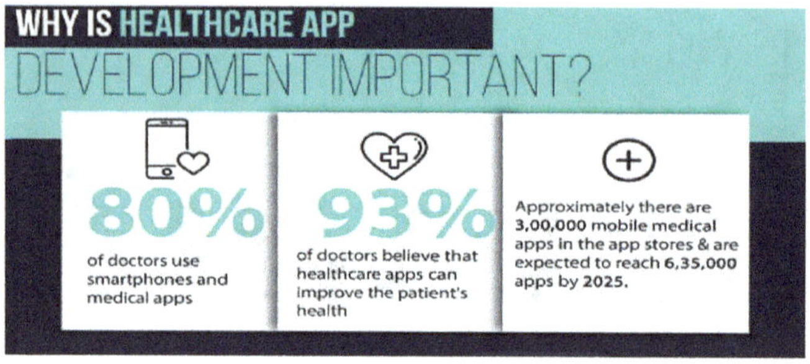

The opportunity to access medical applications on phones and tablets has made Health services available for an abundance of mobile health assets. For certain medical applications, intentions for virtual endorsement, examination and care, executive practice, encoding and paying, and CME or e-learning are available. There is a wide variety of apps that help to identify medical practice and various treatment inquiries, such as clinical reference guides, medical numbers crunchers, medical rules and also other support options, books for courses and searching channels. new smartphone apps are also there that can simulate procedures, or perform basic medical tests, like auditory or visual tests. Most smartphone apps are not intended to replace apps in the office, but instead are intended to enhance them in addition to have an advantage that can improve performance for treatment purposes. The utilization of medical applications has gotten visit and across the board; 70% of medical school HCPs and understudies announced utilizing in any event one medical application consistently, with half utilizing favoured application every day (Wallace et al., 2012).

The essential criteria for decision of application is the cost; clients are most likely to download a free of cost application however, will supplant or update it later, if fundamental, with the one that requires instalment (Murfin, 2013). Some of the costless applications are completely useful, while others are non-functional or somewhat practical except if a membership is purchased. Several popular medical journals and medical reading material can be downloaded as mobile applications after the expense of membership has been incurred (Murfin, 2013).Albeit some medical applications may at first could be exorbitant, they can eventually be savvy if refreshes are included. For model, medical course book applications are regularly refreshed every year, disposing of the need to purchase fresher releases (Murfin, 2013).

One of several HCPs most often use of mobile devices is storage and time planning (Wallace, 2012). Mainstream data processing systems, e.g. Evernote and Remarkableness, allow clients to write notes or to direct them, capture music, store images, and organize content into classifications through an open online archive. Digital library peruse apps, e.g. GoodReader and iAnnotate, allow clients to view, highlight, add, and explain messages in PDF papers (Aungst, 2013).

An extra leniency offered by data storage systems is how these can be more used in blending (Yoo, 2013). For context, GoodReader may be connected with cloud storage, enabling PDF documents to be moved from the server to the peruse program. Like some other data management software, Evernote can also be used in relation to cloud management and per use (Yoo, 2013).

Figure 4. List of apps that are commonly used by healthcare professionals

Information Management	
Evernote	Note-taking and organization
Notability	Note-taking and organization
iAnnotate	PDF viewer
GoodReader	PDF viewer
Box	Cloud storage and file sharing
Dropbox	Cloud storage and file sharing
Google Drive	Cloud storage and file sharing
Communication and Consulting	
Doximity	Social networking site for MDs
Reference and Information Gathering	
Epocrates	Drug and medical reference
Dynamed	Drug and medical reference
Skyscape/Omnio	Drug and medical reference
Micromedex	Drug reference
Dynamed	Medical reference
UpToDate	Medical reference
Medscape	Medical reference
Johns Hopkins Antibiotic Guide	Medical reference
Sanford Guide to Antimicrobial Therapy	Medical reference
Medpage Today	Medical news
Patient Management and Monitoring	
Diagnosaurus	Differential diagnosis
Pocket Lab Values	Laboratory reference
Lab Pro Values	Laboratory reference
Archimedes	Medical calculator
MedCalc	Medical calculator
Mediquations	Medical calculator
Calculate	Medical calculator

It allows a PDF retrieved from the web to be accessed with a peruse, at that point areas of the archive can be reordered into the data management application. Applications are often accessible to facilitate the compilation and retrieval of information, for instance, by entering data into the EHR or EMR of a patient (Mosa et al., 2012). Emergency medical data systems also integrate excerpts that allow EHR and PACS executives to retrieve sufferers information (medical history, health, strategies, test results, x-beams, outputs) securely either internally or externally (Mosa et al., 2012). Often times HCPs utilize mobile applications for time management. This does not call for an uncommon application; local applications that come introduced on mobile gadgets are regularly adequate to sort out and track arrangements, gatherings, call plans, and other clinical obligations. Mobile applications, for example, ZocDoc, it permits patient to see data about and accordingly make meetings with taking an interest specialist, are additionally accessible for the devices like iPhone, Android, and Blackberry (Ozdalga et a;., 2012).

Various applications are additionally accessible for distant review of medical imaging checks. Mobile MIM is a costless application especially for apple devices like iPhone and iPad, affirmed by the Food and Drug Organization, that permits distant review of X-rays and imaging scans when clients can't get to the hospital. This product works with a paid membership or pay-per-use plan utilizing MIMCloud, a HIPAA-agreeable server that permits clients to store and offer medical scans (Ozdalga et a;., 2012). Photos are exportable from the cloud and analysed with the MIMViewer paid application in any setting, in the case of conversations with colleagues or patients. There are even some medical news applications available for instance – "Outbreaks Near Me" apps are available on various platforms such as IOS or Android and provides real time updates regarding the diseases near a user using geo-fencing software. Multiple resources are consulted and checked to gather this information such as online news, eye- witnesses (Mosa et al., 2012).

Smartwatches

A Smartwatch is a famous gadget that is normally worn by competitors and health devotees. As most watches do, it can assist you with telling the time and date. Beside that regular element, a smartwatch comes stacked with applications that offer a great deal of extra features. Some of these highlights are accepting and understanding messages, noting calls, tuning in to music, messing around, and a climate estimate. In the event that you realize where to look, you can modify a smartwatch's usefulness as per your inclinations (Ghanchi, 2019).

Smartwatches are extraordinary devices that can help individuals with their health and wellness objectives. For example, sprinters regularly wear smartwatches that likewise have GPS or Worldwide positioning Framework. GPS enables them in deciding their correct area and makes a magnificent guide in making a day by day course for running. Not just that, however certain applications additionally give their clients better recommendations or alterations that they can add to their exercises and activities. For instance, there are applications in smartwatches that can propose how much calories you have to consume to accomplish your ideal weight (King & Sarrafzadeh, 2017).

Smartwatches are impeccable friends with regards to keeping up your health. Since innovation is consistently improving, you'll be certain that smartwatches will have further developed capacities that help screen our health and wellness. Here are some more reasons and conceivable future applications with respect to why a smartwatch can be gainful for your health (Ghanchi, 2019).

Figure 5. Digital watches used for monitoring health
Source: Tectales,2019

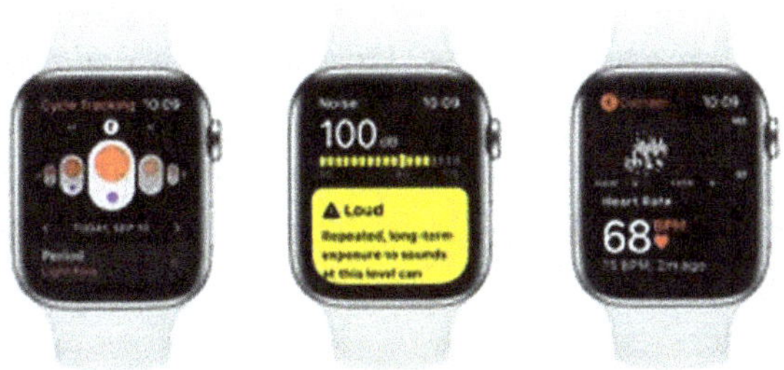

Helps Monitor Heart Rate

Smartwatches are extremely helpful to its client, particularly on following their resting heart rate or RHR. Most of these smartwatches have an incorporated pulse locator or monitoring sensors that helps asses the pulse. Devices, for example, smartwatches are valuable when you realize how much exertion you're applying when you work out. It can you a notice that you have to accomplish more activities, or it can alert you in case you're applying a lot of exertion. Having a smartwatch that can frequently and accurately screen your pulse is an incredible method to abstain from harming yourself (Ghanchi, 2019).

Managing Diabetes

Numerous conditions, including diabetes, depend on the customary and exact taking of prescribed medicines and this is another territory where smartwatches can help. studies have just been done into how a smartwatch can be utilized as a prescription journal: it tells the time, it interfaces with the web, and it's anything but difficult to work. While studies completed so far have been effective, they depend on a ton of manual client input. Wearables are going to need to include blood glucose sensors before this would all be able to be made self-dependent, yet the potential is certainly there and the information would then be able to be cross-referenced with details like every day movement (Ghanchi, 2019).

Speech Therapy

Presently as the technology has enabled us to place a call from our wristwatches in any event – numerous smartwatches are being kitted out with mouthpieces. Those amplifiers can be utilized to determine the status of speech therapy, offering criticism to clients regardless of whether they're rehearsing their speech all alone. One zone where specialists figure this may be valuable is in the treatment of Parkinson's illness. The beginning of the condition can prompt issues with the voice and discourse issue, and smartwatches could make it simpler for patients to remain focused on treatment practices when they're away from the facility.

Seizure Detection

The accelerometers incorporated with smartwatches can possibly be conveyed to identify seizures and tremors, especially with conditions like epilepsy. On account of epilepsy, seizures are activated by exceptional electrical movement in the mind, and the most serious and delayed sorts can keep the cerebrum from oxygen. When epilepsy seizures occur, brisk and viable treatment is a fundamental piece of ensuring the dangers of long term harm to the body are limited. In the event that smartwatches can be utilized to alarm friends, family and healthcare workers about seizures when they occur, can help many people (Ghanchi, 2019).

Figure 6. An example of seizure detection
Source: Gadgetmatch, 2019

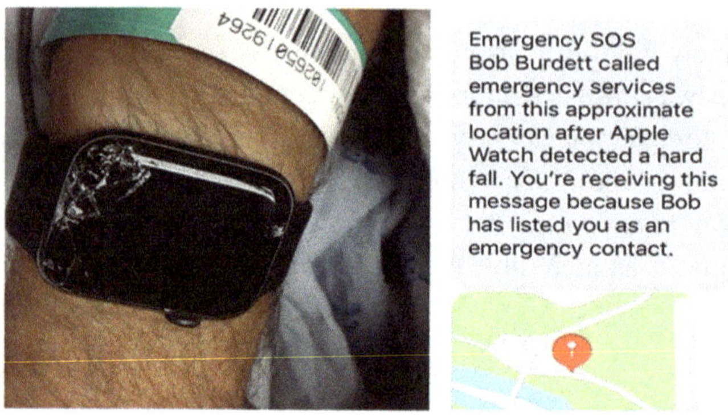

IMPLEMENTATION OF AI IN MHEALTH

Artificial intelligence (AI) in mobile health is the utilization of intricate algorithms and software to copy human insight in the examination of medical information. In particular, artificial intelligence is the capacity of computer algorithms to draw conclusions about the human health without direct human input (Datta et al, 2019)

What makes artificial intelligence different from other traditional or well-known technologies in medical field is its ability to acquire the data, processing the data and then provide a very much characterized yield to the user. AI makes this possible by using machine learning (ML) algorithms. ML algorithms are able to perceive designs from the behaviour and produce its own sense. AI algorithms carry on uniquely in contrast to human behaviour in two different ways:

1. Algorithms are literal: in the event that you set an objective, the algorithm can't change itself and just comprehend what it has been told explicitly.
2. Algorithms are secret elements: algorithms can foresee very exact, however not the reason or the why (Datta., 2019).

Basically, artificial intelligence gadgets are sorted into two: the first is machine learning (ML), as discussed above, which carries out large examinations on the structured data, for instance, hereditary data, imaging data and electrophysiological data (EP). For healthcare applications, ML forms attempt to accumulate patient's uniqueness or comprehend the chance of the sickness impacts. The second is the natural language processing (NLP), which can acquire the data from free or unstructured data, for example, clinical perceptions or wellbeing diaries to improve structured data. The natural language processing forms objects at spinning data towards the machine-reasonable structured records and would then be able to be considered by machine learning strategies. The figure below explains the layout of clinical data making, during natural language processing data improvement and machine learning data examination, to clinical judgment making. In the figure, the layout begins and finishes with clinical exercises. As prevailing as artificial intelligence (AI) systems, they can be enlivened by clinical/human services inconveniences and furthermore be pragmatic to assist the clinical presentation towards the end (Jiang et al., 2017).

Figure 7. Diagram representing the flow of AI and ML
Source: Intechopen, 2019

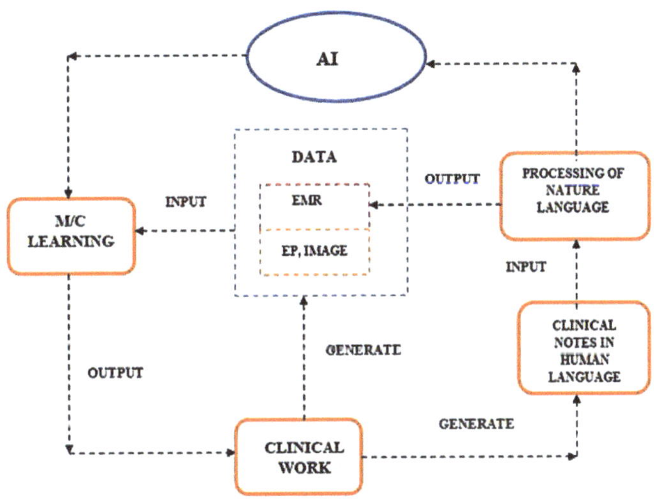

AI in Wearables: AI and machine learning are two essential tools for gathering insights or bits of knowledge. Without an AI engine, the data from a wearable would come up short on any incentive to the vendor just as the client. That is the motivation behind why, wearable application designers are progressively including AI Engine inside wearable health applications and innovative wearable health solutions. Moreover, AI even assisted that data mining is additionally basic to the achievement of an astute healthcare stage that ties numerous smartphones, IoT gadgets, websites and wearables together to accumulate data and return captivating health insights of a person (Shaikh, n.d.).

Wearables for Preventive Health

Google is looking to inject nanobots into the arteries. Don't be afraid yet. If they can find a way to take them out, the next breakthrough in medical technology may be Google X. When implanted through capsules, at the molecular and cellular stage, nanoparticles proactively detect and diagnose disorders, tumours, imminent heart attacks or strokes based on changes in the person's biochemistry.

To receive reading from nanoparticles (nanoparticles are basically IoT devices) the patient will then use a wearable like a wristwatch clamped on his wrist. The wearable then feeds the data to the platform's AI engine and uses its machine learning capabilities to detect irregularities in the wearer's body, if any. Once identified, the wearable indicates a possible disorder such as blocked arteries at a very early stage that may lead to heart attack or cancerous tumour (Shaikh, n.d.).

Wearables for Medical Consultation

The patient can report to their treating physician or an AI doctor on detection of an abnormality. An AI doctor is typically a discrete neural network with a deep learning algorithm, which can detect diseases better than an human doctor can. Deep learning algorithm ensures the application uses a self-learning framework to allow minimum errors and optimal detections. Although the machine learning algorithms share the same data as the application, they are simpler in design, providing comprehensive results (Shaikh, n.d.).

Wearables for Medication Management

AI-based doctor can prescribe medication for you. The neural network that allows AI doctors to diagnose under the surface connects to the platform to capture the medical data needed and administer medicine to the patient. The prescription is then sent to the patients' wearable who may refer to the drug or even order it using the integrated contactless payment system embedded in the wearable with the NFC chip.

Only a smart fitness device will alert you that it's time to take a drug! (Shaikh, n.d.).

Tracking Pulse and Blood Pressure for Stress Monitoring

Wearables and software's for health monitoring help monitor all the things including sleeping habits, heartbeat and a number of other biomarkers. If a patient performs a fitness regime to strengthen his / her health then these devices come very handy. In that case these apps can easily show their enhancement. In addition, patients can make the most of these devices by requesting them for daily walking reminders, heart rate stats, blood pressure, blood glucose, and to monitor their weight. Similarly, the patient's live blood pressure and pulse monitoring alerts them when to take breaks (Shaikh, n.d.).

Figure 8. A smartwatch connected to a smartphone
Source: TheHill, 2020

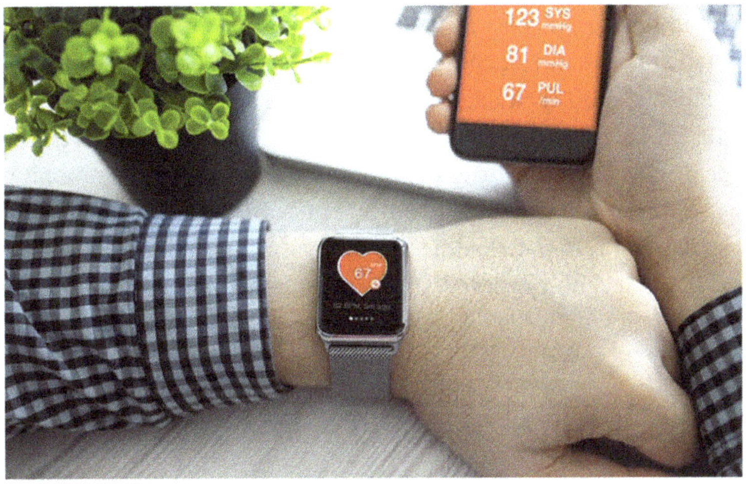

Minute-to-Minute Monitoring of Chronic Disease Conditions

Integrating health and wellness devices with wearable technology may be useful for patients with chronic illnesses. This will help track the patients' medical problems from minute to minute which is almost unimaginable for nurses and physicians. They can show the patient's changes immediately, giving them enough time to respond. A diabetic patient, for example, is indeed vulnerable to the possibility of major changes in their blood sugar levels. Those fluctuations/changes can be tracked using wearable technology, which helps to tailor the insulin treatment with high precision. It optimizes the regulation of diabetes and avoids the dangerous high blood sugar levels. Another critical use is for patients suffering from palpitations. These conditions are so sporadic and short-lived that even advanced instruments for tracking the heart fail to identify them. However, Such tiny and unusual irregularities can be identified with the aid of wearables put on the patients' wrist and linked to a smartphone (Shaikh, n.d.).

DIFFERENCE BETWEEN MHEALTH AND TELEHEALTH

Formally established, telehealth (also widely known as telemedicine) is the use of medical information shared via electronic communications from one location to another, to enhance the clinical health status of a patient. Telemedicine includes a wide range of services and applications that makes the use of two-way videos, e-mails, smart phones, wireless tools and also other forms of telecommunication technology.

Telehealth-related products and services are also part of Healthcare organization's broader investment in either IT industry or medical care delivery. And even in the reimbursement fee structure, there is generally no difference between on-site services and those offered by telemedicine, and often no separate coding needed for remote service billing.

Telehealth also incorporates patient interactions through video conferencing, still picture processing, e-health comprising patient applications, online monitoring of vital signs, continuing medical education, consumer-focused wireless software and nursing call centres.

The definition when it comes to describing mHealth is not quite as straightforward as that. MHealth, as we know is used as an abbreviation for mobile health, referring to the practice of medicine and public health assisted by mobile devices. The term is most widely used in the context of electronic devices, such as smartphones, tablets, computers, and wearable devices. Only since July 2016, the Apple iTunes store already had more than 13,000 healthcare-related features and many more on mobile platforms such as Amazon and Google Play. The most rising mHealth applications are fitness trackers. Other mHealth devices can include heart rate monitors, drug monitors, asthma and diabetes monitoring.

Although there are some ties between Telehealth and mHealth, many physicians still believe that data derived from fitness trackers and other mHealth technology is not reliable enough to be used in diagnostic or patient monitoring. When technology integration and interoperability become more popular, there is likely to be a greater correlation between telehealth and mHealth (Anonymous, 2016).

NEGATIVE EFFECTS OF PHONES AND ELECTRONICS

Mobile telephones produce radio frequencies, Form of non-ionizing electromagnetic radiation which tissues near the telephone will absorb. The radio frequency measurement emitted by a cell phone customer is exposed and depends on various elements such as the telecommunications invention, the distinction between the operator and the consumer, the degree and form of mobile phone used and the distance between the user and the network towers (World Health Organisation[WHO], 2014).

As of today, no relation has been established between continuous mobile usage and brain tumour risk, the expanding utilization of mobile devices and the absence of information for mobile telephone use after some time periods longer than 15 years warrant further research of mobile telephone use and brain disease risk. Specifically, with the ongoing prevalence of mobile telephone use among more young personnel, possibly longer lifetime of presentation, WHO has worked on further research on this gathering and is right now surveying the health effect of RF fields on totally examined endpoints. An association study in Denmark related data charging with brain tumour incidence information from the Danish Metastasis Library from more than 358,000 mobile phone supporters. The investigations found no correlation between the use of cell phones and the glioma, meningioma, or acoustic neuroma incidence, even for individuals who had been influencers of Smartphone for a minimum of 12 years (Naeem, 2014).

Figure 9. Negative rays from mobile
Source: eHealthNetwork, 2018

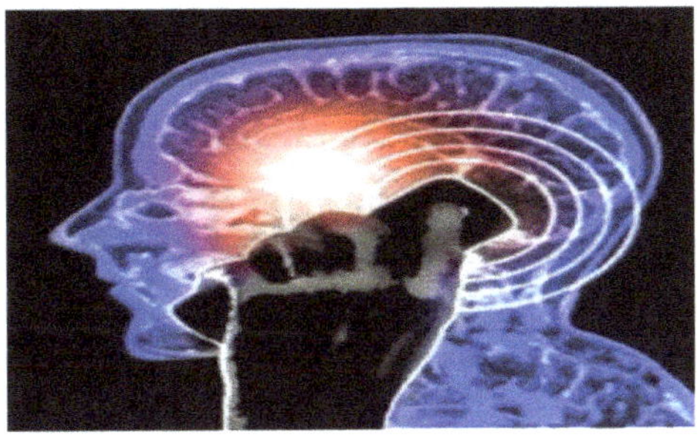

The American Cancer Society (ACS) suggests that now the IARC agreement indicates that there might be a disease-related danger, but the data is not adequately competent to be considered definitive and further work is required. People who are generally concerned about radio frequency exposure may restrict their appearance, including using an ear gadget and limiting the use of mobile phones, chiefly amongst young generation (Naeem, 2014).

Individuals who spend ton of days wearing a Smartwatch often feel like they are insomniac. This particular reaction is likewise basic to cell phone users. It acts as a rule happens in view of the absence of fixation once an individual is utilized to innovation. The productivity likewise continues declining with time. Continuous usage of Smartwatches can also lead to the inception of nausea. A good deal of research work has indicated that EMF radiation prompts comparative outcomes as on account of radiation. On the off chance that an individual faces headache for a large portion of their day, at that point an explanation could be a smartwatch he/she is continuously using. Wearing this watch throughout the day can be a tremendous purpose behind the cerebral pain problem in an individual (Azad, 2019).

Numerous smartwatch clients have now begun encountering the "apparition gadget impact." A circumstance where one gets so joined to their gadget that it starts to control their senses and mental status. many people let these watches become a part of their day to day life, they would urgently check their watch for the time or warnings, yet for a wide scope of data. Their new tech-companion would turn out to be such a natural piece of their life that in any event, when not wearing one, they would feel the urge to check their exposed wrist (Anonymous, 2016).

USE OF MHEALTH IN PANDEMIC

In the current scenario, the whole globe is fighting against the Novel Coronavirus, also known as COVID-19. This is the state of pandemic and many countries have announced a lockdown for the safety of the citizens. So in this pandemic, mHealth is proving to be the technology that is helping the people with their health issues by not compromising the lockdown situation.

mHealth is Being Majorly Used as a Help in the Chronic Diseases: Chronic diseases and conditions with a high risk on quality of life and life expectancy, such as diabetes, heart disorders, asthma, etc., often need continuous care rather than a one-time treatment. These disorders require constant assessment, monitoring and a variety of lifestyle interruptions to keep the condition under control. Hence in these days, mHealth apps are playing a pivotal role in the treatment and management of these disorders.

For instance,

- **Treating Hypertension**: Aside from keeping track of your blood pressure progress calculated on a continuous basis, the mHealth app will include a range of helpful tips, food plans, workout regimens and alternative medicines to keep your hypertension under control.
- **Treating Asthma**: Asthma is another chronic disorder that causes millions of people around the world to suffer. By using a mobile microphone as a spirometer, the mHealth app can assess the condition and provide valuable medications, or it can help the patient get in contact with a renowned specialist in the field.
- **Diabetes Management**: Diabetes is a chronic health condition that is not curable but can only be controlled with a combination of interventions including diet, exercise schedule, yoga, other healthy activities and necessary drugs/medication. Now, some medical IOT devices with their linked mobile apps allow people to monitor blood glucose levels and other metrics. The mHealth app based on these measures can recommend a treatment plan or can even help the patients contact specialists (Rathod, n.d.).

Long Distance Counselling: mHealth helps clinicians to remotely motivate and direct their patients when in-person physical contact is not possible as in the time of pandemic. Normally, during the recovery process of any chronic condition, the patient may become depressed and begin to expect the worst. During such a situation, it is the duty of the doctor to comfort the patient and to ensure that the care given will quickly cure the disease. Using mHealth, a physician can virtually communicate to a patient at any time and can ask whether there is any discrepancy. In the event of a sudden outbreak, like the one we are currently facing, the doctor can immediately warn patients to take evasive action. On the other hand, if the patient discovers that his health is deteriorating quickly and that he needs immediate help, the doctor is just a few clicks away

Hence in the current state, mHealth has opened up a whole new path for patients and caregivers to communicate directly with each other using remote, hand-held devices, no matter how far they are. This technology engulfs all physical barriers and enables both of them to get the best out of the healthcare ecosystem respecting the lockdown situation (Tate, n.d.).

HOW MHEALTH WILL IMPACT LIVES IN THE YEARS TO COME

The technological advancements that we achieve in the next decade or two will charter the course for the medical services will be applied for this century. The rapid improvements in technology and synchronisation abilities have presented many new opportunities to improve and increase the existing healthcare model reach so that more and more people can be helped (The Medical Futurist, 2019).

As we previously discussed, in crisis like the corona virus pandemic the phenomenon of mHealth will play a major role as the number of people being affected by the virus outnumber the medical capacity of the doctors by a very large margin and this is where AI and automated health diagnosis can reduce the pressure on healthcare professionals up to a very large extent. One such example is the application "Aarogya Setu" which uses automation and user information to predict the risk of a person contacting the virus

Figure 10. Depiction of mHealth by an App
Source: Fonearena, 2020

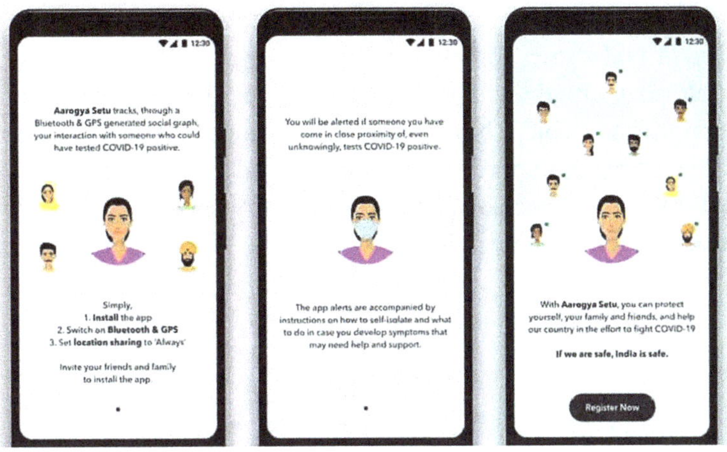

Computerized reasoning can possibly overhaul healthcare totally. Computer based intelligence calculations can draw clinical records, structure treatment designs or make medicates path quicker than any present on-screen character on the healthcare palette including any clinical expert.

Even the government is supporting the measures improving healthcare results in the nation by utilizing new and inventive ways like mHealth arrangements. Various mHealth activities have been begun by the administration. It is additionally working together with driving healthcare organizations and establishments to create answers for improving the healthcare environment in India.

The advancements are huge and the scope for expansion even bigger but the one thing that should be the first priority during this journey is quality precision. If we are counting on machines and algorithms to replace or substitute humans in any scenario we need to make sure that the decisions and diagnostics that are performed are on par if not better than what a human can do, as one small mistake can be fatal and endanger more lives than we can possibly comprehend.

The way to achieve the above stated quality is to carefully select the professionals who will lead the way for automation and develop mHealth solutions as the margin for error in this field is very low and no matter how good the technology gets the top spot in any chain shall be occupied by a human mind (The Medical Futurist, 2019).

CONCLUSION

In conclusion we can say that even though we have made uncountable advancements in the field of mhealth, what we have discovered is just the tip of the iceberg and there might be numerous ways in which mhealth could develop and chances are most of them ways are currently not even thought of.

The current mhealth scenario is dependent majorly on the smartphone acceptance and development which means we are using already existing technology to advance the cause of mhealth. In recent times although health checking sensors have been added to various smartphones to this day it is still widely considered a gimmicky addition with no purpose other than to boast about it.

The margin of error and lack of human connection still makes the mhealth sector far from a viable replacement for doctors and healthcare systems but as we can see in the covid-19 pandemic the healthcare systems can actually benefit and rely upon these technological advancements for various provisions like online consultation and virtual testing appointments.

Even though mhealth is currently unable to replace the existing system it is still very helpful in keeping the system upright and stable. The question still remains, will the advancements in the field of mhealth be able to solve the big problem of automation dependency, the answer is not known to any of us right now but currently it is helping solve various small problems for a large number of people and that is what the development of technology has been all about, To help humanity achieve a better life.

REFERENCES

Anonymous. (2016). *The key differences between Telehealth and mHealth*. https://liveclinic.com/blog/key-differences-telehealth-mhealth/

Anonymous. (2017). *Why mHealth is Essential for Patient Engagement*. https://liquid-state.com/why-mhealth-is-essential-for-patient-engagement/

Aungst, T. D. (2013). Medical applications for pharmacists using mobile devices. *The Annals of Pharmacotherapy*, *47*(7–8), 1088–1095. doi:10.1345/aph.1S035 PMID:23821609

Datta, S., Barua, R., & Das, J. (2019). Application of Artificial Intelligence in Modern Healthcare System. *Alginates - Recent Uses of This Natural Polymer*. https://www.intechopen.com/books/alginates-recent-uses-of-this-natural-polymer/application-of-artificial-intelligence-in-modern-healthcare-system

Ghanchi, J. (2019). 7 Reasons Why A Smartwatch Can Be Beneficial For Your Health With AI. *becominghuman*. https://becominghuman.ai/7-reasons-why-a-smartwatch-can-be-beneficial-for-your-health-with-ai-27e994620b10

Jiang, F., Jiang, Y., Zhi, H., Dong, Y., Li, H., Ma, S., Wang, Y., Dong, Q., Shen, H., & Wong, Y. (2017). Artificial intelligence in healthcare: past, present and future. *Stroke and Vascular Neurology*. https://svn.bmj.com/content/2/4/230

King, C. E., & Sarrafzadeh, M. (2017). A survey of smartwatches in remote health monitoring. *Journal of Healthcare Informatics Research*, *2*(1-2), 1–24. doi:10.100741666-017-0012-7 PMID:30035250

Mechael, P. (2012). mHealth Alliance: A history of mobile & mHealth. *mHealthinsight*. https://mhealthinsight.com/2012/11/24/mhealth-alliance-a-history-of-mobile-mhealth/

Misra, S., Lewis, T. L., & Aungst, T. D. (2013). Medical application use and the need for further research and assessment for clinical practice: Creation and integration of standards for best practice to alleviate poor application design. *JAMA Dermatology*, *149*(6), 661–662. https://pubmed.ncbi.nlm.nih.gov/23783150/. doi:10.1001/jamadermatol.2013.606 PMID:23783150

Mosa, A. S., Yoo, I., & Sheets, L. (2012, Jul 10). A systematic review of health care apps for smartphones. *BMC Med Inform Dec Mak*. https://bmcmedinformdecismak.biomedcentral.com/articles/10.1186/1472-6947-12-67

Murfin, M. (2013). Know your apps: An evidence-based approach to the evaluation of mobile clinical applications. *The Journal of Physician Assistant Education: the Official Journal of the Physician Assistant Education Association, 24*(3), 38–40. doi:10.1097/01367895-201324030-00008 PMID:24261171

Naeem, Z. (2014). Health risks associated with mobile phones use. *International Journal of Health Sciences, 8*(4), V–VI. doi:10.12816/0006077 PMID:25780365

Ozdalga, E., Ozdalga, A., & Ahuja, N. (2012, September 27). The smartphone in medicine: A review of current and potential use among physicians and students. *Journal of Medical Internet Research, 14*(5), e128. doi:10.2196/jmir.1994 PMID:23017375

Rathod, A. (n.d.). Why mHealth is Beneficial for Patients. *Referralmd.* https://getreferralmd.com/2019/04/why-mhealth-is-beneficial-for-patients/

Shaikh, N. (n.d.). Implementing AI in wearable health apps for better tomorrow. *Peerbits.* https://www.peerbits.com/blog/wearable-healthcare-apps-solutions-for-better-tomorrow.html

Singh, K., & Landman, A. B. (2017). Mobile Health. *Key Advances in Clinical Informatics.* https://www.sciencedirect.com/topics/medicine-and-dentistry/mobile-health

Tate, A. (n.d.). Does mHealth Improve The Patient-Provider Connection? *Referralmd.* https://getreferralmd.com/2019/09/does-mhealth-improve-the-patient-provider-connection/

The Medical Futurist. (2019). *How Digital Health Technology Can Help Manage The Coronavirus Outbreak.* https://medicalfuturist.com/how-digital-health-technology-can-help-manage-the-coronavirus-outbreak/

Ventola, C. L. (2014). Mobile Devices and Apps for Health Care Professionals: Uses and Benefits. *PMC: US National Library of Medicine National Institutes of Health, 39*(5), 356–364. https://www.ncbi.nlm.nih.gov/pmc/articles/PMC4029126/

Wallace, S., Clark, M., & White, J. (2012, August 24). 'It's on my iPhone': attitudes to the use of mobile computing devices in medical education, a mixed-methods study. *BMJ Open.* https://bmjopen.bmj.com/content/2/4/e001099

World Health Organisation. (2014). *Electromagnetic fields and public health: mobile phones.* https://www.who.int/news-room/fact-sheets/detail/electromagnetic-fields-and-public-health-mobile-phones

Yoo, J. H. (2013, June 26). The meaning of information technology (IT) mobile devices to me, the infectious disease physician. *Infection & Chemotherapy, 45*(2), 244–251. doi:10.3947/ic.2013.45.2.244 PMID:24265976

Chapter 5
Computational Studies in Breast Cancer

Monika Lamba
The Northcap University, India

Geetika Munjal
Amity University, India

Yogita Gigras
The Northcap University, India

ABSTRACT

Early detection of breast cancer is a worldwide need as many hospitals have appeared in commitment of research pathway. As per WHO (World Health Organisation), early detection of breast cancer boosts the choice of making corrective judgement on medication plan. This corrective choice helps women to save themselves from expensive and unwanted medical test and treatment. Physical observation and medical history play an important role in diagnosing this disease; however, for detailed understanding, some reliable and accurate methods are still required. This chapter reviews existing computational methods and need of novel algorithms that can help in accurately diagnosing this disease. Correct diagnosis and yield results devising treatment strategy. For correct diagnosis micro-array gene expression data is widely used, this chapter highlights various computational studies done on breast cancer microarray data. This review highlights the benefit of computational model being an impressive tool for discovery of cancer along with devising its therapies.

INTRODUCTION

Cancer research is a most important research area in medical field. Among various category of cancer, breast cancer is a cancer of heterogeneous form which take place in different types of cell in women. The second popular leading form of cancer is breast cancer in females. Major cause of women's death is its distant metastasis (Weigelt et al., 2005). Breast cancer is assumed to be the leading reason for death in

DOI: 10.4018/978-1-7998-6527-8.ch005

women as cancerous cells are found in women in form of breast tissue. There are almost twenty partition in breast known as lobes, these lobes are further divided into minute division called lobules. Basically, cancer starts in lobes named lobular carcinoma in women. There exists a slim tube for connection between lobule and lobe called duct (National Cancer Institute). As per clinical research, it is vital to diagnosed breast cancer as early as desirable, so that corrective action regarding prediction of risk (low or high) can help in choosing the appropriate therapy. Patients identified as low risk may be prevented from chemotherapy which is very costly and mainly required in high risk of breast cancer, which results in long term side effects (National institute of Health Consensus Development Panel, 2001). In order to reduce uneasy costs related with therapies, corrective classification of two receptor and prognosis group is required to raise the survival of patients suffering from breast cancer. This can only be done by managing tools that helps precisely in distinguishing the receptor and prognosis group in making right decision timely with treatment already available. Hence, demand is to find out gene expression markers relating with breast cancer supporting in classifying the two-prognosis category of breast cancer.

Breast cancer categorized as malignant shows a different behavior which make it a non-simple from various kind of diseases as cancerous cells can get distributed through breast part to remaining parts of the human body such as lymph, bone etc. (Ries et al., 2006). As many forms of breast cancer exist which respond different to various healing treatment or remedy. It is highly required that correct identification and forecasting of breast cancer in reducing the mortality rate of cancer in women. At an initial stage in women, to recognize breast cancer, mammograms benefit the doctor to give proper mediation to cancer patients. Out of many breast cancer cases, some are like women suffering from cancer that lead to poor rate of survival mostly in last stage and it develop into distantly metastasized. To safeguard women public health, breast cancer research has become the necessity. Micro-array gene expression data has persistently facilitated us to investigate and forecast the medical treatment action of this cancer to certain limit with the support of clinical parameters.

The overview of the chapter is like section 2, defines the clinical parameter in breast cancer followed by various subtypes of breast cancer, different molecular forms of breast cancer and issues related to micro-array gene expression data. Section 3 outlines the data pre-processing of micro-array, feature selection techniques. Section 4 explains the existing approaches with micro-array data. Section 5 defines the experimental results. Section 6 defines pros and cons of swallow learning, followed by Section 7 defines the evaluation of classifier performance. Section 8 conclude the chapter.

BACKGROUND

Clinical Parameters in Breast Cancer

Various pathological factors have important contribution in handling breast cancer patients at various stages. Some of these factors are tumor size, tumor grade, PR (progesterone receptor), HER (human epidermal growth factor receptor), ER (estrogen receptor), and lymph nodes (Golub et al., 1999; Cianfrocca et al., 2004). There also exists a relationship among risk of metastasis and amount of axillary lymph nodes (Donegan, 1997). Breast cancer originates from particular cells where these cells have their intrinsic clinical properties. Measurement regarding tumor size is another necessary and important prognostic factor as probability of the formation of metastasis occurs with change in tumor size. Various clinical parameters in breast cancer are mentioned in Table 1.

Breast Cancer Subtypes

It is stated in various literature that status of receptor is considered for prognosis of breast cancer (Carter et al., 1989; Deroo and Korach, 2006; Gadkar-Sable et al., 2005; Li and O'Malley, 2003; Quenel et al., 1995; Zhou and Hung, 2003; Dalton et al., 1994; Robbins et al., 1995). However, including receptor status, tumor grade is considered to be best in describing the category subtype of breast cancer and its prognosis. Molecular subtypes of breast cancer have dissimilar responses or/and prognosis towards the variety of therapies. Determination of breast cancer is done through measuring level of PR, HER2 and ER.

1. **Estrogen Receptor (ER):** It is a made up of protein molecule and it act on breast cancer tissues. It gets triggered by the hormone; hence it will unite to DNA (deoxyribonucleic acid) and regulate the functioning of miscellaneous genes. ER is known as ER negative (ER-), when the ER is under-exerted and if overexerted, known as ER positive (ER+) breast cancer subtypes. In 70% cases of breast cancer, ERs are overexerted. Estrogen receptor is one of the oldest, but very significant biomarker. In every diagnosed case of breast cancer, measuring the level of ER is compulsory. ER provide prognostic and therapy predictive details, but its better critical objective is as prognostic biomarker for endocrine analysis (Carter et al., 1989).
2. **Progesterone Receptor (PR):** It is a steroid forming a vital class of proteins present in various physiological activity namely, differentiation of cell. Mostly in reproductive tissue, PR has played a fundamental role in pregnancy and ovulation. About 65% cases of ER_positive fall under PR_positive breast cancers, and about 5% cases are monitor as ER_negative and PR_positive breast cancer (Carter et al., 1989; Deroo and Korach, 2006; Gadkar-Sable et al, 2005).
3. **Human Epidermal Growth Factor Receptor 2:** Defines as protein relating to group of trans-membrane receptors namely first HER1, second HER2, third HER3, and fourth HER4, however handle cell proliferation & cell growth. Around thirty percent cases have over expression of the HER2 as HER2 positive gene of breast cancer (Li and O'Malley, 2003; Quenel et al., 1995).
4. **Tumor Grade:** Assigning grade to breast cancer sample is dependent on microscopic likeness of cells as compared to normal breast tissue [3-4]. Assigning grade to tumor is based on 3 microscopic features first is nuclear pleomorphism gland, second is gland formation and third is count of splitting cells. Hence, the particular factors grant a value/score ranging number 1-3 (1 as closest and 3 as the far close to normal breast). The resulting scores are further combined together, if total score is 3-5, called grade_1, if total score is 6 or 7, called grade_2 and if total is 8-9, called as grade 3. But there exist two limitation with grade used for estimating prediction in patients. First, absence of reproducibility in grading among pathologist. Second, massive superiority of tumors is categorized as grade 2 (Zhou and Hung, 2003; Dalton et al., 1994; Robbins et al., 1995).

DIFFERENT MOLECULAR FORMS OF BREAST CANCER

1. **Luminal A**: These are described as PR positive and/or ER positive and low tumor grade. Such cancer indicates best prognosis with low recurrences rate and high survival rates (Mackay et al., 2011).

2. **Luminal B**: These are described as PR positive or/and ER positive and high tumor grade; it is categorized as luminal B type of breast cancer. They have poor prognosis and lesser survival rates when compared with luminal A (Mackay et al., 2011).
3. **HER2+**: Described as PR negative, ER negative, HER2 positive and low tumor grade. Mostly diagnosed among young patients of breast cancer in comparison to other molecular subtypes. It is delicate to periodic redundancy and metastasis.
4. **Basal-Like**: It has PR_negative, ER_negative and HER2_negative. Generally known as TNBC (triple negative breast cancer). Mostly initiate in women at youthful(younger) age. Basal like tumors are dynamic and it shows poor prognosis when seen with luminal A and B types (Sofi et al., 2012).
5. **Normal Breast-Like**: Less common type of breast cancer. These tumors are found small in size and gives good prognosis. Normal breast-like is most common among postmenopausal women when compared with premenopausal women (Suvarchala and Nageswararao, 2011).

As per different behavior of all cancer subtypes, it is pretty necessary to rightly distinguish them. Genes can play a very vital role. Out of millions of genes present in micro-array data, all genes are not strongly associated in classifying the data as cancerous, non-cancerous or cancer subtype. Main task is to identify out the important genes using gene selection process needed to analyze and eliminate duplicates attributes from the datasets that don't contribute to the model of correctness. For high quality of understanding improving the work by performance and reducing the computation requirement of data can be done through selection of genes. Some of the methods are constantly dealing with micro-array datasets (Metzger et al., 2011; Copper, 2001; Alizadeh et al., 2000). Various feature selection algorithms exist nowadays in literature lying in category filter, embedded and wrappers (Alon et al., 1999). Filter method works as not involving any data mining method and by working on parameters like distance, correlation, consistency and dependency. Wrapper methods works as it looks for feature subgroup mainly dependent on classifier and arranging on rank basis using correctness (Lamba et al., 2018).

Table 1. Various clinical parameters help in investigating and forecasting of breast cancer

Parameters	Definition	Category
Age	Defines the age of cancer patient	-
Grade	Defines the grade of cancer	Grade 1,2,3
Size	Defines the size of tumor in centimeter	-
ER	Define Estrogen Receptor status	ER_postive=1, ER_negative = 0
PR	Defines Progesterone Receptor status	PR_postive=1, PR_negative=0
HER	Defines Human Epidermal growth factor status	HER_positive=1, HER_negative=0
Lymph Node	Defines Lymph node assessment	Lymph_postive=1, Lymph_negative=0
Subtype	Defines Molecular category of breast cancer	LuminalA, LuminalB, Normal, Her2 and Basal
Treatment	Defines treatment given or available	Chemo therapy as CT, Hormone therapy as HT, Radiation therapy as RT and none as no therapy needed
DMFS	Defines as distant metastasis free survival	Metastasis_no=0, Metastasis_yes=1
DFS	Defines as recurrence free survival	No_recurrence=0, recurrence=1
RFS	Defines as free survival	Disease_no=0, disease_yes=1
OS	Defines as survival overall	Surviving_no=0, Surviving_yes=1

ISSUES WITH MICROARRAY EXPRESSION DATA

While dealing with the breast cancer data obtained from microarray-based technology, mainly three kind of problems arises namely noise level, dimensionality problem and interrelationship/interaction measurement.

1. **Noise Level**: The data present in microarray form is mostly found noisy (Chudin et al., 2001; Haibe-Kains, 2009) which mostly required numerous steps transforming raw biological data to gene expression data. This noisiness affects the quality of data adversely.
2. **Dimensionality Problem**: Due to production of enormous number of data with support of microarray technology supports in aligning multiple genes parallelly. This results in problem like pattern identification when sample size is too small as compare with the features (Viswanathan et al., 2008). Small sample size with numerous features reduce the performance of various classifier of cancer.
3. **Interrelationship (Correlation) Measurement**: As per the study of microarray-based technology, gene expression is never evaluated alone, they are related sometime directly or not directly to other genes. This interrelation i.e. correlation can be seen with biological pathways containing few to distinct hundred genes answerable for greater interaction of gene expression (Haibe-Kains, 2009; Viswanathan et al., 2008). The pathway is found for the analysis with the support of database which is embellished pathways of signature of genes algorithm.

MICROARRAY DATA PREPROCESSING

To deal with various issues associated with microarray data, pre-processing need to be done in order to eliminate bias if exist and to promote the quality of data at the time of computation. During pre-processing, main steps include dimensionality reduction, normalization and quality controls. Dimensionality reduction is done with two methods namely feature selection and transformation. Both the methods are never performed altogether, subject to the analysis type, any one is used or both may be used but only one followed by other (Haibe-Kains, 2009). Normalization seeks kind of variation to grant differences in technical term among chips, to promote differences among samples. Lots of methods dealing with normalization are proposed targeting gene expression related techniques. Quality controls helps in prior preparation to increase and enhance the quality of data like if chip seems outside the correction limit, then it is neglected (Haibe-Kains, 2009).

In feature transformation, the genes are converted into feature space of lesser dimension without any change in the clinical parameters. Feature selection helps in searching the relevant genes from the available genes present in data giving every possible knowledge needed for its classification (Golub et al., 1999; Devijver and Kittler, 1982). Certain benefits of feature selection are as follows:

It minimizes the complexity and helps in interpreting the model easily. Efficient and scale down the training time of the algorithm. Enhances the accuracy while selecting the correct subset. Minimized the overfitting. Need fewer evaluation and less memory storage. Lot of problems arises while selecting the best subset dealing with correlation between features (Akay, 2009). Variety of methods have been developed for diagnosis of breast cancer in literature (Banaie et al., 2018; Sun et al., 2006; Zheng et al., 2014; Alickovic and Subasi, 2017). Feature selection is mostly categorized into three categories namely filter, embedded and wrapper.

1. **Filter Method:** The strategy work with null data-mining algorithm, it is more like a pre-processing step and is done using statistical test. Mainly factors associated with this approach are information, distance, dependency and consistency. This approach is free from learning algorithm and used for many practical applications due to its uniformity and simplicity. Features having high variance contain more useful knowledge and information then low variance features. Categorized as multivariate and univariate. This approach is robust contrary to overfitting, fastest and scalable. But is abort to pick useful features, prevent dependencies and ignore correlation. Examples are t-test, fisher, correlation, random etc.

Figure 1. Filter method

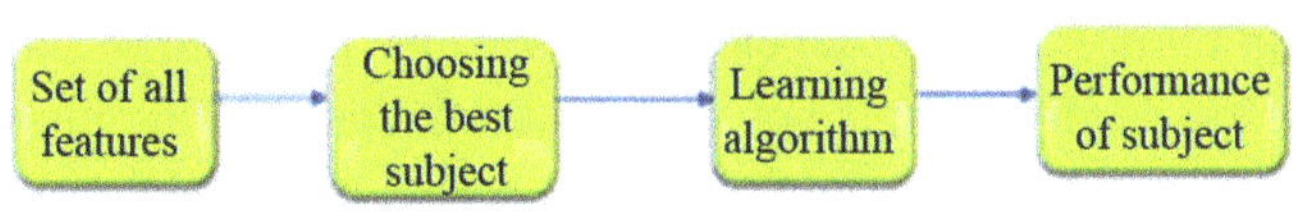

2. **Wrapper Method:** This method finds features based on the classifier and arrange features based on rank using correctness. This method when compared with filter is comparatively computationally expensive. Make use of cross-validation and tried to find best possible set of features based

on performance. Wrapper approach is categorized into randomized and deterministic. It helps in searching most useful features. Defines as simple than embedded and try every possible way to interact with classifier but fails to overcome overfitting (Kohavi and John, 1997; Xiong et al., 2001; Guyon et al., 2002). Examples are best first, greedy, ranker etc.

Figure 2. Wrapper method

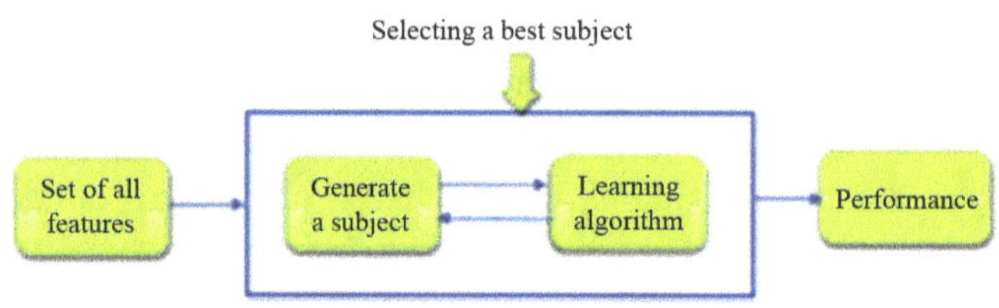

3. **Embedded Method:** This method consists characteristics of filter and wrapper including distinct rating in variety of searches at every stage. It is done using statistical tests and succeed to overcome overfitting (Hastie et al., 2009).

Figure 3. Embedded method

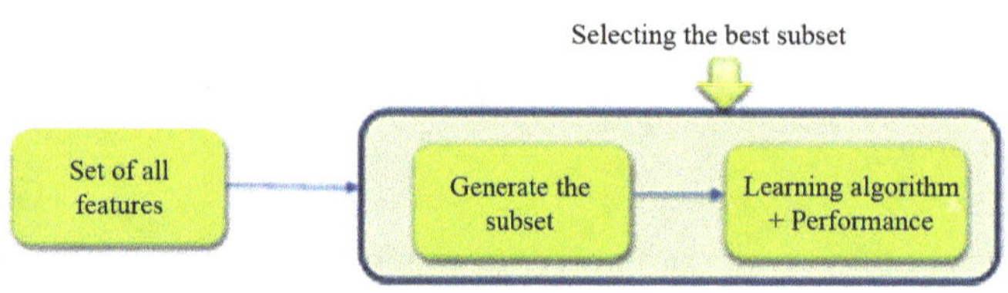

Once the data pre-processing is done, analysis of unsupervised or supervised (Lu and Han, 2003) is carry forward to see the effective change in classification performance and forecast result for breast cancer. Supervised analysis tries to search for relation between input data and output data using algorithm like support vector machine, naïve bayes etc. Unsupervised analysis tries to study the data structure without using any extraneous knowledge like clustering based on same kind of genes. Examples is clustering, k-means, cast etc.

The major goal for classification of cancer in order to correctly predict and forecast the medication of treatment (Gruvberger et al., 2001). Physicians tries to find a way for better understanding of various gene interaction that help them in cancer development because knowledge and information available for cancer is not updated too deeply. As it is not sufficient to judge classification of cancer based on its accuracy, but can lead to information based on statistical results performed using different classifier.

Cancer classifiers are categorized in three categories followed as: first category is based on structure of data without considering its correlation among the data like naïve bayesian (Ahr et al., 2001). Second category is based on interaction among data ignoring the structure of data like cast (cluster-based technique) (Ben-Dor et al., 2000; Zhang et al., 2001). Last category is based on correlation of data with the structure of data like decision tree recursive (Hong and Cho, 2006).

EXISTING APPROACHES DEALING WITH MICROARRAY DATA

An extensive effort has been done by multiple researchers in case of cancer to correctly predict, forecast and prognose the medication treatment. From years, selecting the most relevant genes selection process is carried forward in breast cancer to improve the goodness of classification. This has been improved by microarray technology but the size of the sample creates a huddle to interpret correctness classification straight forward (Boser et al., 1992). Various supervised and unsupervised approaches are discussed in Table 2.

Distinguishing of cancer classes as supervised learning where the output is analyzed from the training data i.e. known data, that helps in predicting the output of test dataset mainly unknown dataset. Cancer based applications such as prognosis, diagnosis and treatment output are a prediction job. There is vital difference among classification of cancer and other methodologies is that huge amount of information investigated at the process of classification. But, data available for cancer is not too advanced that helps researches to aim in depth knowledge of gene interaction and allow biologist to develop information related to cancer. Classification of cancer is not based on accuracy but also on biological data and information obtained from the statistics results, facts and various conclusion from the classifiers. Cancer classifiers is divided into three main category 1) related with classifiers like taken into consideration structure of data not correlation among data. The aim of this classifier is to consider data as the set of distribution while avoiding the real meaning of data and evaluate the classification depending on distribution of dataset. Example network classifier, Naïve Bayes (Gruvberger et al., 2001; Baba and Nakamura, 2002). 2) related to classifiers that take correlation into account avoiding the structure of data. This correlation is taken between the gene value irrespective of data structure. Example SVM, cluster-based technique (Simon, 2003; O'Neill, 1991). 3) last category is based with both correlation and structure of data classifiers tries to develop the relationship among gene which helps biologist a better and deep understanding of correlation of genes and structure of data. Many issues arise with micro array gene expression data that fail to give good accuracy while performing classification, like decision tree recursive (Hong and Cho, 2006).

A lot of work has been done in breast cancer to correctly predict, prognose and diagnose the cancer. Previous studies have used micro-array gene in order to find and search the important genes used for classification of breast cancer. Technology depending on micro-array gene expression data is defined as a tool helps in prognosis, diagnosis and prediction of breast cancer by creating numerous of profiles which make it difficult to interpret micro-array data directly. Multiple unsupervised and supervised approaches are applied on the breast cancer data for prediction, diagnosing and prognosing. They are as follows:

CAST Algorithm

This algorithm is a cluster-based approach that organize the samples into cluster along with increasing the number of related gene data. It uses hierarchical clustering and proposed by Den-Dor (Zhang et al., 2001). Sample data is divided into two groups, one contains majority of samples not suffering from cancer and other as majority of cancer. Main idea is based on similarity and discard the samples/data that are no longer similar with the cluster it is present. It is based on parameter known as threshold helps in controlling the cluster division.

Example: cast algorithm is applied on breast cancer samples containing thousands of gene data having benign and malignant classes. After pre-processing, making clusters using Pearson correlation helps to grouped samples into clusters, used to distinguish benign and malignant types of cancer. Cluster are formed based on the similarity to form the hierarchical tree (Ben-Dor et al., 2000).

BOOSTING

Boosting algorithm is defined as assembled classifiers from collection of various class predicators (Khan et al., 2001). Ben-Dor et al (2000, april) used the algorithm for cancer classification but proves to be a weak classifier. It uses a powerless learning technique to develop classifiers d1, d2, d3,, …, di and use weighted choice. Class can be classified as with test data g:

$$Class\left(g\right) = sign\left(\Sigma_i \omega_i d_i \left(g\right)\right) \tag{1}$$

Here, wi is defined as weight given to the classifiers.

Example: Boosting algorithm is applied on breast cancer data by Hasan (2012). The dataset consists of 286 samples categorize as 106 samples as distant metastasis and 180 samples as free patient to distinguish from metastatic and relapse free patients. The initial data of 22000 genes is reduced to 45 genes as features to identify subtypes of breast cancer.

NEURAL NETWORK

It is a kind of algorithm categorized in artificial intelligence (AI) (White, 1989), having multiple application in vast variety of problem (Shlens, 2014). Khan (2001) used neural network for classification in steps like principal component analysis, gene choice and neural network. Rule based on principal component is reducing the dimensionality just to avoid the overfitting. Followed by neural network can be developed. Helps in making a prediction while dealing classes with micro-array data in reduction, the result produced are biased and failed to achieve good performance. Resulting in removing class label from the dimensionality reduction method, and after this reduction artificial neural network can be established.

This algorithm consists of input nodes with respect to associated principal components and output nodes based on class labels. The author rearranges the input data and split the data into three parts known as 3 ANN, out of three, two were used for training purpose and third one was used for testing. The rearranging was done 1250 times and with each rearranging was done to estimate 3 ANN (Baba and Nakamura, 2002).

Example: On 58 samples, 47 were used for training and 11 for testing consisting of ER+ and ER-. Original size of dataset was 6,728 but after pre-processing the dataset was reduced to 3,389 (Gruvberger et al., 2001).

REGRESSION BASED ALGORITHM

This algorithm is purely based on statistics, helps in finding the relationship among variables. It includes multiple methods consisting of modelling and summarizing variables, identifying dependent and independent variables. Regression aid in understanding the dependency of dependent variable on independent variable. Regression on a large scale is used for foretelling just to know which independent variables are associated to dependent one. Linear, polynomial, logistic etc. Are methods based on regression rule (Yusuff et al., 2012).

Example: out of 176 patients, 130 were used for training and 46 were for testing purpose. In (Meyer and Wien, 2015), logistic regression was performed using variable having skin threatening, mass and calcination. While training, performance was 91.7% accurate and in case of testing it was 67.4% accurate. It showed patient with mass disclosure on mammogram screening, chances of having breast cancer is five times greater, while patient of calcification have 18 times higher chances and patient having skin thickening has very great chances of having breast cancer.

SVM

Vapnik developed support vector machine (SVM) widely used in many data mining application (Simon, 2003; Golub et al., 2003). Majorly used for forecasting and prognosis of cancer. It works by drawing a hyperplane along with maximal margin bounded by the classes. The point lies on the border line called support vector. The area between the margin is defined as the optimum dividing hyperplane (O'Neill, 1991).

Example: The tumor dataset of 314 samples, having 14 dissimilar cancer classes and consisting 16063 gene values. 218 tumors were left after pre-processing process and SVM was applied for binary classification.

DECISION TREE

In classification problem, this algorithm was used on a larger scale known as classification tree. This consist of internal node – defining condition for dividing attribute and leaf nodes – designate as class label.

A cancer classification technique was introduced by Zhang (2001) with the help of gene expression dataset having n sample, individual sample consisting of vector of micro-array gene expression. Classification of the samples was done using recursive partitioning constructing a classifying rule. The tree is established using two-phase method. One phase – if the particular chosen predictor is selected as cut-off value, after that data is divided into smaller/lesser samples. The judgement of choosing predicator and corresponding relative cut-off value are used to clarify the class separation like separating out the normal tissue against cancer tissue of breast, the purity of the sample is determined by function known as entropy defined below:

$$R\log\left(R\right)+\left(1-R\right)\log\left(1-R\right) \tag{2}$$

Where r is defined as normal probability of sample, the function can have maximum value with r = 0 or 1, such that the samples should be of same type, is minimum with r = 0.5, means two samples are fairly dispersed. This entropy function helps in constructing the tree and discover the top suited gene to divide and feasible dividing condition for selecting genes. Second phase is used to trim just to avoid the overfitting.

Example: 62 samples having 22 normal and 40 samples of cancer, consisting of 2000 genes. Zhang, applied recursive partitioning, by checking each 2000 expression genes with their desirable threshold, selecting the best subset of level of gene expression. The algorithm show error according to small size of data, but it will increase as per the increase in size of data as it is dependable on size of input data.

Table 2. Description of various available approaches

Methods	Definition	Advantages	Disadvantages
SVM	Developed in 1995. Widely used for classification of various cancer while training the machine using data containing cancer class details (Guyon et al., 2002).	Handle large numerous features.	Used for binary classification problem but can change multi-class problems to binary class but doesn't result in better performance (Simon, 2003).
Boosting	Defined as a type of accumulated classifier develop various class prediction using superiority (Khan et al., 2001).	It performs proportionate performance in case of classification with other methods Shows good results than decision tree classifiers (Breiman, 1996).	Time-consuming with repetition of training samples to find the accuracy. This algorithm has no superiority while comparing with other machine learning algorithm (Hasan, 2012).
Decision tree as DT	Known as classification trees works like containing nodes as internal shows separating attribute and leaf node as specific class label.	Doesn't dependent on any input parameters. Tree construction is fast. Give good results and performance on increasing the data size.	Sample size for individual class is too low, gives error-prone results (Hong and Cho, 2006).
Artificial Neural Network	In this classification is done in three steps. First principal component analysis -to minimize dimensionality in case of supervised, gene selection and network prediction (Baba and Nakamura, 2002; Ahmed, 2005).	Shows improved result while comparing with regression methods (Dreiseitl and Ohno-Machado, 2002).	Needed many parameters to increase performance. Defines as black box method, difficult to find working of model in the hidden layers. Time consuming and result in overfitting (Khan et al., 2001; Schwarzer et al., 2000; Ahr et al., 2001).
Cast- Clustering based technique	Defines as it adjusts the samples into a cluster with same kind of genes.	Classifies depending on resemblance of gene resulting in little reclining to noise.	Non-scalable with training data. Require more computational time, expensive and inappropriate (Zhang et al., 2001).
Regression	Defines as statistical method finding interrelation among variables- can be dependent or independent.	Provide acceptably fair result by using small data set. Linear regression is easily understandable for forecasting and optimization.	Mostly sensitive to the outliers. Find relationship among dependent and independent variables in linear regression, but required extremes in case of dependent one variable (Yusuff et al., 2012; Meyer and Wien, 2015).

We have summarized our literature survey study in Table 3, where we have depicted the techniques used in breast cancer analysis in past twenty years.

Table 3. Summarized details of Literature Survey

Year and Author Name	Method and Material Used	Contribution
1999 Mariana Nacht	Combined two powerful gene expression profiling technologies including DNA arrays with serial(sequential) scrutiny of gene expression (SAGE) and help to identify route of progression in breast cancer.	Identified genes presented in the breast cancer differentially. Consistency metastatic along with primary tumors with regard to under expressed genes
2001 Sofia Gruvberger	Used Artificial Neural networks, to classify tumor according to ER status. ANN performance based on top finest genes and including ER within.	100 finest ER genes are identified. Result shows that ER_negative and ER_positive tumors demonstrate distinct gene expression phenotypes.
2002 Laura J. van't Veer	Applied supervised classification and unsupervised clustering. Supervised classification is used to find the gene signature. Unsupervised cluster analysis to separate ER_negative and ER_positive samples using agglomerative hierarchical clustering.	Developed 70 genes set, that initially consists of 25000 genes among 117 samples of breast cancer. Identified good and bad prognosis cases.
2003 Christos Sotiriou	Hierarchical clustering used to divide the tumors in two subcategories based on ER status The status is then associated with basal and luminal characteristics.	Identified 485 gene set from 7650 that predict 99 patient's survival. Concluded that Estrogen Receptor is strongly related to gene expression instead of tumor grade. Suggested how gene Profiling help in devising new therapeutic.
2005 Kim M-J	The expression of 22000 transcripts is analyzed using statistical techniques. RNA of tumor against 286 lymph node patients who have not taken any treatment.	76 gene signatures having 16 genes chosen as ERnegative and 60 genes as ER_positive subgroup. Devised a robust tool to identify patient at high risk. Showed specificity as 48% and sensitivity as 93%, independently using testing dataset of 171 lymph node patients.
2006 Anna V. Ivshina	347 tumors of primary breast were investigated on Affymetrix micro-array. Usage of class prediction algorithm to find out 264 powerful grade related markers. Analysis of statistics is used to separate the G2b and G2a subtype, from G1 & G3 subtypes. Used multivariate analysis to find genetic grade like a free prognostic indicator than tumor size and lymph node.	Discovered 264 genes expression markers co-related with tumor grade using 347 main breast cancer samples. Among 264 genes, six classify grade_3 and grade_1 tumor correctly and distinguish tumor grade_2 into category like G2b and G2a. Grade signature showing predictive capacity may be extent to all tumors apart from histologic grade. Integrating the genetic grade analysis with risk factor in order to have better prognosis.
2006 Christos Sotiriou	Developed a set of 128 genes for 189 primary breast cancer patients. Kaplan Meier analysis was used to investigate the relation among gene expression grade index and relapse (deteriorate) the survival of patients.	Discovered grade_3 and grade_1 had recognizable gene expression and grade_2 breast cancer has heterogenous expression profiles. After investigating gene expression with histologic grade, it is analyzed that relapse (weaken) survival is very highly correlated with gene-expression more in comparison to histologic grade. Study helped devising new stratification method for identifying high grade patient.
2009 Ewan K.A Millar	Analysis of gene expression was observed on 60 breast cancer samples. t-test screening and variance-based gene filtering (each evaluated on gene comparing non-recurrence versus recurrences).	Developed gene expression ratio-based signature of gene with the help of training data set of 60 ER positive breast cancer samples. Three gene were discovered for recurrence cases IL17BR, HOXB13 and A1240933 for non-recurrence cases.
2011 Alan Mackay	Define the objective and reproducibility for molecular subtyping using two-way average-linkage (ranked) hierarchical clustering method. Used free-marginal kappa statistics.	No classification system produces perfect agreement (kappa>=.81) among observers. Five distinct genes list generated mainly associated with molecular subtype of breast cancer identified.
2012 Maxime Garcia	Extracted gene signature using interactome–transcriptome integration (ITI) algorithm. ITI distinguish subnetwork of ER negative and ER positive to classify low or high-risk groups of distant metastases.	Produced ER status-specific signatures, validating on individual datasets yielding higher classification accuracy. The classifier obtained seems less sensitive than previous studies It shows higher specificity helps in decision making to avoid unnecessary treatment.
2013 Iman Rezaeian	Introduce a method called gene selection positioned on hierarchical and tree-based model. To choose minimal number of genes using computational experiments. Used Chi2 feature selection and Support Vector Machine.	The approach support gene selection resulting tiny subset of genes with more than 95% accuracy overall. Results show impressive accuracy using 18 genes. The approach can be extended for more refined stratification of patients using small subset of genes.
2014 Ashish Saini	Novel method integrated prognosis risk estimation (IPRE) is proposed for gene selection. Used virtual chromosome score to find the 79 genes to form prognostic gene signature. IPRE algorithm, used to identify progression of breast cancer.	High accuracy achieved in terms of classifying good and bad prognosis. Recommended algorithm shows the possibility to help physician at the beginning stage of breast cancer in treatment decision.
2014 Ashish Saini	Classify breast cancer based on ER subtype to take right treatment that can enhance the lower mortality rate. Author proposed a novel method called RRHGE algorithm using hub topology, Gene signatures extracted from micro-array data to identify ER negative and ER positive subtype.	Achieved good classification performance based on gene interaction network. 471 genes formed gene signature, having 326 ER_positive genes and 145 for ER_ negative genes. Observation show that gene signature based on subnetwork are higher reproducible over datasets. Shows good classification performance compared to non-subnetwork-based gene signatures.
2016 Frank P.Y. Lin	Multidisciplinary team (MDT) helps in decision making for the treatment of adjuvant breast cancer. Standardized medical decision along with machine learning procedures that are designed to forecast MDT about BC treatment.	This approach carries the future possibility to give direct decision support and promote transfer of expertise and boost care quality of patient and cancer conclusion.
2017 Emmanuel S. Adabor	Breast cancer prediction and therapies are supported with deep knowledge of receptor status and hormonal status. Author identified identification of receptors like ER status, HER2 status and PR status using machine learning methods achieving low false- positive rate and high sensitivity. New method-median supplement to distinguish HER2 and hormonal receptor BC patient's status using gene profiling.	Breast Cancer deficient ER, PR and HER2 receptors that are very difficult to examine and treat. The application of author's method allows concurrent inspection of breast cancer patients with saving time and cost.
2017 Fadhl M. Alakwaa	Deep Learning (DL) have reached much importance in genomics and image analysis domains. Author aimed to assess the attainment of feed-forward network, on identifying and classifying breast cancer metabolomics data into ER+/ER-.	DL have shown higher accuracy over other machine learning methods. Deep Learning extracted features are treated as a new novel biomarker like uracil. Using 271 breast cancer tissues, having 204 tissues as ER positive and 67 as ER negative. Deep Learning method results highest prediction accuracy of 0.93. The biological judgement of deep learning's hidden layer acknowledges eight important associated path of breast cancer that are not acquire in comparison from other machine learning algorithms.
2019 David G. P. van Ijendoorn	Selecting set of miRNAs with the help of integration of classification and clustering using wrapper-based feature selection. Fuzzy and rough set were used to understand the overlying, ambiguity and changeableness characteristics of data. Random forest and particle swarm optimization in order to find the set of miRNAs.	To establish the biological significance of miRNA's in breast cancer, biological implication analysis is conducted. The selected miRNAs are authenticated through biological tests and results are statistically important.

Machine learning as part of AI (artificial intelligence), include implementation of algorithm by learning and understanding from the datasets to perform work irrespective of specific instruction. This learning process include analytical acknowledgement of patterns, helps in analyzing the data more correctly to produce exact and correct results. For details study of machine learning technique can refer Nisreen et al., 2017.

EXPERIMENTAL RESULTS

GSM25055 is a microarray-based gene expression dataset collected from NCBI. Various feature selection technique is applied in MATLAB 2019b on this dataset namely, Minimum redundancy Maximum relevance (MRMR), Relief F, FitcLinear and feature selection using neighbour component analysis (FS-RNCA). After applying the feature selection, the results given the ranking of the genes so selecting the TOP 50 genes in each case and applying the classification algorithm Naïve Bayes and Kernel Logistic Regression applied in WEKA 3.9.4. The results achieved in terms of precision are as follows in Table 4.

Table 4. Precision results of four feature selections methods on GSM25055

Machine Learning Algorithm	FITCLINEAR	MRMR	REFIEF F	FSRNCA
Kernel Logistic Regression	0.949	0.829	0.832	0.939
Naïve Bayes	0.936	0.829	0.809	0.965

On selecting a smaller number of genes i.e. 50, FitcLinear and FSRNCA are giving high precision.

On discussing various kind of machine learning algorithms, they are classified as shallow learning methods.

PROS AND CONS

Advantages of Shallow Learning Methods

1. Identification of pattern and trends that can't be easily visible to human beings.
2. Due to self-learning ability of machine learning method helps them to make self-analysis for prediction and make improve on its own.
3. Constant advancement – while gaining experience with time improves correctness.
4. Supervise and handle multi-variety and multi-dimensional data.
5. Machine learning have wide application mostly used as healthcare provider.

Disadvantages of Shallow Learning Methods

1. Data acquisition – massive data of unbiased and good quality is required to train the model.

2. Resources and time – a lot of time is required to develop and learn to attain a definite amount of accuracy and significance.
3. Results analysis – choice of choosing the correct algorithm to correctly describe the results.
4. High error sensitivity – machine learning is independent and autonomous but is deeply sensitive to errors.

Machine learning is too powerful when it is used precisely at right place, it gives an encouraging path in medical field for the correct and accurate detection of cancer. But as in case of Deep Learning require less count of input in order to achieve more processing power and data, help in gaining accurate prognosis and diagnosis of breast cancer (Rauschert et al., 2020). Looking to the great impact shown by the Deep Learning, modelling of variety of data will become simpler and useful for diagnosis in medical field (Anu and Anuja, 2020; Arti et al., 2020).

One model of machine learning that include artificial neural network, Deep Learning (DL) have the ability to allow large dataset to deal with and operate to find the good accuracy while handling performance on diagnosis, prognosis and prediction of breast cancer. DL easily learn complex pattern consisting the dataset for performing classification and making future prediction.

As deep learning needs large amount of data for training purpose, pre-training plays an utmost role to identify the issues arise while training a classifier when whole datasets is not available. Hinton (Russakovsky et al., 2015), perform classification as layer wise pre-training hence, assigning the weight of DBN (deep belief network) along with hidden layers. As a result, it was concluded that pre-training enhances the accuracy. Image net (Oquab er al., 2014) used technique to first train the deep learning model on dataset and then using that model for other work. Apart from training the dataset, weight assigned for identifying original and primitive features like corners, edges and textures that can be used for various work to save model training time and increase the performance of respective model (Shen et al., 2019). Author introduced an algorithm called deep learning for detection of breast cancer correctly making usage of end-to-end training technique on screening mammograms. Lesion definition used for training process and following stages uses image labels, removing dependency on exceptionally possible lesion definition. The performance produce was excellent using convolutional network for distinguishing screening mammograms. Due to deficiency of ROI (region of interest) this end-to-end, technique can be utilized to problems related to medical imaging. Ragab et al. (2019) presented a computer aided detection in two parts a) considering the region of interest (ROI) b) method that make use of region depend and threshold. For feature extraction, technique called convolutional neural network (CNN). SVM was used at the last layer to improve the accuracy.

EVALUATION OF CLASSIFIER PERFORMANCE

Methods used for estimating the efficiency of classifier by dividing the labelled data into subsets as:

1. **Hold Out**: Data is partitioned into two parts, one as training, second as testing. With the help and support of training datasets, a classification model is generated which then estimate the performance of model based on testing datasets, mainly the testing dataset is 20-30% of the original datasets. The division of datasets may vary as increasing the percentage of testing dataset can make the model more prone to error due to less training dataset. But lesser amount of data for testing lead to bias

towards the training dataset. It is classified as simplest form of cross-validation. This method is useful either if size of the datasets is too large or in order to quickly implement validation. Therefore, shortage of training data can lead to overfitting or underfitting for the model used (Kourou et al., 2015).

2. **Cross Validation**: Each sample is passes for the same count of times for training and once for testing within datasets. As a result, it covers the complete original data by both training and testing successfully. In this case resulted accuracy are measured as mean of all different validation cycles. This method helps in removing the bias created by holdout method, using k fold subsets of the datasets. Fold is particular and unique part of data. This method is important as it uses complete dataset for training and testing. Useful in case of small and definite dataset (Kourou et al., 2015).
3. **Random Sampling**: It is similar to holdout but in order to better find out the estimation accuracy, holdout method repeats several times during training and testing samples randomly (Hinton et al., 2006).
4. **Bootstrap**: It is a resampling method; samples are separated with replacement into training and testing sets, that is samples are placed again into the complete dataset after they have been selected for training (Hinton et al., 2006).
5. **Leave– One – Out Cross Validation**: Defined as leave-p-out, it tests the given model by each desirable possibility of p test datapoint. This method finds remarkable estimation of error and easily become extensive for large datasets. The number of iterations is calculated using n_{C_p} with n as total number of points. This grant a model to evaluate as the same number of steps as there are data points. This perform well with small dataset (Kourou et al., 2015).

CONCLUSION

In the review, efforts are made for detailed explanation and comparison of breast cancer based on variety of machine learning. All of the above studies have tried to answer various questions related to breast cancer including i) are the genes considerably correlated with breast cancer ii) if they are associated then, are they correlated with cancerous breast cancer? iii) are the genes reproducible on chosen training set will also work on across different datasets. iv) are genes powerful and robust enough to give similar distribution outcomes for distinct datasets. V) are the identified genes showing the cancer associated pathways for cancer. The performances of methods have individual limitations dependency on training set and controlled biological relevance. The survey also presented objection in utilizing the already available usable data in the best desirable manner, so that it can help in effectively diagnose and prognose breast cancer. To overcome these issues, we have explored deep learning model for breast cancer classification.

REFERENCES

Adabor, E. S., & Acquaah-Mensah, G. K. (2019). Machine learning approaches to decipher hormone and HER2 receptor status phenotypes in breast cancer. *Briefings in Bioinformatics*, *20*(2), 504–514. doi:10.1093/bib/bbx138 PMID:29045694

Ahmed, F. E. (2005). Artificial neural networks for diagnosis and survival prediction in colon cancer. *Molecular Cancer*, *4*(1), 29. doi:10.1186/1476-4598-4-29 PMID:16083507

Ahr, A., Holtrich, U., Solbach, C., Scharl, A., Strebhardt, K., Karn, T., & Kaufmann, M. (2001). Molecular classification of breast cancer patients by gene expression profiling. *The Journal of Pathology: A Journal of the Pathological Society of Great Britain and Ireland, 195*(3), 312-320.

Akay, M. F. (2009). Support vector machines combined with feature selection for breast cancer diagnosis. *Expert Systems with Applications*, *36*(2), 3240–3247. doi:10.1016/j.eswa.2008.01.009

Aličković, E., & Subasi, A. (2017). Breast cancer diagnosis using GA feature selection and Rotation Forest. *Neural Computing & Applications*, *28*(4), 753–763. doi:10.100700521-015-2103-9

Alizadeh, A. A., Eisen, M. B., Davis, R. E., Ma, C., Lossos, I. S., Rosenwald, A., ... Powell, J. I. (2000). Distinct types of diffuse large B-cell lymphoma identified by gene expression profiling. *Nature*, *403*(6769), 503–511. doi:10.1038/35000501 PMID:10676951

Alon, U., Barkai, N., Notterman, D. A., Gish, K., Ybarra, S., Mack, D., & Levine, A. J. (1999). Broad patterns of gene expression revealed by clustering analysis of tumor and normal colon tissues probed by oligonucleotide arrays. *Proceedings of the National Academy of Sciences of the United States of America*, *96*(12), 6745–6750. doi:10.1073/pnas.96.12.6745 PMID:10359783

Baba, Y., & Nakamura, T. (2002). Time dependent principal component analysis. In *Measurement and Multivariate Analysis* (pp. 155–162). Springer. doi:10.1007/978-4-431-65955-6_16

Banaie, M., Soltanian-Zadeh, H., Saligheh-Rad, H. R., & Gity, M. (2018). Spatiotemporal features of DCE-MRI for breast cancer diagnosis. *Computer Methods and Programs in Biomedicine*, *155*, 153–164. doi:10.1016/j.cmpb.2017.12.015 PMID:29512495

Ben-Dor, A., Bruhn, L., Friedman, N., Nachman, I., Schummer, M., & Yakhini, Z. (2000, April). Tissue classification with gene expression profiles. In *Proceedings of the fourth annual international conference on Computational molecular biology* (pp. 54-64). Academic Press.

Boser, B. E., Guyon, I. M., & Vapnik, V. N. (1992). A training algorithm for optimal margin classifiers. In *Proceedings of the Fifth Annual Workshop on Computational Learning Theory*. ACM.

Breiman, L. (1996). Arcing classifiers. *Annals of Statistics*, *26*, 123–140.

Carter, C. L., Allen, C., & Henson, D. E. (1989). Relation of tumor size, lymph node status, and survival in 24,740 breast cancer cases. *Cancer*, *63*(1), 181–187. doi:10.1002/1097-0142(19890101)63:1<181::AID-CNCR2820630129>3.0.CO;2-H PMID:2910416

Chudin, E., Walker, R., Kosaka, A., Wu, S. X., Rabert, D., Chang, T. K., & Kreder, D. E. (2001). Assessment of the relationship between signal intensities and transcript concentration for Affymetrix GeneChip® arrays. *Genome Biology, 3*(1).

Cianfrocca, M., & Goldstein, L. J. (2004). Prognostic and predictive factors in early-stage breast cancer. *The Oncologist*, *9*(6), 606–616. doi:10.1634/theoncologist.9-6-606 PMID:15561805

Cooper, C. S. (2001). Applications of microarray technology in breast cancer research. *Breast Cancer Research*, *3*(3), 158. doi:10.1186/bcr291 PMID:11305951

Dalton, L. W., Page, D. L., & Dupont, W. D. (1994). Histologic grading of breast carcinoma. A reproducibility study. *Cancer*, *73*(11), 2765–2770. doi:10.1002/1097-0142(19940601)73:11<2765::AID-CNCR2820731119>3.0.CO;2-K PMID:8194018

Deroo, B. J., & Korach, K. S. (2006). Estrogen receptors and human disease. *The Journal of Clinical Investigation*, *116*(3), 561–570. doi:10.1172/JCI27987 PMID:16511588

Devijver, P. A., & Kittler, J. (1982). *Pattern recognition: A statistical approach*. Prentice hall.

Donegan, W. L. (1997). Tumor-related prognostic factors for breast cancer. *CA: a Cancer Journal for Clinicians*, *47*(1), 28–51. doi:10.3322/canjclin.47.1.28 PMID:8996077

Dreiseitl, S., & Ohno-Machado, L. (2002). Logistic regression and artificial neural network classification models: A methodology review. *Journal of Biomedical Informatics*, *35*(5-6), 352–359. doi:10.1016/S1532-0464(03)00034-0 PMID:12968784

Gadkar-Sable, S., Shah, C., Rosario, G., Sachdeva, G., & Puri, C. (2005). Progesterone receptors: Various forms and functions in reproductive tissues. *Frontiers in Bioscience*, *10*(2118), 30. doi:10.2741/1685 PMID:15970482

Garcia, M., Millat-Carus, R., Bertucci, F., Finetti, P., Birnbaum, D., & Bidaut, G. (2012). Interactome–transcriptome integration for predicting distant metastasis in breast cancer. *Bioinformatics (Oxford, England)*, *28*(5), 672–678. doi:10.1093/bioinformatics/bts025 PMID:22238264

Golub, T., Mukherjee, S., Ramaswamy, S., Rifkin, R., & Tamayo, P. (2003). *U.S. Patent Application No. 10/294,453*. US Patent Office.

Golub, T. R., Slonim, D. K., Tamayo, P., Huard, C., Gaasenbeek, M., Mesirov, J. P., ... & Bloomfield, C. D. (1999). Molecular classification of cancer: class discovery and class prediction by gene expression monitoring. *Science, 286*(5439), 531-537.

Gruvberger, S., Ringnér, M., Chen, Y., Panavally, S., Saal, L. H., Borg, Å., ... Meltzer, P. S. (2001). Estrogen receptor status in breast cancer is associated with remarkably distinct gene expression patterns. *Cancer Research*, *61*(16), 5979–5984. PMID:11507038

Guyon, I., Weston, J., Barnhill, S., & Vapnik, V. (2002). Gene selection for cancer classification using support vector machines. *Machine Learning*, *46*(1-3), 389–422. doi:10.1023/A:1012487302797

Haibe-Kains, B. (2009). *Identification and assessment of gene signatures in human breast cancer*. Academic Press.

Hasan, A. (2012). Evaluation of Decision Tree Classifiers and Boosting Algorithm for Classifying High Dimensional Cancer Datasets. *International Journal of Modeling and Optimization*, *2*(2), 92–96. doi:10.7763/IJMO.2012.V2.92

Hastie, T., Tibshirani, R., & Friedman, J. (2009). *The elements of statistical learning: data mining, inference, and prediction*. Springer Science & Business Media. doi:10.1007/978-0-387-84858-7

Hinton, G. E., Osindero, S., & Teh, Y. W. (2006). A fast learning algorithm for deep belief nets. *Neural Computation*, *18*(7), 1527–1554. doi:10.1162/neco.2006.18.7.1527 PMID:16764513

Hong, J. H., & Cho, S. B. (2006). The classification of cancer based on DNA microarray data that uses diverse ensemble genetic programming. *Artificial Intelligence in Medicine*, *36*(1), 43–58. doi:10.1016/j.artmed.2005.06.002 PMID:16102956

Ivshina, A. V., George, J., Senko, O., Mow, B., Putti, T. C., Smeds, J., ... Wong, J. E. (2006). Genetic reclassification of histologic grade delineates new clinical subtypes of breast cancer. *Cancer Research*, *66*(21), 10292–10301. doi:10.1158/0008-5472.CAN-05-4414 PMID:17079448

Jain, A., Tayal, D. K., Yadav, D., & Arora, A. (2020). Research Trends for Named Entity Recognition in Hindi Language. In *Data Visualization and Knowledge Engineering* (pp. 223–248). Springer. doi:10.1007/978-3-030-25797-2_10

Khan, J., Wei, J. S., Ringner, M., Saal, L. H., Ladanyi, M., Westermann, F., Berthold, F., Schwab, M., Antonescu, C. R., Peterson, C., & Meltzer, P. S. (2001). Classification and diagnostic prediction of cancers using gene expression profiling and artificial neural networks. *Nature Medicine*, *7*(6), 673–679. doi:10.1038/89044 PMID:11385503

Kohavi, R., & John, G. H. (1997). Wrappers for feature subset selection. *Artificial Intelligence*, *97*(1-2), 273–324. doi:10.1016/S0004-3702(97)00043-X

Kourou, K., Exarchos, T. P., Exarchos, K. P., Karamouzis, M. V., & Fotiadis, D. I. (2015). Machine learning applications in cancer prognosis and prediction. *Computational and Structural Biotechnology Journal*, *13*, 8–17. doi:10.1016/j.csbj.2014.11.005 PMID:25750696

Lamba, M., Munjal, G., & Gigras, Y. (2018). Feature Selection of Micro-array expression data (FSM)-A Review. *Procedia Computer Science*, *132*, 1619–1625. doi:10.1016/j.procs.2018.05.127

Li, X., & O'Malley, B. W. (2003). Unfolding the action of progesterone receptors. *The Journal of Biological Chemistry*, *278*(41), 39261–39264. doi:10.1074/jbc.R300024200 PMID:12893816

Li, Y. (2014). *Sparse machine learning models in bioinformatics*. Academic Press.

Lin, F. P., Pokorny, A., Teng, C., Dear, R., & Epstein, R. J. (2016). Computational prediction of multidisciplinary team decision-making for adjuvant breast cancer drug therapies: A machine learning approach. *BMC Cancer*, *16*(1), 929. doi:10.118612885-016-2972-z PMID:27905893

Lu, Y., & Han, J. (2003). Cancer classification using gene expression data. *Information Systems*, *28*(4), 243–268. doi:10.1016/S0306-4379(02)00072-8

Mackay, A., Weigelt, B., Grigoriadis, A., Kreike, B., Natrajan, R., A'Hern, R., Tan, D. S. P., Dowsett, M., Ashworth, A., & Reis-Filho, J. S. (2011). Microarray-based class discovery for molecular classification of breast cancer: Analysis of interobserver agreement. *Journal of the National Cancer Institute*, *103*(8), 662–673. doi:10.1093/jnci/djr071 PMID:21421860

Metzger Filho, O., Ignatiadis, M., & Sotiriou, C. (2011). Genomic Grade Index: An important tool for assessing breast cancer tumor grade and prognosis. *Critical Reviews in Oncology/Hematology*, *77*(1), 20–29. doi:10.1016/j.critrevonc.2010.01.011 PMID:20138540

Meyer, D., & Wien, F. T. (2015). Support vector machines. *The Interface to libsvm in package e1071, 28.*

Millar, E. K., Graham, P. H., O'Toole, S. A., McNeil, C. M., Browne, L., Morey, A. L., ... Nasser, E. (2009). Prediction of local recurrence, distant metastases, and death after breast-conserving therapy in early-stage invasive breast cancer using a five-biomarker panel. *Journal of Clinical Oncology*, *27*(28), 4701–4708. doi:10.1200/JCO.2008.21.7075 PMID:19720911

Nacht, M., Ferguson, A. T., Zhang, W., Petroziello, J. M., Cook, B. P., Gao, Y. H., ... Madden, S. L. (1999). Combining serial analysis of gene expression and array technologies to identify genes differentially expressed in breast cancer. *Cancer Research*, *59*(21), 5464–5470. PMID:10554019

National Cancer Institute. (n.d.). https://www.cancer.gov/cancertopics

National Institutes of Health Consensus Development Panel. (2001). National Institutes of Health Consensus Development Conference statement: adjuvant therapy for breast cancer, November 1–3, 2000. *JNCI Monographs, 2001*(30), 5-15.

O'Neill, M. C. (1991). Training back-propagation neural networks to define and detect DNA-binding sites. *Nucleic Acids Research*, *19*(2), 313–318. doi:10.1093/nar/19.2.313 PMID:2014171

Oquab, M., Bottou, L., Laptev, I., & Sivic, J. (2014). Learning and transferring mid-level image representations using convolutional neural networks. In *Proceedings of the IEEE conference on computer vision and pattern recognition* (pp. 1717-1724). 10.1109/CVPR.2014.222

Quénel, N., Wafflart, J., Bonichon, F., de Mascarel, I., Trojani, M., Durand, M., Avril, A., & Coindre, J. M. (1995). The prognostic value of c-erbB2 in primary breast carcinomas: A study on 942 cases. *Breast Cancer Research and Treatment*, *35*(3), 283–291. doi:10.1007/BF00665980 PMID:7579499

Ragab, D. A., Sharkas, M., Marshall, S., & Ren, J. (2019). Breast cancer detection using deep convolutional neural networks and support vector machines. *PeerJ*, *7*, e6201. doi:10.7717/peerj.6201 PMID:30713814

Rauschert, S., Raubenheimer, K., Melton, P. E., & Huang, R. C. (2020). Machine learning and clinical epigenetics: A review of challenges for diagnosis and classification. *Clinical Epigenetics*, *12*(1), 1–11. doi:10.118613148-020-00842-4 PMID:32245523

Ries, L. A., Harkins, D., Krapcho, M., Mariotto, A., Miller, B. A., Feuer, E. J., ... Hayat, M. (2006). *SEER cancer statistics review, 1975-2003*. Academic Press.

Robbins, P., Pinder, S., De Klerk, N., Dawkins, H., Harvey, J., Sterrett, G., Ellis, I., & Elston, C. (1995). Histological grading of breast carcinomas: A study of interobserver agreement. *Human Pathology*, *26*(8), 873–879. doi:10.1016/0046-8177(95)90010-1 PMID:7635449

Russakovsky, O., Deng, J., Su, H., Krause, J., Satheesh, S., Ma, S., ... Berg, A. C. (2015). Imagenet large scale visual recognition challenge. *International Journal of Computer Vision*, *115*(3), 211–252. doi:10.100711263-015-0816-y

Saini, A., Hou, J., & Zhou, W. (2014). Breast cancer prognosis risk estimation using integrated gene expression and clinical data. *BioMed Research International*, *2014*, 2014. doi:10.1155/2014/459203 PMID:24949450

Saini, A., Hou, J., & Zhou, W. (2014). RRHGE: A novel approach to classify the estrogen receptor based breast cancer subtypes. *TheScientificWorldJournal, 2014*, 2014. doi:10.1155/2014/362141 PMID:24563630

Schwarzer, G., Vach, W., & Schumacher, M. (2000). On the misuses of artificial neural networks for prognostic and diagnostic classification in oncology. *Statistics in Medicine, 19*(4), 541–561. doi:10.1002/(SICI)1097-0258(20000229)19:4<541::AID-SIM355>3.0.CO;2-V PMID:10694735

Shen, L., Margolies, L. R., Rothstein, J. H., Fluder, E., McBride, R., & Sieh, W. (2019). Deep learning to improve breast cancer detection on screening mammography. *Scientific Reports, 9*(1), 1–12. doi:10.103841598-019-48995-4 PMID:31467326

Shlens, J. (2014). *A tutorial on principal component analysis.* arXiv preprint arXiv:1404.1100

Simon, R. (2003). Diagnostic and prognostic prediction using gene expression profiles in high-dimensional microarray data. *British Journal of Cancer, 89*(9), 1599–1604. doi:10.1038j.bjc.6601326 PMID:14583755

Sofi, G. N., Sofi, J. N., Nadeem, R., Shiekh, R. Y., Khan, F. A., Sofi, A. A., Bhat, H. A., & Bhat, R. A. (2012). Estrogen receptor and progesterone receptor status in breast cancer in relation to age, histological grade, size of lesion and lymph node involvement. *Asian Pacific Journal of Cancer Prevention, 13*(10), 5047–5052. doi:10.7314/APJCP.2012.13.10.5047 PMID:23244108

Sotiriou, C., Neo, S. Y., McShane, L. M., Korn, E. L., Long, P. M., Jazaeri, A., Martiat, P., Fox, S. B., Harris, A. L., & Liu, E. T. (2003). Breast cancer classification and prognosis based on gene expression profiles from a population-based study. *Proceedings of the National Academy of Sciences of the United States of America, 100*(18), 10393–10398. doi:10.1073/pnas.1732912100 PMID:12917485

Sotiriou, C., Wirapati, P., Loi, S., Harris, A., Fox, S., Smeds, J., ... Desmedt, C. (2006). Gene expression profiling in breast cancer: Understanding the molecular basis of histologic grade to improve prognosis. *Journal of the National Cancer Institute, 98*(4), 262–272. doi:10.1093/jnci/djj052 PMID:16478745

Sun, Y., Babbs, C. F., & Delp, E. J. (2006, January). A comparison of feature selection methods for the detection of breast cancers in mammograms: adaptive sequential floating search vs. genetic algorithm. In *2005 IEEE Engineering in Medicine and Biology 27th Annual Conference* (pp. 6532-6535). IEEE.

Suvarchala, S. B., & Nageswararao, R. (2011). Carcinoma breast-histopathological and hormone receptors correlation. *J Biosci Tech, 2*(4), 340–348.

Taneja, A., & Arora, A. (2018). Recommendation research trends: Review, approaches and open issues. *International Journal of Web Engineering and Technology, 13*(2), 123–186. doi:10.1504/IJWET.2018.092831

Van IJzendoorn, D. G., Szuhai, K., Briaire-de Bruijn, I. H., Kostine, M., Kuijjer, M. L., & Bovée, J. V. (2019). Machine learning analysis of gene expression data reveals novel diagnostic and prognostic biomarkers and identifies therapeutic targets for soft tissue sarcomas. *PLoS Computational Biology, 15*(2), e1006826. doi:10.1371/journal.pcbi.1006826 PMID:30785874

Van't Veer, L. J., Dai, H., Van De Vijver, M. J., He, Y. D., Hart, A. A., Mao, M., ... Schreiber, G. J. (2002). Gene expression profiling predicts clinical outcome of breast cancer. *Nature, 415*(6871), 530-536.

Viswanathan, G. A., Seto, J., Patil, S., Nudelman, G., & Sealfon, S. C. (2008). Getting started in biological pathway construction and analysis. *PLoS Computational Biology*, *4*(2), e16. doi:10.1371/journal.pcbi.0040016 PMID:18463709

Wang, Y., Klijn, J. G., Zhang, Y., Sieuwerts, A. M., Look, M. P., Yang, F., ... Jatkoe, T. (2005). Gene-expression profiles to predict distant metastasis of lymph-node-negative primary breast cancer. *Lancet*, *365*(9460), 671–679. doi:10.1016/S0140-6736(05)17947-1 PMID:15721472

Weigelt, B., Peterse, J. L., & Van't Veer, L. J. (2005). Breast cancer metastasis: Markers and models. *Nature Reviews. Cancer*, *5*(8), 591–602. doi:10.1038/nrc1670 PMID:16056258

White, H. (1989). Learning in artificial neural networks: A statistical perspective. *Neural Computation*, *1*(4), 425–464. doi:10.1162/neco.1989.1.4.425

Xiong, M., Fang, X., & Zhao, J. (2001). Biomarker identification by feature wrappers. *Genome Research*, *11*(11), 1878–1887. doi:10.1101/gr.190001 PMID:11691853

Yassin, N. I., Omran, S., El Houby, E. M., & Allam, H. (2018). Machine learning techniques for breast cancer computer aided diagnosis using different image modalities: A systematic review. *Computer Methods and Programs in Biomedicine*, *156*, 25–45. doi:10.1016/j.cmpb.2017.12.012 PMID:29428074

Yusuff, H., Mohamad, N., Ngah, U. K., & Yahaya, A. (2012). Breast cancer analysis using logistic regression. *International Journal of Research and Reviews in Applied Sciences*, *10*(1), 14–22.

Zhang, H., Yu, C. Y., Singer, B., & Xiong, M. (2001). Recursive partitioning for tumor classification with gene expression microarray data. *Proceedings of the National Academy of Sciences of the United States of America*, *98*(12), 6730–6735. doi:10.1073/pnas.111153698 PMID:11381113

Zheng, B., Yoon, S. W., & Lam, S. S. (2014). Breast cancer diagnosis based on feature extraction using a hybrid of K-means and support vector machine algorithms. *Expert Systems with Applications*, *41*(4), 1476–1482. doi:10.1016/j.eswa.2013.08.044

Zhou, B. P., & Hung, M. C. (2003, October). Dysregulation of cellular signaling by HER2/neu in breast cancer. *Seminars in Oncology*, *30*, 38–48. doi:10.1053/j.seminoncol.2003.08.006 PMID:14613025

Chapter 6
The Role of Genetic Data Analysis for Precision Therapy in Cancer:
Personalized Medicine Concept in Cancer Treatment

Sunishtha Singh Yadav
Amity Institute of Biotechnology, Amity University, India

Vandana Chauhan
Amity Institute of Biotechnology, Amity University, India

Vijeta Singh
Amity Institute of Biotechnology, Amity University, India

Svenja Kohler
University of Lübeck, Germany

ABSTRACT

Cancer has been known as a devastating disease that takes thousands of lives every year. And since this is a heterogenous disease, standard treatments, like chemotherapy, radiation, and chemo-radio therapy, are effective in specific patient population subset only. Genetic differences play a very crucial role in defining cancer susceptibility and also in determining the drug's efficacy by affecting regulation, expression, and activity of drug metabolizing enzymes, drug transporters, and drug receptors. This genetic variability of the disease lends itself to the emerging field of precision or personalized medicine. There are some specific ways of acquiring data for precision or personalized medicine approach like genome wide association scan (GWAS). This is basically identification and scanning of biomarkers throughout the complete DNA/genome of several individuals to study any type of genetic variations which are linked with any form of cancer.

DOI: 10.4018/978-1-7998-6527-8.ch006

INTRODUCTION

The term 'oncology' has been derived from two words onco and logy where "onco" defines excessive mass and "logy" is study. Oncology deals with cancer treatment and understanding the genetic predisposition leading to DNA variation and then to the disease ultimately. People probably think of cancer treatment as a modern practice but that is not a true fact as it has it root in ancient Greek. Among manuscript the initial description of this disease and its treatment is mentioned in the book of Edwin Smith Papyrus, back in 3000 BC and described it as "incurable" but with the time it changes. In fact, cancer survival among several years has been increased because of less exposure to life style related habits (like consumption of tobacco/smoking and alcohol) and advancements in the screening methods and treatment regimens (Blackadar, 2019; Jarrell et al., 2020).

The introduction of immunotherapy has driven the cancer care field towards individualization of therapeutic guidelines which ultimately led to basics of personalized medicine approach or precision medicine approach, which is often called precision and personalized medicine (PPM), which is actually customization of therapeutic protocol as per the patient (Kruger et al., 2019; Jarrell et al., 2020). Over the past few decades, it has become apparent that the physiology of cancer is different in different patients and that could be the probably be a reason for difference in the treatment outcome in these patients even after following the same treatment regimen. Therefore, the conventional cancer therapy regimens have been unsuccessful, costly and causes unwanted side effects for patients. A more effective model is based on PPM in order to adjust the conventional and more traditional approach. This viewpoint promotes the creation of personalized therapies for each particular cancer subtype, which utilizes calculation and information related to genetic predisposition and genetic variation data of patients for better and more reliable methods of treatment (Jarrell et al., 2020).

Different forms of cancer have been treated through conventional and more traditional methods for several decades which includes chemotherapy, radiation and surgery. This approach of common treatment protocol for all patients in most of the cases led to deterioration and hazardous damage of healthy, non-malignant tissues and organs as well. The personalized approach or precision medicine approach based on individualization of treatment regimen as per tissues, genetic variations and individual events/factors significant to specific cancer physiology. It helps in determining the appropriate treatment method as per specific malignancy and guides for the novel & targeted treatment protocol which either do not led to any hazards to the healthy tissues/organs or it shall be the minimum harm. Thus, this approach of treatment is more appropriate and safer as compared to others. Moreover, improvements and advancements in the identification of pathways and biomarkers related to cancer, precise and more effective approaches of patient data analysis (Big data); and more accurate high-throughput screening methods will surely lay down a strong base for precision and personalized medicine approach (Jarrell et al., 2020; Fan et al., 2020).

EPIDEMIOLOGY OF CANCER

Genetic Factors

It is a well-known fact that almost all the cancer-causing agents leads to variations in the genetic content. Furthermore, it has been studies by several researchers across the world that variations in the somatic cell's genetic expressions due to mutations finally leads to transformations leading to malignancies. Moreover, for almost all cancer types there exists dominant inheritance which are truly penetrant and called the genetic susceptibility/predisposition. These contributes to approximately 2%-5% of total fatal cancer forms (Bahrami et al., 2018).

Genetic Predisposition/Susceptibility

Several research studies have shown that there are possibilities of any individual not born with a disease but there is a likelihood to acquire it during the life span, this phenomenon is called genetic predisposition or susceptibility. It is not necessary that genetic susceptibility to some specific disease due to any mutation (single gene or multiple genes or combination of alleles) shall lead to some kind of abnormalities. It's been noticed several diseases like cancer, patients inherit genes which has some kind of alteration due to factors such as lifestyle related habits or exposure to different classes of xenobiotics (Allen et al., 2014; Alzu'bi et al., 2019).

Due to genetic predisposition & involvement of several other environmental & related life style factors the genes which suppress tumour formation loses their function and thus give rise to carcinomas or different forms of cancer. It is always suggested to have a knowledge and information about one's genetic predisposition to different disorders/diseases and how is it associated with lifestyle & environmental factors because this will finally explain the increased or decreased incidences for acquiring any potential diseases and its relation to habits like smoking or drinking (Lerman et al., 2015).

Therefore, the basic aim of genetic predisposition is to explain the likelihood of developing certain diseases based on a person's genetic makeup during the course of life span of an individual depending upon the environmental factors & lifestyle related habits one is exposed to. Furthermore, it provides resources for extended information from the World Health Organization and other sources. This phenomenon of genetic susceptibility/ genetic predisposition is basically an outcome of specific genetic variations which could be inherited from the parents. These variations may lead to development of certain disorders or diseases; however, these do not directly cause any specific disease or disorder. There had been certain classical examples within the same family where person with a genetic variation predisposition didn't develop a disease while others did (Allen et al., 2014; Alzu'bi et al., 2019).

Present research scenario focuses on identification of genetic variations which are common in the general population, however these may have lesser impact on diseases or risk of causing any disorder. Individually these variations just have a slight effect on a person's chances of developing any diseases but when combined these significantly increases the risk to develop any disease in an individual. Variations in several genes (which individually are less effective), may therefore explains the susceptibility to the common diseases like different forms of cancer, cardiovascular, vascular disease and mental illness (Allen et al., 2014; Alzu'bi et al., 2019).

In all the cases of genetic predisposition, a number of factors are involved along with an identified genetic variation in defining the risk of disease or likelihood to develop a disease during the course of life. These are often called as modifiers explained as the genetic factors along with lifestyle related habits and environmental factors. There is another category of diseases as well which is called as the multifactorial, these actually are outcome of several factors and their combinations. Though it is not possible to alter an individual's genetic content, however, certain lifestyle related habits and environmentally induced modifications may sometimes lead to increased or decreased incidences as per the individual's genetic predisposition (Lerman et al., 2015).

Environmental Factors

The occurrence of numerous kinds of malignancy shifts extraordinarily between topographical regions. Several variations have been identified through movement from one zone to another having differentiating frequency, variations in occurrence after some pace, & variety inside populaces as indicated by financial status. Along these lines natural components seem to have a noteworthy job in the aetiology of most sorts of malignant growth (Lewandowska et al., 2019).

Infections

16% of the overall frequency of disease is because of contamination. The ratio of percentage for created vs creating nations is 9% vs 21%. The same for Human papillomavirus (HPV) in cervical cancer is 82% vs 91% representing the ratio in created vs creating nations. The strongest evidences are available for HPV type 16 for incidences of liver malignancy 18.81% unending disease with hepatitis B or hepatitis C (Jiang et al., 2018).

Life Style Habits

Alcohol Consumption: The undesired and uncontrolled uptake of alcohol has always been known as an enhancer of several diseases and disorders including some forms of cancer and liver cirrhosis (liver disease) and may add to certain malignant growths of the bosom and enormous gut (Stornetta et al., 2018; Fan et al., 2018).

Smoking: Consumption of tobacco in form of chewing or smoking has been found as an inducer of several forms of cancer of lung, larynx, oral depression and pharynx, throat, pancreas, kidney, and bladder. Use of tobacco leads to 15% (1.1 million new cases for each year) of all disease cases worldwide (25% of cases worldwide in men, 4% in ladies) (Khani ret al., 2018).

Key Discoveries leading to Precision Medicine

The most significant and addressed discoveries which have supported countable progress in the sphere of individualized/personalized or precision medicine approach are single nucleotide polymorphism (SNP) genotyping and biochips/microarray. Some specific variations are as follows (Fig 1):

- **Polymorphism:** Specific stretch on DNA/genome which differs in nucleotides sequence from one individual to another
- **Single Nucleotide Polymorphism (SNP):** This defines variation in the single base in the DNA in comparison to normal base sequence at that very position
- **Copy Number Variant (CNV):** This explains variation in the repeats of DNA sequence at some particular location from one individual to another
- **Indel:** This defines presence of a DNA sequence due to insertion or absence of a DNA sequence due to deletion at a location, which varies from one individual to another

Figure 1. Some specific types of variations

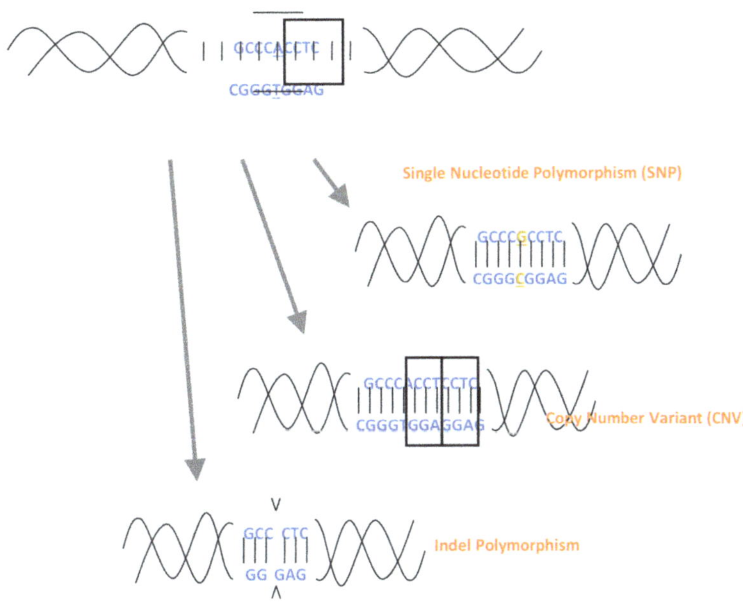

SNPs are basically variations which leads to 90% of all reported variations or polymorphisms. These are actually variations addressed in one/single nucleotide in the sequence of DNA, however, have specific in the specific population. The process leading to exploration of these variations in any population is very critical and specific because these variation or SNPs have genetic susceptibility to certain diseases and treatment outcome to pharmaceuticals in every individual in any specific population. These have also been helpful in separating patients in multitude of research studies and several clinical trials (Yates et al., 2018; Steinke & Holinski, 2019).

Another revolution in the field of PPM was the discovery & introduction of the microarray biochip by providing the ability to store and rapid analysis of entire genome of every patient. This procedure has provided clinicians and researchers across the globe to carry out patients' efficient genotyping of SNPs, and ultimately providing quick introduction and expansion of therapeutics which is protein-based diagnostics (Yates et al., 2018).

Precision or Personalized Medicine Approach (PPM)

Precision care is an evolving method for treating various diseases, it is based on facts that there exists variation in genes in each individual and the expressional outcome of these variations h is affected by environment and lifestyle factors. By having a better understanding of the genetic structure of an individual, including knowledge embedded in their DNA, health-care workers are able to offer a more tailor-made and accurate way to diagnose and treat diseases such as cancer. The aim is that one day, medical imaging will customize cancer treatment to the biological mutations in the cancer cells of each individual. Although treating any diagnosis of cancer using precise treatment is a long way to go in the future, today's precision medicine can be helpful (Aronson et al., 2015; Collins et al., 2015; FDA, 2019; Fan et al., 2020).

Personalized approach is basically customization of treatment to ensure better patient care, with the correct result and the highest margin for safety. By encouraging each patient to seek timely diagnosis, risk assessments and appropriate care, it holds promise to improve health care by also reducing costs.

Precision approach explains refers to adjustments and alterations in the altering the therapeutic care according to each patient's specific characteristics. This doesn't define the introduction and innovation of new drugs or clinical set ups as per individual patient, This does not mean that the development of drugs or medical devices that are specific to a patient, however this facilitates the classification or division of the patients into sub groups of subpopulations with difference in their vulnerability to a particular disease. Furthermore, it considers the differences in the physiology or biology or prognosis of those diseases that they may develop, or the cascade of reactions to a specific treatment. So that different interventions on prevention or therapeutic regimen shall then base on obtaining maximum treatment benefits or outcome with less expenses and almost no side effects. Yet the word 'personalized medicine' is often used to express the sense that this word is often misunderstood as suggesting that it is possible to devise specific treatments for each person (Aronson et al., 2015; Collins et al., 2015; FDA, 2019; Fan et al., 2020).

On the other hand, the usage of the word "precision medicine" will expand to the collection and usage of medications and even include the production of customized medical items for individuals — for example, "a patient-specific tissue or organ and customize medications for various people." Thus, in fact, the concept has very much similarity with personalized medicine that it is sometimes used synonymously.

Personalized or precision medicine (PPM) is basically the implementation and utilization of data generated through screening and diagnostic methods for significant management of an individual patient's predisposition towards a disease. Furthermore, PPM enables hazard assessment/ disease risk evaluation, examination, analysis & interpretation of the symptoms, precautions and execution of treatment regimen specifically designed for individual patient, thus improves the quality of life and public health (Aronson et al., 2015; Collins et al., 2015; FDA, 2019; Fan et al., 2020).

The field of PPM is influenced by pharmacogenetics and pharmacogenomics. Pharmacogenetics explains the effect of particular variation in respective genes which decides how an individual will respond to any discrete drug. Therefore, it is analyzing single drug or multi drugs response in context to specific gene, or group of genes (Juengst et al., 2018).

On the other hand, Pharmacogenomics explains the effect of collective genes which ultimately effects drug response. Furthermore, this helps in identification of genes through genome wide analysis which effects response to a particular drug so that new drug targets and key determinants shall be discovered which will improve the treatment outcome and will decrease the chances of adverse drug reactions (Juengst et al., 2018).

There are number of factors which contribute to these differences in treatment outcomes in context to genetic variation and effect on drug response, these include biological, physical, bio-physical, chemical, bio-chemical, environmental and life style related factors (Aronson et al., 2015; Collins et al., 2015; FDA, 2019).

Aim of Precision Medicine

The aim of cancer precision medicine is to customize the treatment to match the unique genetic constituents and the genetic variations in cancer cells. Precision cancer medicine can include examining the genetic makeup of the cells, or the makeup of the cancer cells if you have cancer (Aronson et al., 2015; Collins et al., 2015; FDA, 2019; Fan et al., 2020). Tests may include:

1. **Testing of the Drug-Genes:** The genes, including those used to treat cancer, will affect the way patient's body handles medications. The oncologist uses genetic test information to decide which medicines and dosages are best suited to specific patient.
2. **Cancer Advanced:** When your cancer persists through treatment, your doctor can recommend you for testing of your cancer cells for their genetic makeup. This method, called tumour sequencing, is used to search for cancer changes or mutations, so your doctor can pick the right treatment for your tumour form.
3. **Family History:** Genetic testing is given to those with a clear family history of the disease for hereditary in certain mutations which may enhance the chances of certain forms of cancer as in case of breast cancer BRCA gene. As compared to the general population, all the individuals who are carrier of this specific gene variation are at increased risk of developing breast cancer. And the same theory is being implemented to the treatment outcome related to specific drugs used for controlling breast cancer (Parp inhibitor). Depending on the family genetics related to different forms of cancer several other new genetic testing methods are available, which gives accurate chances of developing some cancer in future.

Not only breast cancer but many other cancers like lung cancer, colorectal cancer, neuroblastoma and many other malignant tumours are also benefiting from precision medicine treatment.

Artificial Intelligence in Precision Medicine Approach: Technological Advancements Leading to Precision Medicine Approach

Artificial Intelligence provides a fundamental change towards the PM approach. Machine learning techniques are being used for the genomic sequencing and for analysing and interpreting results from the vast quantities of data of patients and medical institutions that are recorded at all the times. Artificial intelligence methods are used in cardiovascular precision medicine to understand the genetic patterns inherited in the existing diseases to improvise them. The patient may need to get a biopsy to find out which genetic variations are present for that specific form of cancer. A biopsy is a test that involves the doctor extracting a cancer sample. This sample will be sent to a special laboratory, where a machine called a DNA sequencer is searching for genetic changes that can cause the cancer to increase. The different methods of studying genetic variations in different cancers includes molecular or tumour profiling, genomic testing and DNA sequencing. The specific methods or the process involves the following:

1. **Microarray Analysis:** In today's era of clinical and translational research, the need of the hour is to analyze huge datasets for functional genomics to derive information from biological experimentation set ups. An example of this is microarray technology which involves studying the expressions of several thousand genes simultaneously in specific conditions. This technology provides enormous quantity of data generated through sequencing thousand genes. Microarray gene expression profiles can be used to relate to external information to get knowledge about the biological events and different related processes which can be further utilized to make new discoveries (Brambilla et al., 2019).
2. **Next Generation Sequencing (NGS):** It is the process to explore, determine and study the nucleotides sequence present on DNA segment. It is high-throughput sequencing process which enables rapid sequencing of DNA & RNA at very low cost as compared to Sanger sequencing. The process

has given new horizons to genomics and molecular biology studies. This includes Illumina (Solexa) sequencing (emission of fluorescent signal by DNA based), Roche 454 sequencing (based on pyro-sequencing) and Ion Torrent: Proton / PGM sequencing (based on measuring direct release of H+) (Morash et al., 2018). Lin and co-workers (2020) suggested that the next generation sequencing strategy should be considered in precision medicine by applying it in triple-negative breast cancer patients receiving platinum and PARP inhibitors treatment.

Precision Medicine/Personalized Medicine Approach in Cancer Treatment

The disruptive approach which consider both variations in an individual and population specific characteristics to provide personalized or individualized care is called Precision medicine (PM). It is a disruptive approach which helps in widening the molecular & biological expertise and helps in exploring the great genetic diversity of patients (Malone et al., 2020; Lin et al., 2020).

This approach is based on individualization or customization of treatment regimen and other healthcare according to an individual on the basis of data procured from molecular and the genetic analysis at individual level. And it also utilizes the data and information obtained from the rest of the population (Stockley et al., 2016; Krebs & Milani, 2019; Hockings et al., 2020). Hence, personalized or precision medicine depends on molecular & genetic analysis and population statistics to form the platform for tailored and individualized healthcare. The most important aim of precision medicine is to provide personalized & accurate interventions to patients by utilizing the understanding of biology, to be précised molecular and genetic analysis. The strategies utilized for precision medicine includes crucial decision-making steps and processes which are based on biomarker-driven approaches comprises of genes, different gene products (like transcripts. Proteins etc.) and metabolites. Based on the diversity in biomarkers at both molecular and genetic level, omics technologies provide an increased high-throughput and thus presents outstanding opportunities to represent the full view of biological systems and mechanisms in a very unbiased & hypothesis free mode. However, holistic approach shall be applied to different steps & levels of biological information so that a deep understanding of diseases, mechanisms and processes should be acquired (Mantere et al., 2019; Lin et al., 2020).

The dynamic understanding of interactions of gene and environment (on individual & population levels) leads to forecast of any normal or pathological conditions in the patients. Thus, this new concept of system medicine is very specific and targeted and depends on global & integrative approaches necessary for better outcome-based orientation for patient care (Wynn et al., 2018). Furthermore, a biological system can only be fully understood by considering the space & time parameters. Figure 2 gives an overview of the multi-scale perspective of precision medicine approach over conventional approach.

Different forms of cancer lead to death in the major population of India and other countries across the world. The reason behind this is the heterogeneity of the disease. The malignant tumours may have versatile genetic and molecular which will lead to difference in the expression of proteins in different patients with same cancer form. The field of personalized or precision medicine evolved due to this inherent variability. With the implementation of personalized/precision medicine approach, it is possible to characterize tumours on the molecular basis (Krzyszczyk et al., 2018). This approach may result in immense patient benefits in different forms of cancer (Grinnell, 2020).

Figure 2. An overview of the multi-scale perspective of precision medicine approach over conventional approach.

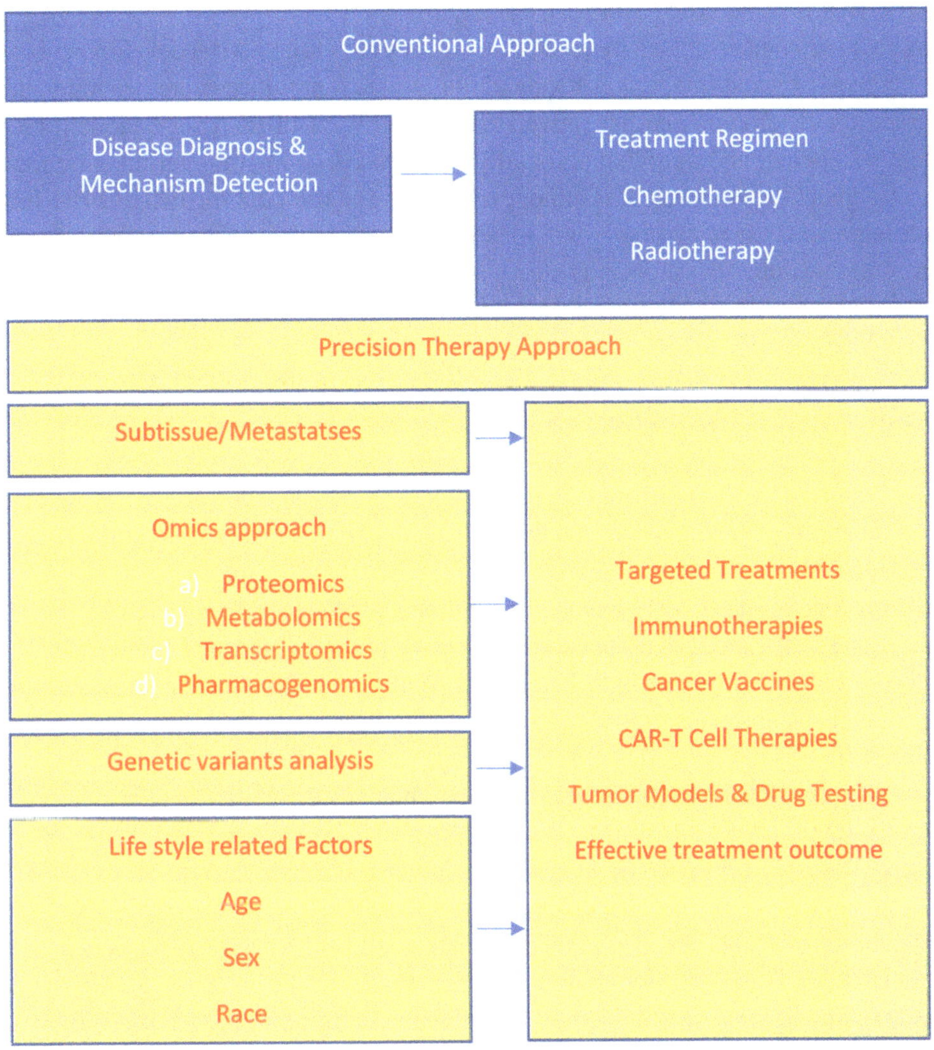

The knowledge of all the complicated elaborated cascade of formation and development of cancer & furtherance has been upgraded with the interventions of novel and innovative laboratory-based techniques which include different procedures, processes and mechanisms like DNA sequencing, gene expression profiling, proteomics, DNA methylation etc. Certain projects like International Cancer Genome Consortium & Cancer Genome Atlas have characterized genetic variations in tumours and have also disclosed molecular pathways & functional key mutations involved in carcinogenesis & cell proliferation. These mechanisms & processes have significant impact on the different steps during clinical diagnosis, medical prognosis & therapeutic regimen of cancer patients and thus have supported the customization of anti-tumour therapy in routine oncological practices. Such inventions and innovations actually have significant suggestions for persons with increased risk to develop certain malignant tumours by identification and categorization of patients receiving benefit from intensive screening and follow-ups.

For instance, women with mutation in tumour suppressor genes BRCA1 or BRCA2 are susceptible to develop ovarian, breast and other forms of cancer and are therefore, prospects for specialized screening programmes (Richards et al., 2015; Mukherjee et al., 2019).

Furthermore, the advancements in molecular techniques, was followed by developments and innovations in the diagnosis related imaging & histopathology which provided more accurate and appropriate characterization of tumours and have given specialized ways of tracking treatment response. For instance, the development and introduction of FISH (fluorescence in situ hybridisation technique) for the purpose of clinical examination of routine testing of breast tumours for ERBB2 (HER2/neu) gene amplification in patients. Several factors like identification of common genetic variations in tumours, introduction of high-throughput molecular diagnostics and cost-effective etc., are leading the way to the personalized or individualized treatment in many diseases like different forms of cancer (Richards et al., 2015; Mukherjee et al., 2019).

Benefits of Precision Medicine

1. **Improve Diagnosis and Treatment:** Precision cancer medicine allows cancer diagnosis and other illnesses more precise and assesses the unique genetic structure of their tumours to pick the most appropriate and safe therapies for them.
2. **Benefits to other Cancers Also:** It is used in treatment of other cancers like lung cancer, leukaemia, sarcoma, colorectal cancer, neuroblastoma and many other malignant tumours.
3. **Improved Predictability of which Therapies Will Work Best for Specific Patients:** Use of precision medicine approach allows doctors to apply best therapies to their cancer patients with best approach.
4. **Improve Disease Detection:** Precision medicine improves the ability of researchers to detect the disease easily.
5. **Customize Disease Prevention Strategies:** It helps to customize the strategies available for disease prevention.
6. **The Efficiency of Care:** Precision medicine makes decisions based on particular factors which affect their health. Today decision-making on treatments is on the patients' shoulders, because only doctors know no better how a single person and their condition would be affected by one form of treatment. Health facilities should prepare for personalized care methodologies for each of their patients with specificity, thereby increasing the chances of cure.
7. **Limit Cost:** Targeted treatment based on genetic mapping, with more knowledgeable treatment decisions, will reduce the cost of care and has a greater chance of being successful. The cost is significantly lower with a focus on preventive care rather than disease treatment.
8. **Population Health:** Studying genetic variations in a population as a whole and as parts may help identify causes and improve treatment for specific diseases. Genetic analysis of parts of a population can predict disease probability and early detection.

Limitations of Precision Medicine

1. **Legal Problems:** A lot of genomic data must be obtained from a large number of people from the population representing each and every segmentation in order to achieve epitome efficacy. It

is legally uncertain who controls the data when and where such a huge data is obtained. The government does not own the data; FDA has blocked individuals from corporate access to their own genetic records. The problem here is that it's the responsibility of whoever owns the data and it may be costly.

2. **The Relevance of Information:** Data from one million volunteers will be gathered for genomic research, according to President Obama 's proposal. It is highly likely that certain parts of the population that 'drop out' or insufficient samples of some disorder, or even over-representation of some other form of disorder.
3. **Infrastructure Requirements:** Precision medicine has the potential to have a significant effect on healthcare, but it needs substantial investment in infrastructure and time for implementation. Fundamental improvements to the system and process of data collection, storage, and sharing have to be made to incorporate precision medicine. The federal budget earmarked for precision medicine production does not cover the cost and it is uncertain who will have to invest the balance of the money.
4. **Healthcare Cost:** Ideally, effective treatment can avoid repetitive attempts, readmission, and help take preventive measures against illness, preventing the haemorrhage of health care funds. But in order to achieve this point, it needs significant investment in infrastructure for information processing, storage and sharing as well as security infrastructure to protect the data and other associated expenses may prove a burden.

Precision medicine essentially uses modern technology and methods to figure out and classify the causes for treating health and illness, and to avoid disease and promote wellness. It holds high expectations but the drawbacks weigh it down.

The promise it holds is too big for these drawbacks to hold it back for a long time, healthcare providers, government and IT professionals are working together to develop a solution to overcome these short-term drawbacks.

Side Effects of Precision Medicine

Scientists have expected précised cancer therapies to be less harmful than conventional chemotherapy medications, since cancer cells are more target-dependent than normal cells. Yet targeted cancer treatments may have thoughtful side effects. Side effects hinge on on the medication a patient takes for the precision medicine therapy. Some common side effects of it are:

1. Skin problems as well as rashes and strong itching
2. Sensitive reactions like dizziness, tightness in chest, trouble in breathing and inflammation in the lips or tongue
3. Raised up levels of liver enzymes
4. Fatigue
5. Constipation and diarrhea
6. Poor blood clotting and wound healing
7. High blood pressure
8. Low blood cell counts
9. Gastrointestinal perforation

Some side effects of such targeted therapies were related to improved patient outcomes. For example, patients who develop acneiform rash (acne-like skin eruptions) while being treated with the erlotinib or gefitinib signal transduction inhibitors, both of which target the receptor of the epidermal growth factor, appeared to react to these drugs better than patients who do not develop the rash. Similarly, patients who experience elevated blood pressure when receiving the angiogenesis inhibitor have typically had better outcomes. The few targeted treatments approved for use in children, including immunosuppression and reduced sperm output, may have different side effects in children than adults.

Genome Wide Association Scan (GWAS)

Genome-wide association scan/study involves expeditious scanning of biomarkers across the whole genome or the DNA of several individuals to explore genetic variations and their association with a specific disease. After identification of novel variations and their association with specific disease, the researchers then utilize this data to develop crucial approach to identify, determine, treat or prevent the disorder/disease. These methods and studies based on the methods are actually useful in exploring gene variations which leads to common but complex diseases such as different forms of cancer, asthma, heart disease, diabetes & mental illnesses. After completion of major projects like Human Genome Project in 2003 & International HapMap Project in 2005, the scientists, researchers and clinicians now have different research tools with which the contribution of gene variations to common diseases can be studied. These tools include computerized databases with references from human genome sequence, a quick map of human genetic variation and a set of new and advanced technologies approaches which shall rapidly and more accurately do the analysis of genetic variations across the whole genome samples and thus can contribute to the onset of disease or a disorder (Massard et al., 2017, Forman & Sotelo, 2019).

The furious pace of technological advances, such as DNA sequencing and genotyping technologies, has begun to enhance our understanding of human diversity in pharmacologic traits. Meanwhile, methodological advances, such as the genome-wide association scan/study (GWAS) approach, have facilitated the discovery of genetic variation with considerable clinical relevance. The *sine qua non of* (an essential condition or requirement) the rapidly developing field of pharmacogenomics is the translation of genomic information from these convergent developments into individualized patient care. Exciting promises of the new science abound, including the possibilities of optimized drug therapy, adverse-effect risk prediction, and improved drug discovery and development (Nattestad et al., 2018; DeLeonardis el al., 2019).

Benefit of GWAS

- The impact of GWAS on healthcare and practice of medicine is potentially substantial. The data generated through genome-wide association scan studies will lay down the platform and groundwork for the personalized medicine approach and therefore introduction of more customized strategies will take place.
- After improvisation in the efficiency and cost of GWAS and incorporation of other innovative technologies, the medical practitioners & health care professionals will definitely be able to utilize these for providing patients with customized and individualized information regarding the facts related to their risk of acquiring certain diseases during their life span.
- The information generated through GWAS will enable the medical practitioners & health care professionals to follow and implement prevention programs like tailored unique genetic makeup

of an individual. Furthermore, in the best-case scenario if there shall be no illness occurred in the individual then the information generated through these protocols shall be utilized for the selection of the treatment methods which will be more effective and least adverse reaction causing in the patient's group. In such methods, there are two groups one consists of individuals with the disease and the other group which is health and do not have the disease. The sample is obtained from both the groups to study the genetic variations (Richards et al., 2015; Mukherjee et al., 2019).

GWAS Protocol/ Procedure

- The protocol is based on identification of participants, making groups of participants one consists of people with the disease and another group consist of individuals without the disease. Then DNA sample is obtained from sample collected from each individual in both the groups (sampling methods include either drawing a blood sample or by rubbing a cotton swab along the inside of the mouth to harvest cells).
- The whole genome or DNA is first isolated and purified from blood sample or the other cells, and then tiny chips and after which scanning takes place on an automated laboratory machine.
- The automated machine rapidly examines the genome from each sample for the targeted strategical biomarkers of genetic variation know as single nucleotide polymorphisms (SNPs).
- If the results of the scanning show significant frequency of certain genetic variation in the sample of an individual with some disease as compared to others without any disease, then such variations are known to be "associated" or "linked" with that disease. These associated or linked genetic variations are very crucial pointers to the disease-causing problem which resides in the specific region of human genome. Important thing is, these linked variations may sometime not lead to the disease, however, these may just be "tagging along" with the actual causal variants.
- Because of above mentioned reasons, the scientists, the medical practitioners & health care professionals have to follow different methods like DNA sequencing in the specific region of the genome, to study the actual genetic variation involved in the disease.

GWAS Data Access

The National Centre for Biotechnology Information (NCBI), a part of NIH's National Library of Medicine, has developed databases for scientists/researchers, the medical practitioners & health care professionals. All the records of data generated from GWAS on a number of diseases, disorders and all such conditions have already been presented on NCBI Web site, called the Database of Genotype and Phenotype (dbGaP).

CONCLUSION

Genetic diversity explored through SNPs, CNVs or Indel along with certain environmental exposures contributes to both disease susceptibility or predisposition and variation in drug response. On identification of new or unreported genetic associations, the information is utilized to explore best possible ways to explore, analyse, treat or prevent the disease or disorder. It suggests that precision and personalized medicine approach has potential to enhance effective treatment outcome rate by adopting pharmacogenomics testing prior the treatment regimen to decrease rate of adverse drug reactions (ADRs) (Ginsburg

& Phillips, 2018; Krebs & Milani, 2019; Hockings et al., 2020). As the clinical researchers have noticed that specific variants of a gene are responsible for increased risk of ADRs in context to some categories and combinations of drugs. Therefore, integration & application PPM into clinical practises will surely allow spectrum for drug dosage and drug combination selection as per the individual patients genomics so that the treatment outcome shall be improved and more effective in every patient and furthermore, this will also reduce the chances of drug-induced morbidity and death (Ginsburg & Phillips, 2018; Krebs & Milani, 2019; Hockings et al., 2020).

Personalized or precision medicine can help in the prediction of an individual's likelihood to develop certain diseases during life span. Due to the ongoing advancement and upgradation in the field of PPM, the researchers, clinicians & medical practitioners continue to discover novel methods, tools and technologies to support programmes based on identification of patients at who are at higher risk for developing devitalizing disease. While researchers are making progress on a daily basis, for most patients, the precision medicine approach to cancer treatment is still not part of routine care. Many new drugs intended to address a particular shift are being studied in clinical trials in precision medicine right now. Some clinical trials support patients suffering from different forms and cancer stages. Others support patients who have various forms and stages of cancer. The tumour must have some genetic modification that can be activated by a drug being studied to be eligible for precision medicine trials.

Precision medicine allows doctors to choose medications based on the patient's genetic understanding of the condition, and to establish customized care plans. Patients have genetic variations that allow cancer to develop and spread and these are somewhat different across various periods for each patient. Treatment can usually be a combination of surgery, chemotherapy, radiation, and immunotherapy, depending on the form, size, and stage of cancer. Precision medicine can help with genetic variations and analysis to determine particular tailored treatment plans, with some medications being more appropriate for different genetic profile.

REFERENCES

Allen, N. L., Karlson, E. W., Malspeis, S., Lu, B., Seidman, C. E., & Lehmann, L. S. (2014). Biobank participants' preferences for disclosure of genetic research results: Perspectives from the OurGenes, OurHealth, OurCommunity project. *Mayo Clinic Proceedings*, *89*(6), 738–746. doi:10.1016/j.mayocp.2014.03.015 PMID:24943692

Alzu'bi, A. A., Zhou, L., & Watzlaf, V. J. M. (2019, April 1). Genetic Variations and Precision Medicine. *Perspectives in Health Information Management*, 16. PMID:31019429

Aronson, S. J., & Rehm, H. L. (2015, October 15). Building the foundation for genomics in precision medicine. *Nature*, *526*(7573), 336–342. doi:10.1038/nature15816 PMID:26469044

Bahrami, A., Hasanzadeh, M., Shahidsales, S., Farazestanian, M., Hassanian, S. M., Moetamani Ahmadi, M., Maftouh, M., Gharib, M., Yousefi, Z., Kadkhodayan, S., Ferns, G. A., & Avan, A. (2018). Genetic susceptibility in cervical cancer: From bench to bedside. *Journal of Cellular Physiology*, *233*(3), 1929–1939. doi:10.1002/jcp.26019 PMID:28542881

Blackadar, C. B. (2016). Historical review of the causes of cancer. *World Journal of Clinical Oncology*, *7*(1), 54–86. doi:10.5306/wjco.v7.i1.54 PMID:26862491

Brambilla, D., Chiari, M., Gori, A., & Cretich, M. (2019). Towards precision medicine: the role and potential of protein and peptide microarrays. *The Analyst, 144*.

Collins, S. F., & Varmus, H. (2015). A New Initiative on Precision Medicine. *The New England Journal of Medicine*, *372*(9), 793–795. doi:10.1056/NEJMp1500523 PMID:25635347

DeLeonardis, K., Hogan, L., Cannistra, S. A., Rangachari, D., & Tung, N. (2019, September). When Should Tumor Genomic Profiling Prompt Consideration of Germline Testing? *Journal of Oncology Practice / American Society of Clinical Oncology*, *15*(9), 465–473. doi:10.1200/JOP.19.00201 PMID:31509718

Fan, X., Peters, B. A., Jacobs, E. J., Gapstur, S. M., Purdue, M. P., Freedman, N. D., Alekseyenko, A. V., Wu, J., Yang, L., Pei, Z., Hayes, R. B., & Ahn, J. (2018). Drinking alcohol is associated with variation in the human oral microbiome in a large study of American adults. *Microbiome*, *6*(1), 59. doi:10.118640168-018-0448-x PMID:29685174

Fan, Y., Guo, L., Zheng, H., Ji, C., Wang, W., & Sun, H. (2020, January). BMP-9 is a novel marker for colorectal tumorigenesis undergoing the normal mucosa-adenoma-adenocarcinoma sequence and is associated with colorectal cancer prognosis. *Oncology Letters*, *19*(1), 271–282. PMID:31897139

FDA. (n.d.). *Novel drug approvals for 2019*. https://www.fda.gov/drugs/new-drugs-fda-cders-new-molecular-entities-and-new-therapeutic-biological-products/novel-drug-approvals-2019

Forman, A., & Sotelo, J. (2019, September 30). Tumor-Based Genetic Testing and Familial Cancer Risk. *Cold Spring Harbor Perspectives in Medicine*. Advance online publication. doi:10.1101/cshperspect.a036590 PMID:31570381

Ginsburg, G. S., & Phillips, K. A. (2018). Precision Medicine: From Science to Value. *Health Affairs (Project Hope)*, *37*(5), 694–701. doi:10.1377/hlthaff.2017.1624 PMID:29733705

Grinnell, F. (2020). Biomedical ethics 2.0: Redefining the meaning of disease, patient and treatment. *Nature Reviews. Molecular Cell Biology*, *10*(8), 1038. doi:10.103841580-020-0247-7 PMID:32303721

Hockings, J. K., Pasternak, A. L., Erwin, A. L., Mason, N. T., Eng, C., & Hicks, J. K. (2020). Pharmacogenomics: An evolving clinical tool for precision medicine. *Cleveland Clinic Journal of Medicine*, *87*(2), 91–99. doi:10.3949/ccjm.87a.19073 PMID:32015062

Jarrell, D. K., Drake, S., & Brown, M. A. (2020). Advancing Therapies for Cancer—From Mustard Gas to CAR T. *Sci*, *2*(2), 42. doi:10.3390ci2020042

Jiang, M. Y., Feng, R. M., & Wang, L. (2018). Performance of Combined Liquid Based Cytology and HPV Nucleic Acid Test for Detecting Cervical Precancer Among Women Attending Screening. *Zhonghua Zhong Liu Za Zhi*, *40*(10), 750–756. PMID:30392339

Juengst, E., & McGowan, M. (2018). Why Does the Shift from 'Personalized Medicine' to 'Precision Health' and 'Wellness Genomics' Matter? *AMA Journal of Ethics*, *20*(9), e881–e890. doi:10.1001/amajethics.2018.881 PMID:30242820

Khani, Y., Pourgholam-Amiji, N., Afshar, M., Otroshi, O., Sharifi-Esfahani, M., Sadeghi-Gandomani, H., Vejdani, M., & Salehiniya, H. (2018). Tobacco Smoking and Cancer Types: A Review. *Biomedical Research and Therapy*, *5*(4), 2142–2159. doi:10.15419/bmrat.v5i4.428

Krebs, K., & Milani, L. (2019). Translating pharmacogenomics into clinical decisions: Do not let the perfect be the enemy of the good. *Human Genomics, 13*(1), 39. doi:10.118640246-019-0229-z PMID:31455423

Kruger, S., Ilmer, M., Kobold, S., Cadilha, B. L., Endres, S., Ormanns, S., Schuebbe, G., Renz, B. W., D'Haese, J. G., Schloesser, H., Heinemann, V., Subklewe, M., Boeck, S., Werner, J., & von Bergwelt-Baildon, M. (2019). Advances in cancer immunotherapy. *Journal of Experimental & Clinical Cancer Research, 38*(1), 268. doi:10.118613046-019-1266-0 PMID:31217020

Krzyszczyk, P., Acevedo, A., Davidoff, E. J., Timmins, L. M., Marrero-Berrios, I., Patel, M., White, C., Lowe, C., Sherba, J. J., Hartmanshenn, C., O'Neill, K. M., Balter, M. L., Fritz, Z. R., Androulakis, I. P., Schloss, R. S., & Yarmush, M. L. (2018). The growing role of precision and personalized medicine for cancer treatment. Technology. *Singap World Sci, 6*(3-4), 79–100. PMID:30713991

Lerman, C., Schnoll, R. A., Hawk, L. W. Jr, Cinciripini, P., George, T. P., Wileyto, E. P., Swan, G. E., Benowitz, N., Heitjan, D. F., & Tyndale, R. F. (2015). Use of the Nicotine Metabolite Ratio as a Genetically Informed Biomarker of Response to Nicotine Patch or Varenicline for Smoking Cessation: A Randomised, Double-Blind Placebo-controlled Trial. *The Lancet. Respiratory Medicine, 3*(2), 131–138. doi:10.1016/S2213-2600(14)70294-2 PMID:25588294

Lewandowska, A. M., Rudzki, M., Rudzki, S., Lewandowski, T., & Laskowska, B. (2019). Environmental risk factors for cancer – review paper. *Annals of Agricultural and Environmental Medicine, 26*(1), 1–7. doi:10.26444/aaem/94299 PMID:30922021

Lin, P. H., Chen, M., Tsai, L. W., Lo, C., Yen, T.-C., Huang, T. Y., Chen, C.-K., Fan, S.-C., Kuo, S.-H., & Huang, C.-S. (2020). Using next-generation sequencing to redefine BRCAness in triple-negative breast cancer. *Cancer Science, 111*(4), 1375–1384. doi:10.1111/cas.14313 PMID:31958182

Malone, E. R., Oliva, M., Sabatini, P. J. B., Stockley, T. L., & Siu, L. L. (2020). Molecular profiling for precision cancer therapies. *Genome Medicine, 12*(1), 8. doi:10.118613073-019-0703-1 PMID:31937368

Mantere, T., Kersten, S., & Hoischen, A. (2019). Long-read sequencing emerging in medical genetics. *Frontiers in Genetics, 10*, 426. doi:10.3389/fgene.2019.00426 PMID:31134132

Massard, C., Michiels, S., Ferte, C., Le Deley, M. C., Lacroix, L., Hollebecque, A., Verlingue, L., Ileana, E., Rosellini, S., Ammari, S., Ngo-Camus, M., Bahleda, R., Gazzah, A., Varga, A., Postel-Vinay, S., Loriot, Y., Even, C., Breuskin, I., Auger, N., ... Soria, J.-C. (2017). High-throughput genomics and clinical outcome in hard-to-treat advanced cancers: Results of the MOSCATO 01 trial. *Cancer Discovery, 7*(6), 586–595. doi:10.1158/2159-8290.CD-16-1396 PMID:28365644

Morash, M., Mitchell, H., Beltran, H., Elemento, O., & Pathak, J. (2018). The Role of Next-Generation Sequencing in Precision Medicine: A Review of Outcomes in Oncology. *J Pers Med., 17*(8), 30.

Mukherjee, S. (2019, October). Genomics-Guided Immunotherapy for Precision Medicine in Cancer. *Cancer Biotherapy & Radiopharmaceuticals, 34*(8), 487–497. doi:10.1089/cbr.2018.2758 PMID:31314580

Nattestad, M., Goodwin, S., Ng, K., Baslan, T., Sedlazeck, F. J., Rescheneder, P., Garvin, T., Fang, H., Gurtowski, J., Hutton, E., Tseng, E., Chin, C.-S., Beck, T., Sundaravadanam, Y., Kramer, M., Antoniou, E., McPherson, J. D., Hicks, J., McCombie, W. R., & Schatz, M. C. (2018). Complex rearrangements and oncogene amplifications revealed by long-read DNA and RNA sequencing of a breast cancer cell line. *Genome Research*, *28*(8), 1126–1135. doi:10.1101/gr.231100.117 PMID:29954844

Richards, S., Aziz, N., Bale, S., Bick, D., Das, S., Gastier-Foster, J., Grody, W. W., Hegde, M., Lyon, E., Spector, E., Voelkerding, K., & Rehm, H. L. (2015). Standards and guidelines for the interpretation of sequence variants: A joint consensus recommendation of the American College of Medical Genetics and Genomics and the Association for Molecular Pathology. *Genetics in Medicine*, *17*(5), 405–423. doi:10.1038/gim.2015.30 PMID:25741868

Steinke-Lange, V., & Holinski-Feder, E. (2019, August). Genetic Screening and Personalized Prevention in Colorectal Cancer. *Visceral Medicine*, *35*(4), 226–230. doi:10.1159/000501941 PMID:31602383

Stockley, T. L., Oza, A. M., Berman, H. K., Leighl, N. B., Knox, J. J., Shepherd, F. A., Chen, E. X., Krzyzanowska, M. K., Dhani, N., Joshua, A. M., Tsao, M.-S., Serra, S., Clarke, B., Roehrl, M. H., Zhang, T., Sukhai, M. A., Califaretti, N., Trinkaus, M., Shaw, P., ... Bedard, P. L. (2016). Molecular profiling of advanced solid tumors and patient outcomes with genotype-matched clinical trials: The Princess Margaret IMPACT/COMPACT trial. *Genome Medicine*, *8*(1), 109. doi:10.118613073-016-0364-2 PMID:27782854

Stornetta, A., Guidolin, V., & Balbo, S. (2018). Alcohol-derived acetaldehyde exposure in the oral cavity. *Cancers (Basel)*, *10*(1), 20. doi:10.3390/cancers10010020 PMID:29342885

Wynn, R., Adams, K., Kowalski, R. L., Shivega, W. G., Ratwani, R. M., & Miller, K. E. (2018). R. The Patient in Precision Medicine: A Systematic Review Examining Evaluations of Patient-Facing Materials. *Journal of Healthcare Engineering*, *2018*, 1–10. doi:10.1155/2018/9541621 PMID:30250657

Yates, L. R., Seoane, J., Le Tourneau, C., Siu, L. L., Marais, R., Michiels, S., Soria, J. C., Campbell, P., Normanno, N., Scarpa, A., Reis-Filho, J. S., Rodon, J., Swanton, C., & Andre, F. (2018). The European Society for Medical Oncology (ESMO) precision medicine glossary. *Annals of Oncology: Official Journal of the European Society for Medical Oncology*, *29*(1), 30–35. doi:10.1093/annonc/mdx707 PMID:29140430

Chapter 7
The Role of E-Health Interventions in Improving Clinical Outcomes and Overall Health for Prostate Cancer Patients:
A Review

Donovan Anthony McGrowder
Faculty of Medical Sciences, The University of the West Indies, Jamaica

Fabian G. Miller
https://orcid.org/0000-0002-5821-1711
Faculty of Education, The Mico University College, Jamaica

Jabari G. Brown
Faculty of Medical Sciences, The University of the West Indies, Jamaica

Cameil Wilson-Clarke
https://orcid.org/0000-0002-9475-9637
Faculty of Medical Sciences, The University of the West Indies, Jamaica

Lennox Anderson-Jackson
https://orcid.org/0000-0002-9712-0214
Faculty of Medical Sciences, The University of the West Indies, Jamaica

ABSTRACT

Globally, prostate cancer is a major healthcare problem. It is among the most frequently diagnosed malignancies and is the primary cancer in males in North America and the Caribbean, Europe, and some parts of Africa. Mobile health interventions afford prostate cancer patients in following prostate specific antigen results including trends, getting a better understanding of the severity of their disease and evaluate carefully the benefits and risks of the available treatment options. This review will examine the use of mobile health applications in prostate cancer research particularly in (1) clinical decision of selecting best treatment option or active surveillance, (2) monitoring disease- and treatment-related symptoms, (3) oncological and supportive care, (4) treatment decisions, and (5) health literacy and promotion of physical exercise. The benefits of telemedicine are discussed. Challenges will be examined and

DOI: 10.4018/978-1-7998-6527-8.ch007

recommendations given for the development and efficient use of mobile health applications by prostate cancer patients and healthcare providers.

INTRODUCTION

The Epidemiology of Prostate Cancer

Globally, lung cancer is the most frequent malignancy in men followed by prostate cancer. In 2018, GLOBOCAN estimates that there were 1,276,106 new cases of prostate cancer worldwide with 358,989 recorded deaths from the disease (Bray et al., 2018). The incidence of prostate cancer rises with age, and rates differs across populations and regions (Ferlay et al., 2018). Ferlay et al. reported in 2018 an age standardized rate of 79.1 per 100,000 people for Oceania followed closely by 73.7 per 100,000 people for North America and 62.1 per 100,000 people for Europe (Ferlay et al., 2018). The disease is more frequently diagnosed among older men and worldwide the mean age is 66 years (Perdana et al., 2016; Panigrahi et al., 2019). It is reported that approximately 1 in 350 men below the age of 50 years will be diagnosed with the disease while in those within the 50 - 59 age group, the incidence rate increases to 1 in 50 men, and those over 65 years, 3 in 5 men (Perdana et al., 2016). Notably the incidence rate differs among ethnic groups with the highest observed in African American men with 157.6 per 100,000 people compared with 93.9 per 100,000 in Caucasian men (SEER Cancer Statistics Review, 2016). The differences in incidence rates could be attributed to genetic makeup, environmental factors which influences the etiology of the disease and variances in screening methods involving prostate specific antigen (PSA) testing as well as inequalities in healthcare access (Chu et al., 2011).

The well known risk factors of prostate cancer are family history, advancer age over 65 years old, ethnicity, genetic factors and other associated factors such as unbalanced diet, obesity, physical inactivity, infections, inflammation, and environmental contact with ionizing radiation or cancer-causing chemicals (Wilson et al., 2012; Markozannes et al., 2016). Approximately 20% of prostate cancer patients indicated a family history and hereditary genetic background is concomitant with elevated risk for the disease, with a contribution of approximately 5% (Gallagher et al., 1998; Sridhar et al., 2010). Dietary factors may have a crucial role in the progression of prostate cancer. Studies have reported a positive association between fat and dairy products, and prostate cancer mortality (Armstrong et al., 1975). A review of epidemiological and experimental studies showed that diets rich in saturated animal fat are associated with increased growth of prostate cancer cells due to higher levels of androgens (Vankateswaran and Klot, 2010). On the converse, Brassica vegetables have shown evidence for a protective effect against prostate cancer, and decreased risk have been observed with consumption of green tea and soy (Joseph et al., 2004; Fujiki et al., 1998).

The epidemiology of prostate cancer has been transformed due to the identification of biomarkers such as prostate specific antigen that are positively associated with the diagnosis of prostate cancer (Filella et al., 2018). Furthermore, there is increased survival among prostate cancer patients due to effective treatments, improved supportive care and advances in cancer detection. However, there are disease-specific and treatment-related side-effects which may negatively impact the health-related quality of life and well-being of prostate cancer patients (Lin et al., 2009).

BACKGROUND

Electronic Health (eHealth) and Mobile Health (mHealth) - Definitions and Applications

Electronic health (eHealth) is the protected and cost-effective usage of information communication technology (ICT) in a productive manner which is supportive of organizations, professionals, and patients in healthcare fields (Catan et al., 2015). In this fashion information is enriched and distributed via the internet and allied technologies to support areas in health-related fields such as health education and research, healthcare and health investigation (Pagliari et al., 2005). There are a number of benefits that eHealth offers to healthcare professionals such as reduction in workload as communications with patients can be simplified and streamlined. In addition, patients can be educated, trained and their treatment managed by the healthcare professionals from a distance. Electronic health also seeks to afford patients with services such as remote diagnosis of disease, treatment, consultation in their home environment and self-care management at home. In this manner patients are empowered (Dahlke et al., 2015; Kondylakis et al., 2013).

The European Commission in 2020 issued an eHealth Action Plan 2012 - 2020 that explain the role of eHealth in personalized medicine and to encourage healthcare professionals and patients to increasingly engage the use of technological devices in the delivery of healthcare (European Commission, 2012). The European Commission is of the opinion that the effective application of eHealth can results in the delivery of personalized healthcare that is well-organized, effective and inclusive. Possible outcomes of the personalized healthcare are patient empowerment, decrease patient morbidity and mortality, reduce length of hospitalization, improved quality of life, and greater access to services (European Commission, 2012). On-going technical developments in medical informatics, public health, the internet and associated technologies in this dynamic environment will globally advance healthcare and its delivery.

Developments in wireless technology have led to the growth of mobile health (mHealth). Mobile health is a subdivision of eHealth and is the use of mobile technology such as mobile phones and associated communication devices such as personal digital assistants, tablet computers and smart watches in the provision of healthcare (Lewis et al., 2016). Mobile health offers the opportunity of shared health information between healthcare professionals and patients thus resulting in faster diagnosis, more effective monitoring of health status, improved access to therapy and rehabilitation, reduction in time for the receipt of prescription and training in self-management (Kondylakis et al., 2017).

There is growing use and acceptance of mobile health in healthcare fields as it is viewed as a valued tool in patient-centered care or personalized medicine which is the objective of modern healthcare schemes (Ventola, 2014). Furthermore, the clinical application of mobile health is useful for decision-making support, gathering of clinical health data for patient care and research, education and collaboration of healthcare professionals, real-time monitoring of patients, track chronic diseases such as diabetes mellitus and cancer and monitoring public health (Pereira-Azevedo et al., 2018).

In the last decade there have being increasing use of mHealth applications (apps) tablets and smartphone with features such as Bluetooth and cameras in medical care. It is noted that there are approximately 300,000 mHealth apps accessible in the Google Play Store and Apple App Store (Byambasuren et al., 2018). Some of the most well-known categories of mHealth apps are recommended to patients for the diagnosis of disease, self-care management and treatment of health conditions include pregnancy, chronic illnesses such as diabetes mellitus, hypertension and obesity (Rowland et al., 2020). There are other apps that are associated with physical activity and fitness, nutrition and health behavior (Statista, 2019). However, it is important to note that only a limited number of mHealth apps have been technically reviewed and/or deemed appropriate for use by the USA Food and Drug Administration and European Medicines Agency (Pelletier, 2012).

mHealth apps are highly applicable to the treatment of chronic conditions such as cancer and health management (Mahmood et al., 2019). Research have demonstrated the advantages of using mHealth apps to aid patients with cancers including better-quality of life and emotional well-being, greater physical activity and weight reduction, decreased depression and anxiety and extending cost-effective care (Pope et al., 2019). According to a study conducted in February 2016, there were approximately 599 iOS and Androids–related apps for breast cancer in the United States which generally provide information on the disease, treatment and management (Giunti et al., 2018). Interestingly, the Mobile Application Rating Scale (MARS) has been found to be a useful methodology to analyze the quality of smartphone apps available on the Android and iOS platforms for patients diagnosed with genitourinary cancers including prostate cancer (Amor-Garcia et al., 2020).

Chow et al. reported the implementation of a novel mobile app-based intervention called iCanThrive that provides coping skills with telephone coaching and improve the well-being of breast cancer survivors (Chow et al., 2020). Likewise, Lidington et al. documented a randomized controlled trial with breast cancer patients with early staged disease where the effectiveness of the mobile app called OWise Breast Cancer will be evaluated for self-management of care and monitoring of symptoms (Lidington et al., 2020). A recently conducted quasi-experimental interventional clinical trial examined the viability and applicability of a mHealth app tailored to differentiated thyroid cancer patients and found significantly enhanced quality of life and patient education, increased remote monitoring and improved disease self-management (Giannoula et al., 2020).

Telemedicine has a number of applications in gynecology and women's health (Lee and Hitt, 2020) and disease management and treatment of children diagnosed with cancer (Kermani et al., 2020). Tele medicine can be applied to screening programs, and psycho-oncological care in breast cancer patients. Marino et al. describes a telemedicine screening program among 321 patients who undergo breast cancer screening (Marino et al., 2020) while a web-based psycho-oncological intervention training platform was effective in providing strategies for managing disease-related burden to breast cancer patients in need of psychological care (Ringwald et al., 2019). In addition, telemedicine allows the provision of radiation oncology consultations to prostate cancer patients located regionally and remotely with high level of satisfaction (Hamilton et al., 2018).

In urology, an important review of apps in December 2017 revealed 176 in Google Play Store and Apple App Store of which 20 were related to prostate cancer (Pereira-Azevedo, 2018). There are documented mHealth/eHealth apps in the literature relating to prostate cancer. Three noted examples are the Follow MyPSA app for males on active surveillance for prostate cancer, the Prostate Cancer Research International Active Surveillance (PRIAS) which utilized a mobile apps by males with low-risk disease, and Rotterdam Prostate Cancer Risk Calculator (RPCRC) where algorithms predicting risk are generated via the use of a smartphone app (Pereira-Azevedo, 2018).

Electronic health and mobile health applications are increasing used by health professionals and prostate cancer patients. Studies have shown that there has been timely diagnosis of prostate cancer, improvements in shared-decision making of treatment options, improved treatment adherence, enhanced communication between patient and provider and overall better-quality health care. This review will examine the use of electronic health and mobile health applications in prostate cancer research particularly in (i) risk assessment and clinical decision of treatment or active surveillance in early localized prostate cancer (ii) monitoring disease- and treatment-related symptoms, (iii) oncological and supportive care, (iv) health literacy and user satisfaction and (v) promotion of physical exercise. The benefits of telemedicine will be discussed. Challenges will be examined and recommendations given for the development and efficient use of electronic health and mobile health applications by prostate cancer patients and healthcare providers.

IMPLEMENTATION OF MOBILE HEALTH SYTEMS

Implementation Strategy of mHealth Systems Among Primary Care Patients

There has been a substantial increase in studies on mHealth systems including those examining their use in primary care. Quanbeck et al. reported the implementation of an evidence-based mHealth system called *Seva* that integrate treatment of patients with alcohol use disorder in primary care (Quanbeck et al., 2018). Seva provided patients with a discussion board and collaborative modules relating to self-regulation and problem solving to manage difficult situations as well as tools such as cognitive behavioral therapy, relaxation exercises and health tracking. It also offers clinicians with a Web portal comprising a Clinical Report generated by self-reported data from patients concerning their well-being and alcohol use (Quanbeck et al., 2018). The implementation strategy of *Seva* at each clinical site involved four phases which were (1) train key clinical staff involved in substance abuse, (2) organize a comfortable working environment for persons involved in *Seva*, (3) assess progress of previous phases and perform rapid-cycle tests of concepts, and (4) employ technology that should be easy to use and accepted by staff and patients (Quanbeck et al., 2018). In another study, Shiferaw et al. designed and implemented a mHealth technology for maternity services in a financially-constraints setting (Shiferaw et al., 2018). This technology was aimed at assisting health care professionals with midlevel training to offer improved maternal health care services to patients by an automated data collection system and electronic decision making process. The implementation strategy of this mHealth system comprise (1) staff recruitment including health care and information technology professionals, and capacity building, (2) mHealth system design which include front end component employed as a mobile-based apps and a back-end module implemented as web-based application, (3) collection and reporting of data, (4) electronic health records and decision support and (5) health care professionals providing general and specialized education along the continuum of service comprising antenatal, delivery and postnatal care (Shiferaw et al., 2018).

In an earlier study, Mirkovic et al. implemented and evaluated the usefulness of the Connect Mobile app in supporting patients with cancer in the management of health-related issues in a randomized clinical trial with prostate- and breast-cancer patients (Mirkovic et al., 2014). The implementation of the Connect mHealth system comprise (1) recruit cancer patients and health care professionals, (2) utilize Connect via a Web browser using laptop or desk computers using a JQuery Mobile framework and (3) patient employ the assessment, symptom self-management support, information, messaging, communication and diary modules. The assessment of the Connect mobile app involved examining both an Asus Transformer tablet computer and mobile phone versions of the app (Mirkovic et al., 2014).

The implementation of a mHealth system can increase care among patients with chronic diseases in primary care settings. However, there are challenges involving the availability of human and technological resources (Folaranmi, 2014) which must be overcome in order to have an effective and sustainable mHealth system.

MOBILE HEALH, SCREENING, DIAGNOSIS AND TREATMENT OF PROSTATE CANCER

Mobile Health in Risk Assessment and Clinical Decision of Treatment or Active Surveillance

Mobile health applications are increasingly used in urologic care by medical practitioners and their patients and a number of potential prostate cancer prediction models have been documented in the literature (Louie et al., 2015). These prediction models utilize risk factors such as family history, age and ethnicity along with PSA values to produce an index of prostate cancer risk and a suitable algorithm to manage the patient's diagnosis and prognosis (Louie et al., 2015). The web-based RPCRC was redesigned into an application (smartphone app) using similar algorithms in order to increase its use and accessibility among urologists and patients. Pereira-Azevedo et al. tested the usability of mobile phone app of the RPCRC among 92 participants comprising of general practitioners, urologists and medical students via the Post-Study System Usability Questionnaire (PSSUQ) (Pereira-Azevedo et al., 2017). The RPCRC smartphone app was instrumental in predicting prostate cancer risk and diagnosing clinical significant disease with scores for informational quality of 78-92%. The mobile phone app's interface is well designed as scores ranging from 80-95% were obtained for interface quality and 88-99% for system usefulness (Pereira-Azevedo et al., 2017; Table 1). Notably, a systematic review of the performance of prostate cancer risk calculator apps using the validated user version of the Mobile Application Rating Scale found that they enhanced clinical decision-making and were beneficial in providing counselling intervention for patients at risk for prostate cancer (Adam et al., 2018).

The Prostate Cancer Research International Active Surveillance (PRIAS) study was implemented in 2006 and is completely web-based. It sought to improve clinical decision making of urologist and their patients with low-risk prostate cancer regarding whether active surveillance or active treatment is more appropriate (van den Bergh et al., 2007). The entry of demographic, PSA measurement and PSA-doubling time in the online website by physicians results in an automatic recommendation on whether the patient with low-risk prostate cancer should remain on active surveillance or change to restorative treatment (Bokhorst et al., 2016). Furthermore, prostate cancer patients using a mobile app called Follow myPSA are able to document and tract their PSA test and other clinical results, and physicians are able to view in real-time the clinical information of their patient (Venderbos and Roobol, 2017).

In a prospective cohort study of 500 men across 8 countries with low-risk prostate cancer enrolled in the PRIAS study and followed for a median time of 6.5 years, more than one-half (65%) switched from active surveillance to invasive treatment within 2.3 years (Drost et al., 2018; Table 1). In another report of the PRIAS study comprising of 5,302 low-risk prostate cancer patients across 18 countries and followed for 10 years, 48% of the subjects remained on active surveillance after 5 years and 27% after 10 years (Bokhorst et al., 2016). These studies indicate that the PRIAS study has a simple protocol that is easy to use in daily clinical practice and there are limitations regarding the use of active surveillance in decreasing the adverse effects of over-diagnosis in low-risk prostate cancer patients (Drost et al., 2018; Bokhorst et al., 2016).

Table 1. Mobile health apps used in decision-making for diagnosis, active surveillance or treatment of prostate cancer patients

References	Study Population	mHealth/eHealth Application	Outcome of mHealth Application
Draisma et al., 2003	ERSPC study (enrolled 42,376 men with 1498 cases of prostate cancer)	Stimulation model based on results of the Rotterdam section of ERSPC study	Lead time estimate support prostate cancer screening for more than one year
Roobol et al., 2012	ERSPC Rotterdam risk calculator population: 3624 men (886 prostate cancer cases) and 2896 men (547 prostate cancer cases)	Development of DRE-Base Risk Calculator	RPCRC identified most prostate cancer cases and prevented 30 -35% biopsies
van Vugt et al., 2012	Multi-centre randomized control study of 443 prostate cancer patients (55-75 years) in 5 Dutch hospitals	ERSPC Risk Calculator use to assess urologist and patient compliance with recommendation	Urologists and patients complied with the RC recommendation in 368 of 443 (83%) cases
Pereira-Azevedo et al., 2017	Study of 92 participants comprising urologists, general practitioners, and medical students	Algorithms generated from ERSPC Risk Calculator	App received high scores for usefulness, information quality and interface quality
Bokhorst et al., 2016	PRIAS Study – 10 year including 5,302 men with low-risk prostate cancer across 18 countries	Web-based simple protocol – PSA tests, prostate biopsies and DREs	Low prostate cancer mortality for men on active surveillance
Drost et al., 2018	PRIAS Study – 500 men enrolled in 8 countries	Web-based study with analysis of PSA tests, DREs and prostate biopsies	More than half of men switched to invasive treatment within 2.3 years
Gulati et al., 2014	Population-based study of patients with localized prostate cancer	Calibrated microsimulation model - with age, PSA and Gleason score	In the age group 50 – 69 years the risk of over-diagnosis of prostate cancer was estimated as 5% - 44%

Use of Web-based PROMS and mHealth Applications to Monitor Symptoms

The treatment options offered to prostate cancer patients include prostatectomy and radiotherapy (Tyson et al., 2017). Patient undergoing radiotherapy may experience symptoms such as pain, bowel and urinary symptoms which are associated with both the disease and treatment (Liberman et al., 2014). The equality and content of clinical advice from physicians on managing these symptoms during radiotherapy and after prostatectomy differ greatly. Patients have used many different approaches to relieve the symptoms with diverse outcomes (Blomberg et al., 2016). Over the past ten years there have been the introduction of more technology some of which are mobile-based or web-based for offering advice on supportive care, monitoring symptoms of patients with cancer and meeting other needs albeit social, physical and emotional (Ruland et al., 2013; Maguire et al., 2015).

The comprehensive care and support for prostate cancer patients should encompass early monitoring of symptoms and signs, tailored care planning, training in self-care, and daily use of patient-reported outcome measures (PROMs) in clinical practice (Field et al., 2019). There are a number of studies that have utilized web-based PROMs which involved patient-reporting of the multi-dimensional aspects of health-related quality of life as well as signs and symptoms of disease (Chen et al., 2013). Web-based PROMs have been shown to contribute to better patient management as there is prompt detection of symptoms and side effects during treatment, improved patient satisfaction, better quality of life and well-being and increased clinician-patient satisfaction (Valderas et al., 2008; Jensen et al., 2014). Borosund et al. conducted a large randomized large randomized controlled trial of 325 prostate and breast cancer patients using a Web-based system. They found that 63.6% of the participants were regular users. Prostate cancer patients with elevated levels of symptom distress were more likely to use the discussion forum, participate in symptom assessments, and readily sought advice from healthcare provider (Boround et al., 2013).

There are reports of the use of smartphones for the collection of PROMS (Maguire et al., 2015) and the development of an interactive app on a smartphone or tablet coupled with an ICT platform, called Interaktor (Olsson et al., 2015; Langius-Eklöf et al., 2017). Interaktor is a health care management app that: (i) allow patients to assess and document the incidence, regularity and distress level of symptoms which is available in real-time to the healthcare provider, (ii) enables the healthcare provider via a web interface to monitor the patient's data and health status, (iii) possess a risk assessment model which alert the healthcare provider via text messages based on the severity of symptoms, (iv) provide links to relevant websites with health information and uninterrupted access to evidence-based self-care instruction, and (v) generate graphs of the patients' history of reported symptoms which is reviewed by patient and healthcare provider (Olsson et al., 2015; Langius-Eklof et al., 2017).

Langius-Eklöf and colleagues evaluated adherence to reporting, behavior and experience of 66 prostate cancer patients using Interaktor to monitor their symptoms during radiotherapy. There was significant self-management and care among participants with 87% adhering to daily reporting of symptoms (Ann Langius-Eklof et al., 2017). Through the use of Interaktor there was effective self-management of symptoms on a routine basis during radiotherapy, increase patient well-being, and improved patient-centered care for healthcare survivors (Langius-Eklöf et al., 2017). In a non-randomized controlled study of 64 patients in the control group and 66 patients in an intervention group that uses Interaktor, the later reported lower levels of nausea and fatigue at the end of radiation treatment (Sunberg et al., 2017). Moreover, the intervention group had lower burden in insomnia, urinary-related symptoms and emotional functioning (Sunberg et al., 2017).

Patients with prostate cancer may experience pain, a most distressing symptom that could be associated with significant levels of psychological distress and physical disability (Shi et al., 2011). There is the use of mHealth in pain management where video-conferencing technology was used to provide coping skills intervention to patients experiencing cancer pain (Somers et al., 2015). Furthermore, some patients with prostate cancer undergo radiotherapy which is associated with a number of side effects such as diarrhoea, rectal bleeding, painful bowel movements, blood in the urine, and frequent urination and urinary leakage (Gay et al., 2018). The symptoms related to radiotherapy can lead to decreased quality of life, increased cost and hospitalisation and low treatment adherence particularly if there is ineffective patient management (van Tol-Geerdink et al., 2013; Zelefsky et al., 2013). Langius-Eklot et al. reported a prospective, randomized controlled trial that will be implemented involving men with locally advanced prostate cancer undergoing curative radiotherapy treatment. In this trial, patients in the intervention group will report daily via smartphone apps symptoms experienced during treatment and up to 3 weeks subsequent to the treatment (Langius-Eklof et al., 2017). The authors are of the view that information on outcome measures such as quality of life, health costs, symptom burden, disease progress and health literacy will increase our understanding of how to develop a personalized care for prostate cancer patients using mobile technology (Langius-Eklof et al., 2017).

MOBILE HEALTH, SUPPORTIVE CARE, PHYSICAL ACTIVITY AND USER SATISFACTION

mHealth in Oncological and Supportive Care, and Promotion of Physical Activity

A diagnosis of cancer presents emotional challenges and it is reported that approximately 30 - 40% of patients experience psychological distress such as depression and anxiety symptoms (Mitchell et al., 2011). The emotional distress experienced by prostate cancer patients is associated with reduced quality of life (Roth et al., 2008). General health-related quality of life (HRQoL) and disease-specific HRQoL (such as urinary and bowel function) are affected by prostate cancer and its management (Eton and Lepore, 2002). Mobile phone health apps can be useful management tools for oncological care as they can assist both healthcare professionals and patients in monitoring symptoms, improve communication and follow up, provide specific cancer information and support drug adherence (Wang et al., 2014). Rincon et al. conducted a systematic review of the effect of mobile app use on the quality of life and well-being of prostate cancer patients (Rincon et al., 2017). The study found that there is a deficiency of rigorous clinical trials involving cancer-focused mobile phone apps and assessment of quality of life and/or wellbeing (Rincon et al., 2017). In the few studies identified, there was no association between mobile phone apps intervention and quality of life, and well-being of prostate cancer patients (Rincon et al., 2017).

Prostate cancer patients need supportive care and patient-reported outcomes (PROs) are increasing used by healthcare providers as they have been shown to improve patient engagement and self-care, evaluate pain and distress, increase communication between patients and providers, and overall better health outcomes (Basch et al., 2017; Segal et al., 2013). Tran et al. evaluated the practicality and suitability of obtaining electronic PROs remotely using validated HRQoL tools for prostate cancer (Tran et al., 2020). Using the Strength Through Insight App and validated HRQoL tools, the researchers found that the smartphone app was an acceptable and feasible manner of collecting electronic PROs (Tran et al., 2020). In another study that investigated the use of mobile health application to collect PROs and guide postoperative care of prostate cancer patients after robot-assisted radical prostatectomy, the majority of the participants (75%) found the app easy to use and understand. The results suggest that the implementation of mobile apps can improve the compliance of prostate cancer patients with perioperative instructions and facilitate the collection of PROs with little resource utilization (Belarmino et al., 2019).

Unmet psychological and functional supportive care needs during and after treatments have been reported by prostate cancer patients (Hyde et al., 2017). Supportive care is important as it assist with patient's adaptation and coping with the disease, improve knowledge and understanding, increase health-related quality of life, lessen functional declines and apprise decision making (Chambers et al., 2017). A systematic review of 16 studies including 10 randomized control trials (comprising 2,446 men) investigated the suitability, acceptability and effectiveness of online supportive care interventions (decision aids, patient support, medical records/follow-up) at improving the lives of prostate cancer survivors (Forbes et al., 2019). The researchers found primary evidence of online supportive care among prostate cancer survivors.

However, most of the studies had small sample size and insufficient acceptability measures which indicate the need for larger trials and more emphasis on translation of operational intervention (Forbes et al., 2019). An earlier study reported the use of Composite Holistic Assessment Tool-Prostate (CHAT-P), an online prostate-specific holistic needs assessment (HNA) tool that facilitates the self-management of prostate cancer patients. This online tool provided links to trustworthy sources of advice and support relating the disease process and treatment (Nanton et al., 2017). The HNA tool was accessed via a secured login system and CHAT-P generated an output which summarizes the patient's needs and a proposed care plan that can be reviewed by the patient and health care provider (Nanton et al., 2017). Moreover, Bogaert et al. described an eHealth tool called CHESS (Comprehensive Health Enhancement Support System) which comprised a series of interactive tools aimed at supporting the needs of prostate cancer survivors and their partners (Bogaert et al., 2012). The findings from this formative study were used to improve user satisfaction and design a series of navigational features and collaborative tools for the CHESS prostate cancer computer-mediated system (Bogaert et al., 2012). Similarly, a randomized control trial involving an internet-based couple counseling program was as effective as traditional sexual counseling in improving sexual outcomes of prostate cancer patients with localized disease, and their partners (Schover et al., 2012).

Different treatment option for prostate cancer patients may cause symptoms such as dysfunction of the bowel, urinary incontinence and erectile dysfunction (Roth et al., 2008). These symptoms may negatively impact the mental health of prostate cancer patients so there is need for psychological intervention by mental health professionals (Parahoo et al., 2015). Internet-based psychological interventions may be useful in providing support to men with prostate cancer, allowing easy access to key health information specific to care, support for those in rural areas, and bridging gaps in the delivery of care (Anderson and Cuijper, 2008).

Lange et al. examined the usefulness of guided chat room groups in providing psychosocial care post-treatment for prostate cancer patients (Lange et al., 2017). Using a quasi-experimental design and 5 web-based chat-group sessions the study found that the intervention group had higher scores on coping with the disease, reduction in depression and improvement in the physical component of quality of life (Lange et al., 2017). In a randomized control trial reported by Wootten et al. a self-guided online psychological intervention called My Road Ahead combined with online peer discussion forum was used to assess psychological distress of 142 prostate cancer patients with localized disease. There were significant improved reductions in psychological distress within the intervention group post-treatment (Wootten et al., 2015). Furthermore, a technology assisted cognitive-behavioral stress management intervention effectively reduced depressive symptoms and improved health-related quality of life in prostate cancer patients with advanced disease (Yanez, et al., 2015). However, a randomized control longitudinal study involving an online educational support network did not observe any noteworthy improvements in quality of life of patients with prostate cancer (Osei et al., 2013). These studies suggests that larger randomized control trials should be performed to evaluate the efficacy of eHealth technology coupled with established psychological intervention tools on improving the health-related quality of life and psychological care of prostate cancer patients.

mHealth and Treatment Decisions, Physical Activity and Health Literacy

Treatments for localized prostate cancer includes expectant management which comprise observation or active surveillance, radical prostatectomy, radiation therapy, cryotherapy, hormone therapy and chemotherapy (Mottet et al., 2016). Despite these treatment options, the best decision have not yet being established although the American Urological Association Clinical Guidelines suggest that active surveillance is a practical choice for patients diagnosed with early, localized prostate cancer (Middleton et al., 1995).

Primary care practitioners usually work with the prostate cancer patient in arriving at the best decisions regarding therapy (Schapira et al., 1997). In a study by Holmboe et al. comprising 100 men newly diagnosed localized prostate cancer (from hospital and community-based urology practice groups), patients' decision regarding treatment were based on their understanding and belief of the essential characteristics of each treatment option and the possible side effects (Holmboe et al., 2000). There is a recent study that investigated the practicability of The Staying Strong And Healthy protocol, an intervention delivered via telephone to lessen metabolic and cardiovascular risks related to androgen deprivation therapy (Manson et al., 2019).

Moreover, a study that examined the readability of 62 websites for prostate cancer patients with information regarding treatment options found that only few website had online resources that were written lower than a high school reading level (Ellimoottil et al., 2012). In 2017, a prospective multicentre and cluster-randomized control trial called the EasiPRO3 study that involves a comprehensive on-line programme (Prostana) commenced among prostate cancer patients in Germany. The study seeks to evaluate the satisfaction of primary care patients exposed to cross specialties, with their treatment decision (Vosgerau et al., 2017). The authors are of the view that the findings from the study may be able to provide insight into how inventive online-based programs support prostate cancer patients, their families and clinicians in making treatment decisions (Vosgerau et al., 2017).

Physical activity can have a positive effect on clinical outcomes of prostate cancer patients such as improvements in health-related quality of life and cardiorespiratory fitness, reduced cancer-specific morbidity and mortality, and decreased treatment related side effects such as depression, psychological distress, anxiety, pain and fatigue (Bourke et al., 2015; Santa et al., 2014). Electronic health tools such as web-based and mobile apps have shown potential for the promotion of physical exercise in patients with chronic diseases (Walsh et al., 2018). In a prospective study which sought the opinions of colorectal, breast and prostate cancer survivors on the use of smartphone apps to produce physical activity, the majority of the participants were receptive to the use of smartphone apps to promote physical activity (Roberts et al., 2019).

Trinh et al. examined the usefulness of a 12-week web-based intervention called Rise Tx to increase moderate to vigorous physical activity and decrease sedentary behavior among 46 prostate cancer survivors. The web-based intervention was highly accessible, effectively reduced sedentary behavior and significantly increased moderate to vigorous activity among prostate cancer survivors (Trinh et al., 2018). Furthermore, there is the implementation of a computer-tailored physical activity intervention called

OncoActive by Golsteijn et al. which seeks to increase the level of physical activity among colorectal and prostate cancer survivors in The Netherlands (Golsteijn et al., 2017). The efficacy of the OncoActive intervention is assessed in a randomized control trial consisting of 428 patients over a 12-month period (Golsteijn et al., 2017). The authors suggests that if the findings show that the OncoActive intervention is effective, it could be implemented nationwide and extended to other cancer types (Golsteijn et al., 2017).

The increasing accessibility of electronic health programs and health information available online affords prostate cancer patients and their families to improve their knowledge of their health condition and probably better overall health (Nagler et al., 2010). However, the actual use of the available heath resource is contingent on the patient's eHealth literacy. A study by Bender et al. comprising 1,362 prostate cancer patients in four Canadian provinces sought to determine patterns and factors related with internet use of health-related information as well as essential information and features in a website (Bender et al., 2019). The majority (two-thirds) of the prostate cancer patients used the internet to access health information about prostate cancer and to make important health decisions (Bender et al., 2019). In an earlier study, Schaffer et al. develop a prostate cancer electronic health tutorial aimed at assessing user satisfaction and to support the decision making process between patients and their physicians. The findings indicate that user satisfaction with the eHealth tutorial was high particularly among prostate cancer patients with localized disease (Schaffert et al., 2018). The participants also indicated that access and the quality of online health information was good and they were empowered to make better decisions regarding treatment (Schaffert et al., 2018).

Other support for eHealth literacy among prostate cancer patients came from Le et al. who reported that incorporating SMS text messages in an education intervention conducted among African American men was feasible and reasonable accepted by the participants. The authors suggest that incorporating SMS text messages in interventions is a promising avenue to support these men in making informed decision about prostate cancer screening, treatment and their overall health (Le et al., 2016). Furthermore, a cross-sectional exploratory study of 142 partners of newly diagnosed prostate cancer patients with localized disease was conducted using a telephone survey. There were high levels of electronic health literacy among the partners that was concomitant with their knowledge of treatment options, reliance on social network for additional health information which was disease specific and their involvement in obtaining a second opinion (Song et al., 2017).

TELEMEDICINE AND PROSTATE CANCER

Telemedicine-Interventions Used in Supportive Care of Prostate Cancer Patients

Telemedicine, also commonly called telehealth is the use of technology such as video platform, mobile phones, web and telephone to deliver healthcare services to patients in remote locations (Sood et al., 2007). There is the exchange of critical health resources via electronic communications between healthcare providers and patients in the comfort of their homes, allowing for possible cost savings and improved patient management (Stroetmann, 2013).

Telemedicine have been incorporated in different aspect of the supportive care of prostate cancer patients through different technological platforms. In this manner it affords urologic care to men in remote locations, provides access to specialty care follow up and facilitates telephone or web-based interventions which may reduce psychological distress (Ellimoottil et al., 2016). ProsCan, a peer-based telephone support for prostate cancer patients and their partners within a trial design was evaluated in 20 couples who received sessional intervention. There was reduction in psychological distress among the prostate cancer survivors although sexual relations of couples did not improve (Chambers et al., 2013; Table 2). Likewise, in a nationwide study of 292 prostate cancer patients including those from remote locations, survivorship care was provided through telemedicine platforms that facilitate partner involvement. Using validated psychological tools it was found that there were significantly lower levels of psychological distress in married prostate cancer survivors who experience good partner support (Karmen et al., 2015; Table 2).

Telemedicine enhances psychological care by allowing healthcare providers to support patients who live in remote locations between visits (Maheu and Gordon, 2000). Michel et al. carried out a randomized controlled trial where 239 men with prostate cancer in the intervention group received psychological intervention by telephone while the control group received standard care. Prostate cancer survivors in the intervention group improved in problem solving and cognitive framing (Michel et al., 2002). There were also reductions in the number and intensity of side effects and significant improvement in sexual satisfaction from baseline to 4 months (Michel et al., 2002; Table 2).

In clinical research telemedicine can be used to increase samples size and individuals of different representations particular those in various remote geographical regions. Scurrey et al. found that telemedicine via telephone interviews was effective in recruiting prostate cancer patients in rural areas and permit increase access and greater convenience. Although participants reported an overall positive experience, sound quality and better access for patients who face challenges with commuting to telemedicine location are areas for improvement (Scurrey et al., 2019)

Web-based intervention for prostate cancer patients facilitate a multidisciplinary approach particularly when all the healthcare providers are not at the same healthcare centre, and overcome mobility and geographical challenges (Roland et al., 2013). A retrospective study of 171 patients with urologic diseases of which 14% was prostate cancer was conducted by Chu and colleagues. It was reported that web-based prostate cancer program was affordable and successfully used to assess the wide range of urologic conditions including prostate cancer in remote clinic (Chu et al., 2015; Table 2). Likewise, a Web-based survey was conducted to examine the perceptions and peruse acceptance of remote video visit technology in a urological patient population. The level of participation in among the patients in the video visit technology group was high which suggests that telemedicine may assist urologists in reaching diverse population in remote areas via this technology (Viers et al., 2015a; Table 2).

Telemedicine delivery tools such as video technology can be used by healthcare professionals to improve the quality of care to patients in their environments without the time and pressure constraints of a clinic visit (Somers et al., 2015). In a randomized control trial Viers et al. investigated the use of video technology by prostate cancer patients following radical prostatectomy. Prostate cancer survivors in the intervention group experience similar satisfaction, comparable efficiency and lesser cost compared to office visits (Viers et al., 2015b). Likewise, support for telemedicine using video technology in an outpatient urology clinic is noted in a study by Andino et al. who conducted an on-site survey among patients where access to technology required for video visit was assessed. The majority of patients across all age groups were highly interested and possess the technology required to participate in video visits (Andino et al., 2017). The authors suggests that video visits have the potential to increase patient experience especially those who live in remote areas and travel long distances during visits to specialty clinics (Andino et al., 2017; Table 2).

Table 2. Telemedicine applications and outcomes of prostate cancer patents

Reference	Study Population	Telemedicine Applications	Outcomes of Telemedicine Application
Chambers et al., 2013	Focus group of twenty couples with male having localized prostate cancer	Peer-delivered telephone support with DVD education (eight session intervention)	Couples received adequate support with decrease in stress but no improvement in unmet sexuality needs
Karmen et al., 2015	A randomized controlled trial of 292 prostate cancer survivors enlisted by 9 Community Clinical Oncology Program sites in the USA	Telephone calls involving prostate cancer patients and partners	Decreased psychological distress of patients and partners in intervention group
Michel et al., 2002	Clinical trial of 105 African-American and 134 Caucasian prostate cancer patients after radiation therapy or surgical intervention	Psychoeducational intervention via weekly telephone calls over an 8-week period	Improvement in problem solving, cognitive framing, control of incontinence and satisfaction with sexual functioning
Viers et al., 2015a	Randomized control study of 55 prostate cancer patients	Video visit technology and traditional office visit	Patients in video visit technology intervention group incurred lower travel time, costs and distance travelled. High level of urologist satisfaction.
Viers et al., 2015b	Study of 1,378 prostate cancer patients who participated in a web-based survey	Web-based survey that evaluating patient's acceptance of video visit	Reduced costs and increasing quality and access to health care services
Andino et al., 2017	On-site survey of urologic patients including 108 prostate cancer survivors at an outpatient urology clinic over a 3-month period	Evaluation of importance and value of video visits by patients before implementation of telemedicine program	The majority of patients possess video technology and express interest in video visit
Chu et al., 2015	Retrospective study 171 patients with urologic diseases including prostate cancer (14%)	Urologic care delivered via telemedicine clinics over a 6-month period	Patients including those with prostate cancer saves time and cost per visit
Scurrey et al., 2019	A study of 20 patients with cancer of which 8 had prostate cancer	Telephone interviews	The majority of the patients embrace telehealth as a viable option as it allow greater access to healthcare, more convenience and personal interactions

CHALLENGES AND FUTURE RESEARCH DIRECTIONS

Studies including randomized control trials have shown that mHealth improves the lives of prostate cancer patients. The clinical application of mHealth in urologic care provides improves access to screening, diagnostic and treatment decision support, increased patient compliance, social support, psychological care and cancer-specific health information. A few studies that examined user attitude towards mHealth have shown that most prostate cancer patients reported an overall good satisfaction, and view it as an opportunity for enhanced self-efficacy and provider-driven clinical management.

Nevertheless, there is a need to make available mHealth tools that are more accessible and understandable to men of ethnic minorities, lesser socioeconomic status as well as those living in remote areas. Also noteworthy are the challenges to the employment of mHealth technologies in medical practice settings due to apprehensions regarding confidentiality, privacy, data security and ownership issues, geographical, organizational and cultural obstacles that may be present within the clinical practice setting, and the integration into electronic health record platforms present at the clinician office or healthcare institution. There are also concerns regarding poorly validate health information, lack of current data, little or no quality control and absence of regulations to ensure that these health apps are accurate, user-friendly and efficient.

With the continued expansion of mHealth technology these concerns need to be urgently addressed and to create a delicate balance between usability and privacy protection. Strategies that could be employed in addressing these issues include the involvement of the healthcare team including urologists in the development, review and verification of app contents, and apps subscribing to evidence-based protocols. Furthermore, healthcare organizations should create standard guidelines regarding the identification, evaluation, selection and clinical use of these mobile apps to make the most of their usefulness and safety.

Despite the prospective effectiveness of mHealth applications for supporting the care of prostate cancer patients, documented interventions in this area of research are few compared to those for breast cancer, diabetes management, nutrition and fitness, and physical exercise adherence. In addition it is observed that some studies such as those utilizing web-based interventions have a small number of participants in the intervention and control groups, and therefore the study design do not have satisfactory power to test the null hypothesis. Therefore there is need for employing large randomized control trials in the evaluation of existing and new mobile health interventions in accessing user satisfaction and patient related outcomes concomitant with person-centered management of prostate cancer patients.

CONCLUSION

Mobile health provides opportunities and health resources for patients and providers to promote shared decision making on diagnosis and treatment for improved health outcomes and overall health. It also assist prostate cancer patients to have a better understanding of their disease severity, track critical health information, evaluate the benefits and risks of the different treatment, and greater access to psychological care. The delivery of telemedicine in supportive care to prostate cancer patient in remote locations is acceptable, feasible, economical and effective particularly for those who are cared for by multidisciplinary teams. The use of electronic PROs on digital platforms provide innovative ways for effective collection of data, with possibly greater person-centered management of prostate cancer patients.

REFERENCES

AAMC Reporter. (2012, Oct.). Available online: https://www.aamc.org/newsroom/reporter/october2012/308516/health-care-apps.html

Adam, A., Hellig, J. C., Perera, M., Bolton, D., & Lawrentschuk, N. (2018). Prostate Cancer Risk Calculator' mobile applications (Apps): A systematic review and scoring using the validated user version of the Mobile Application Rating Scale (uMARS). *World Journal of Urology*, *36*(4), 565–573. doi:10.100700345-017-2150-1

Amor-García, M. Á., Collado-Borrell, R., Escudero-Vilaplana, V., Melgarejo-Ortuño, A., Herranz-Alonso, A., Arranz Arija, J. Á., & Sanjurjo-Sáez, M. (2020). Assessing apps for patients with genitourinary tumors using the Mobile Application Rating Scale (MARS): Systematic search in app stores and content analysis. *JMIR mHealth and uHealth*, *8*(7), e17609. doi:10.2196/17609

Andersson, G., & Cuijpers, P. (2008). Pros and cons of online cognitive-behavioural therapy. *The British Journal of Psychiatry*, *193*(4), 270–271. doi:10.1192/bjp.bp.108.054080

Andino, J. J., Guduguntla, V., Weizer, A., Roberts, W. W., Wittmann, D., Miller, D., Morgan, T. M., & Ellimoottil, C. (2007). Examining the value of video visits to patients in an outpatient urology clinic. *Urology*, *110*, 31–35. doi:10.1016/j.urology.2017.07.050

Andriole, G. L., Crawford, E. D., Grubb, R. L. III, Buys, S. S., Chia, D., Church, T. R., Fouad, M. N., Gelmann, E. P., Kvale, P. A., Reding, D. J., Weissfeld, J. L., Yokochi, L. A., O'Brien, B., Clapp, J. D., Rathmell, J. M., Riley, T. L., Hayes, R. B., Kramer, B. S., Izmirlian, G., ... Berg, C. D. (2009). Mortality results from a randomized prostate-cancer screening trial. *The New England Journal of Medicine*, *360*(13), 1310–1319. doi:10.1056/NEJMoa0810696

Armstrong, B., & Doll, R. (1975). Environmental factors and cancer incidence and mortality in different countries, with special reference to dietary practices. *International Journal of Cancer*, *15*(4), 617–631. doi:10.1002/ijc.2910150411

Basch, E., Deal, A. M., Dueck, A. C., Scher, H. I., Kris, M. G., Hudis, C., & Schrag, D. (2017). Overall survival results of a trial assessing patient-reported outcomes for symptom monitoring during routine cancer treatment. *Journal of the American Medical Association*, *318*(2), 197–198. doi:10.1001/jama.2017.7156

Belarmino, A., Walsh, R., Alshak, M., Patel, N., Wu, R., & Hu, J. C. (2019). Feasibility of a mobile health application to monitor recovery and patient-reported outcomes after robot-assisted radical prostatectomy. *Eur. Urol. Oncol.*, *2*(4), 425–428. doi:10.1016/j.euo.2018.08.016

Bender, J. L., Feldman-Stewart, D., Tong, C., Lee, K., Brundage, M., Pai, H., Robinson, J., & Panzarella, T. (2019). Health-related internet use among men with prostate cancer in Canada: Cancer registry survey study. *Journal of Medical Internet Research*, *21*(11), e14241. doi:10.2196/14241

Blomberg, K., Wengström, Y., Sundberg, K., Browall, M., Isaksson, A. K., Nyman, M. H., & Langius-Eklöf, A. (2016). Symptoms and self-care strategies during and six months after radiotherapy for prostate cancer - scoping the perspectives of patients, professionals and literature. *European Journal of Oncology Nursing*, *21*, 139–145. doi:10.1016/j.ejon.2015.09.004

Bokhorst, L. P., Valdagni, R., Rannikko, A., Kakehi, Y., Pickles, T., Bangma, C. H., & Roobol, M. J. (2016). A decade of active surveillance in the PRIAS Study: An update and evaluation of the criteria used to recommend a switch to active treatment. *European Urology*, *70*(6), 954–960. doi:10.1016/j.eururo.2016.06.007

Borosund, E., Cvancarova, M., Ekstedt, M., Moore, S. M., & Ruland, C. M. (2013). How user characteristics affect use patterns in web-based illness management support for patients with breast and prostate cancer. *Journal of Medical Internet Research*, *15*(3), e34. doi:10.2196/jmir.2285

Bourke, L., Boorjian, S. A., Briganti, A., Klotz, L., Mucci, L., Resnick, M. J., Rosario, D. J., Skolarus, T. A., & Penson, D. F. (2015). Survivorship and improving quality of life in men with prostate cancer. *European Urology*, *68*(3), 374–383. doi:10.1016/j.eururo.2015.04.023

Bray, F., Ferlay, J., Soerjomataram, I., Siegel, R. L., Torre, L. A., & Jemal, A. (2018). Global cancer statistics 2018: GLOBOCAN estimates of incidence and mortality worldwide for 36 cancers in 185 countries. *CA: a Cancer Journal for Clinicians*, *68*(6), 394–424. doi:10.3322/caac.21492

Byambasuren, O., Sanders, S., Beller, E., & Glasziou, P. (2018). Prescribable mHealth apps identified from an overview of systematic reviews. *NPJ Digital Medicine*, *1*(1), 12. doi:10.103841746-018-0021-9

Catan, G., & Espanha, R., Veloso, Mendes, R., Toren, O. & Chinitz, D. (2015). The impact of eHealth and mHealth on doctor behavior and patient involvement: An Israeli and Portuguese comparative approach. *Studies in Health Technology and Informatics*, *210*, 813–817.

Chambers, S. K., Hyde, M. K., Smith, D. P., Hughes, S., Yuill, S., Egger, S., O'Connell, D. L., Stein, K., Frydenberg, M., Wittert, G., & Dunn, J. (2017). New challenges in psycho-oncology research III: A systematic review of psychological interventions for prostate cancer survivors and their partners: clinical and research implications. *Psycho-Oncology*, *26*(7), 873–913. doi:10.1002/pon.4431

Chambers, S. K., Schover, L., Halford, K., Ferguson, M., Gardiner, R. A., Occhipinti, S., & Dunn, J. (2013). ProsCan for Couples: A feasibility study for evaluating peer su pport within a controlled research design. *Psycho-Oncology*, *22*(2), 475–479. doi:10.1002/pon.2110

Chen, J., Ou, L., & Hollis, S. J. (2013). A systematic review of the impact of routine collection of patient reported outcome measures on patients, providers and health organizations in an oncologic setting. *BMC Health Services Research*, *13*(1), 21. doi:10.1186/1472-6963-13-211

Chow, P. I., Drago, F., Kennedy, E. M., & Cohn, W. F. (2020). A novel mobile phone app intervention with phone coaching to reduce symptoms of depression in survivors of women's cancer: Pre-post pilot study. *JMIR Cancer*, *6*(1), e15750. doi:10.2196/15750

Chu, L. W., Ritchey, J., Devesa, S. S., Quraishi, S. M., Zhang, H., & Hsing, A. W. (2011). Prostate cancer incidence rates in Africa. *Prostate Cancer*.

Chu, S., Boxer, R., Madison, P., Kleinman, L., Skolarus, T., Altman, L., Bennett, C., & Shelton, J. (2015). Veterans affairs telemedicine: Bringing urologic care to remote clinics. *Urology*, *86*(2), 255–260. doi:10.1016/j.urology.2015.04.038

Chui, P. L. (2019). Cancer- and chemotherapy-related symptoms and the use of complementary and alternative medicine. *Asia-Pacific Journal of Oncology Nursing*, *6*(1), 4–6. doi:10.4103/apjon.apjon_51_18

Dahlke, D. V., Fair, K., & Hong, Y. A. (2015). Apps seeking theories: Results of a study on the use of health behavior change theories in cancer survivorship mobile apps. *JMIR mHealth and uHealth*, *3*(1), e31. doi:10.2196/mhealth.3861

Davis, T. L., DiClemente, R., & Prietula, M. (2016). Taking mHealth forward: Examining the core characteristics. *JMIR mHealth and uHealth*, *4*(3), e97. doi:10.2196/mhealth.5659 de Koning, H. J., Gulati, R., Moss, S. M., Hugosson, J., Pinsky, P. F., Berg, C. D., Auvinen, A., Andriole, G. L., Roobol, M. J., Crawford, E. D., Nelen, V., Kwiatkowski, M., Zappa, M., Luján, M., Villers, A., de Carvalho, T. M., Feuer, E. J., Tsodikov, A., Mariotto, A. B., ... Etzioni, R. (2018). The efficacy of prostate-specific antigen screening: Impact of key components in the ERSPC and PLCO trials. *Cancer*, *124*(2), 1197–1206. doi:10.1002/cncr.31178

Draisma, G., Boer, R., Otto, S. J., van der Cruijsen, I. W., Damhuis, R. A. M., Schroder, F. H., & de Koning, H. J. (2003). Lead times and over-detection due to prostate-specific antigen screening: Estimates from the European Randomized Study of Screening for Prostate Cancer. *Journal of the National Cancer Institute*, *95*(12), 868–878. doi:10.1093/jnci/95.12.868

Drost, F.-J. H., Rannikko, A., Valdagni, R., Pickles, T., Kakehi, Y., Remmers, S., van der Poel, H. G., Monique, C. H., & Roobol, J. (2018). PRIAS study group. Can active surveillance really reduce the harms of over-diagnosing prostate cancer? A reflection of real life clinical practice in the PRIAS Study. *Translational Andrology and Urology*, *7*(1), 98–105. doi:10.21037/tau.2017.12.28

Ellimoottil, C., Polcari, A., Kadlec, A., & Gupta, G. (2012). Readability of websites containing information about prostate cancer treatment options. *The Journal of Urology*, *188*(6), 2171–2175. doi:10.1016/j.juro.2012.07.105

Ellimoottil, C., Skolarus, T., Gettman, M., Boxer, R., Kutikov, A., Lee, B. R., Shelton, J., & Morgan, T. (2016). Telemedicine in urology: State of the art. *Urology*, *94*, 10–16. doi:10.1016/j.urology.2016.02.061

Eton, D. T., & Lepore, S. J. (2002). Prostate cancer and health-related quality of life: A review of the literature. *Psycho-Oncology*, *11*(4), 307–326. doi:10.1002/pon.572

European Commission. (2012). *eHealth Action Plan 2012-2020: Innovative healthcare for the 21st century*. Available online: https://ec.europa.eu/digital-single-market/en/news/ehealth-action-plan-2012-2020-innovative-healthcare-21st-century

Ferlay, J. E. M., Lam, F., Colombet, M., Mery, L., Pineros, M., Znaor, A., Soerjomataram, I., & ... . (2011). *Global cancer observatory: cancer today*. International Agency for Research on Cancer. Available from https://gco.iarc.fr/today

Field, J., Holmes, M. M., & Newell, D. (2019). PROMs data: Can it be used to make decisions for individual patients? A narrative review. *Patient Related Outcome Measures*, *10*, 233–241. doi:10.2147/PROM.S156291

Filella, X., Fernández-Galan, E., Fernández Bonifacio, R., & Foj, L. (2018). Emerging biomarkers in the diagnosis of prostate cancer. *Pharmacogenomics and Personalized Medicine*, *11*, 83–94. doi:10.2147/PGPM.S136026

Folaranmi, T. (2014). mHealth in Africa: Challenges and opportunities. *Perspectives in Public Health*, *134*(1), 14–15. doi:10.1177/1757913913514703

Forbes, C. C., Finlay, A., McIntosh, M., Siddiquee, S., & Short, C. E. (2019). A systematic review of the feasibility, acceptability, and efficacy of online supportive care interventions targeting men with a history of prostate cancer. *Journal of Cancer Survivorship: Research and Practice*, *13*(1), 75–96. doi:10.100711764-018-0729-1

Fujiki, H., Suganuma, M., Okabe, S., Sueoka, N., Komori, A., Sueoka, E., Kozu, T., Tada, Y., Suga, K., Imai, K., & Nakachi, K. (1998). Cancer inhibition by green tea. *Mutation Research*, *402*(1-2), 307–310. doi:10.1016/S0027-5107(97)00310-2

Gallagher, R. P., & Fleshner, N. (1998). Prostate cancer: 3. Individual risk factors. *Canadian Medical Association Journal*, *159*(7), 807–813.

Gay, H. A., & Michalski, J. M. (2018). Radiation therapy for prostate cancer. *Missouri Medicine*, *115*(2), 146–150.

Giannoula, E., Iakovou, I., Katsikavelas, I., Antoniou, P., Raftopoulos, V., Chatzipavlidou, V., Papadopoulos, N., & Bamidis, P. (2020). A mobile app for thyroid cancer patients aiming to enhance their quality of life: Protocol for a quasi-experimental interventional pilot study. *JMIR Research Protocols*, *9*(3), e13409. doi:10.2196/13409

Giunti, G., Giunta, D., Guisado-Fernandez, E., Bender, J., & Fernandez-Luque, L. (2018). A biopsy of breast cancer mobile applications: State of the practice review. *International Journal of Medical Informatics*, *110*, 1–9. doi:10.1016/j.ijmedinf.2017.10.022

Golsteijn, R. H. J., Bolman, C., Volders, E., Peels, D. A., de Vries, H., & Lechner, L. (2017). Development of a computer-tailored physical activity intervention for prostate and colorectal cancer patients and survivors: OncoActive. *BMC Cancer*, *17*(1), 446. doi:10.118612885-017-3397-z

Gulati, R., Inoue, L. Y., Gore, J. L., Katcher, J., & Etzioni, R. (2014). Individualized estimates of overdiagnosis in screen-detected prostate cancer. *Journal of the National Cancer Institute*, *106*(2), 1–5. doi:10.1093/jnci/djt367

Hamilton, E., Van Veldhuizen, E., Brown, A., Brennan, S., & Sabesan, S. (2018). Telehealth in radiation oncology at the Townsville Cancer Centre: Service evaluation and patient satisfaction. *Clin. Transl. Radiat. Oncol.*, *15*, 20–25. doi:10.1016/j.ctro.2018.11.005

Holmboe, E. S., & Concato, J. (2000). Treatment decisions for localized prostate cancer: Asking men what's important. *Journal of General Internal Medicine*, *15*(10), 694–701. doi:10.1046/j.1525-1497.2000.90842.x

Howell, D., Molloy, S., Wilkinson, K., Green, E., Orchard, K., Wang, K., & Liberty, J. (2015). Patient-reported outcomes in routine cancer clinical practice: A scoping review of use, impact on health outcomes, and implementation factors. *Annals of Oncology: Official Journal of the European Society for Medical Oncology*, *26*(9), 1846–1858. doi:10.1093/annonc/mdv181

Hyde, M. K., Newton, R. U., Galvão, D. A., Gardiner, R. A., Occhipinti, S., Lowe, A., Wittert, G. A., & Chambers, S. K. (2017). Men's help-seeking in the first year after diagnosis of localized prostate cancer. *European Journal of Cancer Care*, *26*(2), e12497. doi:10.1111/ecc.12497

Jain, S., Loblaw, A., Vesprini, D., Zhang, L., Kattan, M. W., Mamedov, A., Jethava, V., Sethukavalan, P., Yu, C., & Klotz, L. (2015). Gleason upgrading with time in a large prostate cancer active surveillance cohort. *The Journal of Urology*, *194*(1), 79–84. doi:10.1016/j.juro.2015.01.102

Jensen, R. E., Snyder, C. F., Abernethy, A. P., Basch, E., Potosky, A. L., Roberts, A. C., Loeffler, D. R., & Reeve, B. B. (2014). Review of electronic patient-reported outcomes systems used in cancer clinical care. *Journal of Oncology Practice / American Society of Clinical Oncology*, *10*(4), e215–e222. doi:10.1200/JOP.2013.001067

Joseph, M. A., Moysich, K. B., Freudenheim, J. L., Shields, P. G., Bowman, E. D., Zhang, Y., Marshall, J. R., & Ambrosone, C. B. (2004). Cruciferous vegetables, genetic polymorphisms in glutathione S-transferases M1 and T1, and prostate cancer risk. *Nutrition and Cancer*, *50*(2), 206–213. doi:10.120715327914nc5002_11

Kamen, C., Mustian, K. M., Heckler, C., Janelsins, M. C., Peppone, L. J., Mohile, S., McMahon, J. M., Lord, R., Flynn, P. J., Weiss, M., Spiegel, D., & Morrow, G. R. (2015). The association between partner support and psychological distress among prostate cancer survivors in a nationwide study. *Journal of Cancer Survivorship: Research and Practice*, *9*(3), 492–499. doi:10.100711764-015-0425-3

Kermani, F., Orooji, A., & Sheikhtaheri, A. (2020). Teleoncology for children with cancer: A scoping review on applications and outcomes. *International Journal of Medical Informatics*, *139*, 104–118. doi:10.1016/j.ijmedinf.2020.104118

Kessel, K. A., Vogel, M. M., Schmidt-Graf, F., & Combs, S. E. (2016). Mobile apps in oncology: A survey on health care professionals' attitude toward telemedicine, mHealth, and oncological apps. *Journal of Medical Internet Research*, *18*(11), e312. doi:10.2196/jmir.6399

Kondylakis, H., Koumakis, L., Hänold, S., Nwankwo, I., Forgó, N., Marias, K., Tsiknakis, M., & Graf, N. (2017). Donor's support tool: Enabling informed secondary use of patient's biomaterial and personal data. *International Journal of Medical Informatics*, *97*, 282–292. doi:10.1016/j.ijmedinf.2016.10.019

Kondylakis, H., Koumakis, L., & Tsiknakis, M. (2013). Smart recommendation services in support of patient empowerment and personalized medicine *BT*. In G. A. Tsihrintzis, M. Virvou, & L. C. Jain (Eds.), *Multimedia services in intelligent environments: Recommendation services* (pp. 39–61). Springer International Publishing. doi:10.1007/978-3-319-00375-7_4

Kranse, R., Roobol, M., & Schröder, F. H. (2008). A graphical device to represent the outcomes of a logistic regression analysis. *The Prostate*, *68*(15), 1674–1680. doi:10.1002/pros.20840

Lange, L., Fink, J., Bleich, C., Graefen, M., & Schulz, H. (2017). Effectiveness, acceptance and satisfaction of guided chat groups in psychosocial aftercare for outpatients with prostate cancer after prostatectomy. *Internet Interventions: the Application of Information Technology in Mental and Behavioural Health*, *9*, 57–64. doi:10.1016/j.invent.2017.06.001

Langius-Eklöf, A., Christiansen, M., Lindström, V., Blomberg, K., Hälleberg Nyman, M., Wengström, Y., & Sundberg, K. (2017). Adherence to report and patient perception of an interactive app for managing symptoms during radiotherapy for prostate cancer: Descriptive study of logged and interview data. *JMIR Cancer*, *3*(2), e18. doi:10.2196/cancer.7599

Langius-Eklöf, A., Crafoord, M. T., Christiansen, M., Fjell, M., & Sundberg, K. (2017). Effects of an interactive mHealth innovation for early detection of patient-reported symptom distress with focus on participatory care: Protocol for a study based on prospective, randomized, controlled trials in patients with prostate and breast cancer. *BMC Cancer*, *17*(1), 466. doi:10.118612885-017-3450-y

Le, D., Holt, C. L., Saunders, D. R., Wang, M. Q., Coriolan, A., Savoy, A. D., Slade, J. L., Muwwakkil, B., & Atkinson, N. L. (2018). Feasibility and acceptability of SMS text messaging in a prostate cancer educational intervention for African American men. *Health Informatics Journal*, *22*(4), 932–947. doi:10.1177/1460458215598636

Leslie, S. W., Soon-Sutton, T. L., Sajjad, H., & Siref, L. E. (2020). Prostate cancer. In *StatPearls*. StatPearls Publishing.

Lewis, J., Ray, P., & Liaw, S.-T. (2016). Recent worldwide developments in eHealth and mHealth to more effectively manage cancer and other chronic diseases - a systematic review. *Yearbook of Medical Informatics*, *1*, 93–108.

Liberman, D., Mehus, B., & Elliott, S. P. (2014). Urinary adverse effects of pelvic radiotherapy. *Translational Andrology and Urology*, *3*(2), 186–195.

Lidington, E., McGrath, S. E., Noble, J., Stanway, S., Lucas, A., Mohammed, K., van der Graaf, W., & Husson, O. (2020). Evaluating a digital tool for supporting breast cancer patients: A randomized controlled trial protocol (ADAPT). *Trials*, *21*(1), 86. doi:10.118613063-019-3971-6

Lin, D. W., Porter, M., & Montgomery, B. (2009). Treatment and survival outcomes in young men diagnosed with prostate cancer: A Population-based Cohort Study. *Cancer*, *115*(13), 2863–2871. doi:10.1002/cncr.24324

Louie, K. S., Seigneurin, A., Cathcart, P., & Sasieni, P. (2015). Do prostate cancer risk models improve the predictive accuracy of PSA screening? A meta-analysis. *Annals of Oncology: Official Journal of the European Society for Medical Oncology*, *26*(5), 848–864. doi:10.1093/annonc/mdu525

Maguire, R., Ream, E., Richardson, A., Connaghan, J., Johnston, B., Kotronoulas, G., Pedersen, V., McPhelim, J., Pattison, N., Smith, A., Webster, L., Taylor, A., & Kearney, N. (2015). Development of a novel remote patient monitoring system: The advanced symptom management system for radiotherapy to improve the symptom experience of patients with lung cancer receiving radiotherapy. *Cancer Nursing*, *38*(2), E37–E47. doi:10.1097/NCC.0000000000000150

Maheu, M. M., & Gordon, B. L. (2000). Counseling and therapy on the internet. *Professional Psychology, Research and Practice*, *31*(5), 484–489. doi:10.1037/0735-7028.31.5.484

Mahmood, A., Kedia, S., Wyant, D. K., Ahn, S., & Bhuyan, S. S. (2019). Use of mobile health applications for health-promoting behavior among individuals with chronic medical conditions. *Digital Health*, *5*. Advance online publication. doi:10.1177/2055207619882181

Manson, A., Myers, J., Billinger, S., Ward, J., Parker, W., Hamilton-Reeves, J., Michel, C., & Maliski, S. L. (2019). Feasibility of an intervention for men on androgen deprivation therapy: A research protocol. *Research in Nursing & Health*, *42*(5), 324–333. doi:10.1002/nur.21977

Marino, M. M., Rienzo, M., Serra, N., Marino, N., Ricciotti, R., Mazzariello, L., Leonetti, C. A., Ceraldi, M. P., Casamassimi, A., Capocelli, F., Martone, G., & Caracciolo, A. L. (2020). Mobile screening units for the early detection of breast cancer and cardiovascular disease: A pilot telemedicine study in Southern Italy. *Telemedicine Journal and e-Health*, *26*(3), 286–293. doi:10.1089/tmj.2018.0328

Markozannes, G., Tzoulaki, I., Karli, D., Evangelou, E., Ntzani, E., Gunter, M. J., Norat, T., Ioannidis, J. P., & Tsilidis, K. K. (2016). Diet, body size, physical activity and risk of prostate cancer: An umbrella review of the evidence. *European Journal of Cancer (Oxford, England)*, *69*, 61–69. doi:10.1016/j.ejca.2016.09.026

Middleton, R. G., Thompson, I. M., Austenfeld, M. S., Cooner, W. H., Correa, R. J., Gibbons, R. P., Miller, H. C., Oesterling, J. E., Resnick, M. I., Smalley, S. R., & Wasson, J. H. (1995). Prostate Cancer Clinical Guidelines Panel Summary report on the management of clinically localized prostate cancer. The American Urological Association. *The Journal of Urology*, *154*(6), 2144–2148. doi:10.1016/S0022-5347(01)66718-1

Mirkovic, J., Kaufman, D. R., & Ruland, C. M. (2014). Supporting cancer patients in illness management: Usability evaluation of a mobile app. *JMIR mHealth and uHealth*, *2*(3), e33. doi:10.2196/mhealth.3359

Mishel, M. H., Belyea, M., Germino, B. B., Stewart, J. L., Bailey, D. E., Robertson, C., & Mohler, J. (2002). Helping patients with localized prostate carcinoma manage uncertainty and treatment side effects: Nurse-delivered psychoeducational intervention over the telephone. *Cancer*, *94*(6), 1854–1866. doi:10.1002/cncr.10390

Mitchell, A. J., Chan, M., Bhatti, H., Halton, M., Grassi, L., Johansen, C., & Meader, N. (2011). Prevalence of depression, anxiety, and adjustment disorder in oncological, haematological, and palliative-care settings: A meta-analysis of 94 interview-based studies. *The Lancet. Oncology*, *12*(2), 160–174. doi:10.1016/S1470-2045(11)70002-X

Mottet, N., Bellmunt, J., & Briers, E. (2016). *Guidelines on prostate cancer*. https://urowcb.org/wp-content/uploads/EAU-Guidelines

Nagler, R. H., Gray, S. W., Romantan, A., Kelly, B. J., DeMichele, A., Armstrong, K. et al. (2010). Differences in information seeking among breast, prostate, and colorectal cancer patients: results from a population-based survey. *Patient Educ. Couns.*, *81*, S54-S62.

Nanton, V., Appleton, R., Loew, J., Ahmed, N., Ahmedzai, S., & Dale, J. (2017). Men don't talk about their health, but will they CHAT? The potential of online holistic needs assessment in prostate cancer. *BJU International*, *121*(4), 494–496. doi:10.1111/bju.14114

Olsson, C. E., Alsadius, D., Pettersson, N., Tucker, S. L., Wilderäng, U., Johansson, K. A., & Steineck, G. (2015). Patient-reported sexual toxicity after radiation therapy in long-term prostate cancer survivors. *British Journal of Cancer*, *113*(5), 802–808. doi:10.1038/bjc.2015.275

Osei, D. K., Lee, J. W., Modest, N. N., & Pothier, P. K. (2013). Effects of an online support group for prostate cancer survivors: A randomized trial. *Urologic Nursing*, *33*(3), 123–133. doi:10.7257/1053-816X.2013.33.3.123

Pagliari, C., Sloan, D., Gregor, P., Detmer, D., Kahan, J. P., Oortwijn, W., & MacGillivray, S. (2005). What is eHealth (4): A scoping exercise to map the field. *Journal of Medical Internet Research, 7*(1), 9. doi:10.2196/jmir.7.1.e9

Panigrahi, G. K., Praharaj, P. P., Kittaka, H., Mridha, A. R., Black, O. M., Singh, R., Mercer, R., van Bokhoven, A., Torkko, K. C., Agarwal, C., Agarwal, R., Abd Elmageed, Z. Y., Yadav, H., Mishra, S. K., & Deep, G. (2019). Exosome proteomic analyses identify inflammatory phenotype and novel biomarkers in African American prostate cancer patients. *Cancer Medicine, 8*(3), 1111–1123. doi:10.1002/cam4.1885

Parahoo, K., McDonough, S., McCaughan, E., Noyes, J., Semple, C., Halstead, E. J., Neuberger, M. M., & Dahm, P. (2015). Psychosocial interventions for men with prostate cancer: A Cochrane systematic review. *BJU International, 116*(2), 174–183. doi:10.1111/bju.12989

Pelletier, S. G. (2012). Explosive growth in health care apps raises oversight questions. *AAMC Reporter*. Available at https://www.aamc.org/newsroom/reporter/october2012/308516/health-care-apps.html

Perdana, N. R., Mochtar, C. A., Umbas, R., & Hamid, A. R. (2016). The risk factors of prostate cancer and its prevention: A literature review. *Acta Medica Indonesiana, 48*(3), 228–238.

Pereira-Azevedo, N., Osório, L., Fraga, A., & Roobol, M. J. (2017). Rotterdam Prostate Cancer Risk Calculator: Development and usability testing of the mobile phone app. *JMIR Cancer, 3*(1), e1. doi:10.2196/cancer.6750

Pereira-Azevedo, N. M., & Venderbos, L. (2018). eHealth and mHealth in prostate cancer detection and active surveillance. *Translational Andrology and Urology, 7*(1), 170–181. doi:10.21037/tau.2017.12.22

Pope, Z., Lee, J. E., Zeng, N., Lee, H. Y., & Gao, Z. (2019). Feasibility of smartphone application and social media intervention on breast cancer survivors' health outcomes. *Translational Behavioral Medicine, 9*(1), 11–22. doi:10.1093/tbm/iby002

Quanbeck, A., Gustafson, D. H., Marsch, L. A., Chih, M. Y., Kornfield, R., McTavish, F., Johnson, R., Brown, R. T., Mares, M. L., & Shah, D. V. (2018). Implementing a mobile health system to integrate the treatment of addiction into primary care: A hybrid implementation-effectiveness study. *Journal of Medical Internet Research, 20*(1), e37. doi:10.2196/jmir.8928

Rincon, E., Monteiro-Guerra, F., Rivera-Romero, O., Dorronzoro-Zubiete, E., Sanchez-Bocanegra, C. L., & Gabarron, E. (2017). Mobile phone apps for quality of life and well-being assessment in breast and prostate cancer patients: Systematic review. *JMIR mHealth and uHealth, 5*(12), e187. doi:10.2196/mhealth.8741

Ringwald, J., Gerstner, L., Junne, F., Ziser, K., Schäffeler, N., Wallwiener, M., Hautzinger, M., Bäuerle, A., Brucker, S., Zipfel, S., & Teufel, M. (2019). Mindfulness and skills based distress reduction in oncology: Das Webbasierte Psychoonkologische Make It Training. *Psychotherapie, Psychosomatik, Medizinische Psychologie, 69*(9-10), 407–412. doi:10.1055/a-0835-6905

Roberts, A. L., Potts, H. W., Koutoukidis, D. A., Smith, L., & Fisher, A. (2019). Breast, prostate, and colorectal cancer survivors' experiences of using publicly available physical activity mobile apps: Qualitative study. *JMIR mHealth and uHealth, 7*(1), e10918. doi:10.2196/10918

Roobol, M. J., van Vugt, H. A., Loeb, S., Zhu, X., Bul, M., Bangma, C. H., van Leenders, A. G. L. J. H., Steyerberg, E. W., & Schröder, F. H. (2012). Prediction of prostate cancer risk: The role of prostate volume and digital rectal examination in the ERSPC risk calculators. *European Urology*, *61*(3), 577–583. doi:10.1016/j.eururo.2011.11.012

Roth, A. J., Weinberger, M. I., & Nelson, C. J. (2008). Prostate cancer: Psychosocial implications and management. *Future Oncology (London, England)*, *4*(4), 561–568. doi:10.2217/14796694.4.4.561

Rowland, S. P., Fitzgerald, J. E., Holme, T., Powell, J., & McGregor, A. (2020). What is the clinical value of mHealth for patients? *NPJ Digital Medicine*, *3*(1), 4. doi:10.103841746-019-0206-x

Ruland, C. M., Andersen, T., Jeneson, A., Moore, S., Grimsbo, G. H., Borosund, E., & Ellison, M. C. (2013). Effects of an Internet support system to assist cancer patients in reducing symptom distress a randomized controlled trial. *Cancer Nursing*, *36*(1), 6–17. doi:10.1097/NCC.0b013e31824d90d4

Ruland, C. M., Maffei, R. M., Borosund, E., Krahn, A., Andersen, T., & Grimsbø, G. H. (2013). Evaluation of different features of an eHealth application for personalized illness management support: Cancer patients' use and appraisal of usefulness. *International Journal of Medical Informatics*, *82*(7), 593–603. doi:10.1016/j.ijmedinf.2013.02.007

Santa Mina, D., Guglietti, C. L., Alibhai, S. M., Matthew, A. G., Kalnin, R., Ahmad, N., Lindner, U., & Trachtenberg, J. (2014). The effect of meeting physical activity guidelines for cancer survivors on quality of life following radical prostatectomy for prostate cancer. *Journal of Cancer Survivorship: Research and Practice*, *8*(2), 190–198. doi:10.100711764-013-0329-z

Schaffert, R., Dahinden, U., Hess, T., Bänziger, A., Kuntschik, P., Odoni, F., Spörri, P., Strebel, R. T., Kamradt, J., Tenti, G., Mattei, A., Müntener, M., Subotic, S., Schmid, H.-P., & Rüesch, P. (2018). Evaluation of a prostate cancer E health tutorial: Development and testing of the website prostata-information. *Der Urologe. Ausg. A*, *57*(2), 164–171. doi:10.100700120-017-0552-8

Schapira, M. M., Nattinger, A. B., Katz, D. A., & Lawrence, W. (1997). Information seeking and satisfaction with treatment decision in patients with clinically localized prostate cancer. *Medical Decision Making*, *17*, 544.

Schover, L. R., Canada, A. L., Yuan, Y., Sui, D., Neese, L., Jenkins, R., & Rhodes, M. M. (2012). A randomized trial of internet-based versus traditional sexual counseling for couples after localized prostate cancer treatment. *Cancer*, *118*(2), 500–509. doi:10.1002/cncr.26308

Scurrey, S., Garland, S. N., Thoms, J., & Laing, K. (2019). Evaluating the experience of rural individuals with prostate and breast cancer participating in research via telehealth. *Rural and Remote Health*, *19*(3), 5269. doi:10.22605/RRH5269

SEER Cancer Statistics Review 1975-2013. (n.d.). *National Cancer Institute, Bethesda, MD*. Available from: https://seer.cancer.gov/csr/1975_2015/

Segal, C., Holve, E., Sabharwal, R., & Seer, C. X. (2013). *Collecting and using patient-reported outcomes (PRO) for comparative effectiveness research (CER) and patient-centered outcomes research (PCOR): Challenges and opportunities.* http://citeseerx.ist.psu.edu/viewdoc/download?doi=10.1.1.831.9388&rep=rep1&type=pdf

Shi, Q., Smith, T. G., Michonski, J. D., Stein, K. D., Kaw, C., & Cleeland, C. S. (2011). Symptom burden in cancer survivors 1 year after diagnosis: A report from the American Cancer Society's Studies of Cancer Survivors. *Cancer, 117*(12), 2779–2790. doi:10.1002/cncr.26146

Shiferaw, S., Workneh, A., Yirgu, R., Dinant, G. J., & Spigt, M. (2018). Designing mHealth for maternity services in primary health facilities in a low-income setting - lessons from a partially successful implementation. *BMC Medical Informatics and Decision Making, 18*(1), 96. doi:10.118612911-018-0704-9

Somers, T. J., Abernethy, A. P., Edmond, S. N., Kelleher, S., Wren, A. A., & Sams, G. P. (2015). A pilot study of a mobile health pain coping skills training protocol for patients with persistent cancer pain. *Journal of Pain and Symptom Management, 50*(4), 553–558. doi:10.1016/j.jpainsymman.2015.04.013

Song, L., Tatum, K., Greene, G., & Chen, R. C. (2017). eHealth literacy and partner involvement in treatment decision making for men with newly diagnosed localized prostate cancer. *Oncology Nursing Forum, 44*(2), 225–333.

Sood, S., Mbarika, V., Jugoo, S., Dookhy, R., Doarn, C. R., Prakash, N., & Merrell, R. C. (2007). What is telemedicine? A collection of 104 peer-reviewed perspectives and theoretical underpinnings. *Telemedicine Journal and e-Health, 13*(5), 573–590. doi:10.1089/tmj.2006.0073

Sridhar, G., Masho, S. W., Adera, T., Ramakrishnan, V., & Roberts, J. D. (2010). Association between family history of prostate cancer. *J. M. H., 7*, 45–54.

Statista. (2019). *Number of apps available in leading app stores as of 3rd quarter 2019*. https://www.statista.com/statistics/276623/number-of-apps-available-in-leading-app-stores/

Stroetmann, K. A. (2013). Achieving the integrated and smart health and wellbeing paradigm: A call for policy research and action on governance and business models. *International Journal of Medical Informatics, 82*(4), e29–e37. doi:10.1016/j.ijmedinf.2012.05.008

Sundberg, K., Wengström, Y., Blomberg, K., Hälleberg-Nyman, M., Frank, C., & Langius-Eklöf, A. (2017). Early detection and management of symptoms using an interactive smartphone application (Interaktor) during radiotherapy for prostate cancer. *Supportive Care in Cancer, 25*(7), 2195–2204. doi:10.100700520-017-3625-8

Tran, C., Dicker, A., Leiby, B., Gressen, E., Williams, N., & Jim, H. (2020). Utilizing digital health to collect electronic patient-reported outcomes in prostate cancer: Single-arm pilot trial. *Journal of Medical Internet Research, 22*(3), e12689. doi:10.2196/12689

Trinh, L., Arbour-Nicitopoulos, K. P., Sabiston, C. M., Berry, S. R., Loblaw, A., Alibhai, S. M., Jones, J. M., & Faulkner, G. E. (2018). RiseTx: Testing the feasibility of a web application for reducing sedentary behavior among prostate cancer survivors receiving androgen deprivation therapy. *The International Journal of Behavioral Nutrition and Physical Activity, 15*(1), 124. doi:10.118612966-018-0757-2

Tyson, M. D., Penson, D. F., & Resnick, M. J. (2017). The comparative oncologic effectiveness of available management strategies for clinically localized prostate cancer. *Urologic Oncology, 35*(2), 51–58. doi:10.1016/j.urolonc.2016.03.021

Valderas, J., Kotzeva, A., Espallargues, M., Guyatt, G., Ferrans, C., Halyard, M. Y., Revicki, D. A., Symonds, T., Parada, A., & Alonso, J. (2008). The impact of measuring patient-reported outcomes in clinical practice: A systematic review of the literature. *Quality of Life Research: An International Journal of Quality of Life Aspects of Treatment, Care and Rehabilitation*, *17*(2), 179–193. doi:10.100711136-007-9295-0

Van Bogaert, D., Hawkins, R., Pingree, S., & Jarrard, D. (2012). The development of an eHealth tool suite for prostate cancer patients and their partners. *The Journal of Supportive Oncology*, *10*(5), 202–208. doi:10.1016/j.suponc.2012.02.003

van den Bergh, R. C., Roemeling, S., Roobol, M. J., Roobol, W., Schröder, F. H., & Bangma, C. H. (2007). Prospective validation of active surveillance in prostate cancer: The PRIAS study. *European Urology*, *52*(6), 1560–1563. doi:10.1016/j.eururo.2007.05.011

van Tol-Geerdink, J. J., Leer, J. W., van Oort, I. M., van Lin, E. J., Weijerman, P. C., Vergunst, H., Witjes, J. A., & Stalmeier, P. F. (2013). Quality of life after prostate cancer treatments in patients comparable at baseline. *British Journal of Cancer*, *108*(9), 1784–1789. doi:10.1038/bjc.2013.181

van Vugt, H. A., Roobol, M. J., Busstra, M., Kil, P., Oomens, E. H., de Jong, I. J., Bangma, C. H., Steyerberg, E. W., & Korfage, I. (2012b). Compliance with biopsy recommendations of a prostate cancer risk calculator. *BJU International*, *109*(10), 1480–1488. doi:10.1111/j.1464-410X.2011.10611.x

van Vugt, H. A., Roobol, M. J., van der Poel, H. G., van Muilekom, E. H. A. M., Busstra, M., Kil, P., Oomens, E. H., Leliveld, A., Bangma, C. H., Korfage, I., & Steyerberg, E. W. (2012b). Selecting men diagnosed with prostate cancer for active surveillance using a risk calculator: A prospective impact study. *BJU International*, *110*(2), 180–187. doi:10.1111/j.1464-410X.2011.10679.x

Venderbos, L. D., & Roobol, M. J. (2017). m-PRIAS: An e-health technology for men on active surveillance for prostate cancer. *Quality of Life Research: An International Journal of Quality of Life Aspects of Treatment, Care and Rehabilitation*, *26*(1), 99.

Venkateswaran, V., & Klotz, L. H. (2010). Diet and prostate cancer: Mechanisms of action and implications for chemoprevention. *Nature Reviews. Urology*, *7*(8), 442–453. doi:10.1038/nrurol.2010.102

Ventola, C. L. (2014). Mobile devices and apps for health professionals: Uses and benefits. *P&T*, *39*(5), 356–364.

Viers, B. R., Lightner, D. J., & Rivera, M. E. (2015b). Are Patients Willing to Engage in Telemedicine for Their Care: A Survey of Preuse Perceptions and Acceptance of Remote Video Visits in a Urological Patient Population. *Urology*, *85*(6), 1233–1239. doi:10.1016/j.urology.2014.12.064

Vosgerau, S., Urbanski, D., Kollenbach, P., Schöne, M., Gedamke, M., Donatz, V., Bültmann, O., & Amelung, V. (2017). Easipro3-Enhancing satisfaction with prostate cancer treatment decision with the mobile health program Prostana: A multicenter randomized controlled trial. Easipro3. *Value in Health*, *20*(9), A504. doi:10.1016/j.jval.2017.08.598

Walsh, D. M., Moran, K., Cornelissen, V., Buys, R., Cornelis, N., & Woods, C. (2018). Electronic health physical activity behavior change intervention to self-manage cardiovascular disease: Qualitative exploration of patient and health professional requirements. *Journal of Medical Internet Research*, *20*(5), e163. doi:10.2196/jmir.9181

Wang, J., Wang, Y., Wei, C., Yao, N. A., Yuan, A., Shan, Y., & Yuan, C. (2014). Smartphone interventions for long-term health management of chronic diseases: An integrative review. *Telemedicine Journal and e-Health*, *20*(6), 570–583. doi:10.1089/tmj.2013.0243

Wilson, K. M., Giovannucci, E. L., & Mucci, L. A. (2012). Lifestyle and dietary factors in the prevention of lethal prostate cancer. *Asian Journal of Andrology*, *14*(3), 365–374. doi:10.1038/aja.2011.142

Wootten, A. C., Abbott, J. A., Meyer, D., Chisholm, K., Austin, D. W., Klein, B., McCabe, M., Murphy, D. G., & Costello, A. J. (2015). Preliminary results of a randomized controlled trial of an online psychological intervention to reduce distress in men treated for localized prostate cancer. *European Urology*, *68*(3), 471–479. doi:10.1016/j.eururo.2014.10.024

Yanez, B., McGinty, H. L., Mohr, D. C., Begale, M. J., Dahn, J. R., Flury, S. C., Perry, K. T., & Penedo, F. J. (2015). Feasibility, acceptability, and preliminary efficacy of a technology-assisted psychosocial intervention for racially diverse men with advanced prostate cancer. *Cancer*, *121*(24), 4407–4415. doi:10.1002/cncr.29658

Zelefsky, M. J., Lee, W. R., Zietman, A., Khalid, N., Crozier, C., Owen, J., & Wilson, J. F. (2013). Evaluation of adherence to quality measures for prostate cancer radiotherapy in the United States: Results from the Quality Research in Radiation Oncology (QRRO) Survey. *Practical Radiation Oncology*, *3*(1), 2–8. doi:10.1016/j.prro.2012.01.006

KEY TERMS AND DEFINITIONS

Active Surveillance: A means of closely monitoring localized (early) prostate cancer, but not providing treatment unless there are changes in the prostate specific antigen and/or other test results that show that the disease is getting worse.

Electronic Health: The protected and cost-effective usage of information communication technology in a productive manner that is supportive of healthcare.

Health Literacy: The ability of an individual to obtain, read, understand and to communicate basic health information in a manner that appropriate health decisions can be made and good health is both maintained and promoted.

Mobile Health: The use of mobile technology such as mobile phones and associated Communication devices such as personal digital assistants, tablet computers and smart watches in the provision of healthcare.

Prostate Cancer: A type of cancer that develops in the prostate gland and is diagnosed by prostate-specific antigen blood test, digital rectal examination followed by transrectal ultrasound guided biopsy.

Symptom: A subjective evidence of a disease or disorder that is apparent to the patient and includes nausea, pain, or weakness.

Telemedicine: The use of technology such as video platform, mobile phones, web, and telephone to deliver healthcare services to patients in remote locations.

Chapter 8
Incautious Usage of Social Media:
Impact on Emotional Intelligence and Health Concerns

Vrinda Kharbanda
https://orcid.org/0000-0002-9349-3953
J. C. Bose University of Science and Technology, India

Rosy Madaan
Manav Rachna International Institute of Research and Studies, India

Komal Kumar Bhatia
J. C. Bose University of Science and Technology, India

ABSTRACT

The purpose of this chapter is to examine the incautious usage of social media and its impact on emotional intelligence and health. After a brief introduction to the emotional intelligence and the conceptualisation and evaluation of this construct, this chapter discusses a variety of studies that shed light on the social media, emotional intelligence and health relationships. The idea of emotional intelligence (EI) is of unmatched enthusiasm for both the literature and inside scholarly world. This chapter discusses emotional intelligence and focuses on the evolution of EI by examining the different models. This chapter lists some applications of emotional intelligence in our daily life. The chapter also discusses how the abilities correlate with emotional intelligence and helps individuals cope with unsettling emotions effectively and encourage pleasurable emotions to facilitate personal development and well-being.

INTRODUCTION

Emotions are the incredible leaders of one's life and without acknowledgment, Emotions derive an individual. The world is as the mind sees and feels it; the world is as the mind considers it (Grades, 2019).

DOI: 10.4018/978-1-7998-6527-8.ch008

Uncontrolled emotions can however affect an individual, making users prone to anxiety and depression. If someone is unable to manage their emotions, they are probably not managing their stress either. This can lead to serious health problems. So to control emotions, to distinguish feelings, to understand them, and to manage them is basically what emotional intelligence is. As a center develops in conventional psychology, emotional intelligence has risen. With the help of this, one can understand emotions and know when and how to use them. Knowledge about the reaction in any particular situation will help the user to handle and manage their actions in a better manner. It can help individuals overcome and deal with social media instigated issues (self-doubt, anxiety, depression, low self-esteem) efficiently. Suicides, digital - addictions, etc. caused by social media games can be stopped, and it will also enable the user to get the most out of technology without being abused by various social media tactics.

BACKGROUND

Emotional intelligence has been a significant matter of interest both in intellectual world and in the general masses since 1995. But one may trace the historical origins of emotional and psychological intelligence back to the 19th century. Charles Darwin published first ever known work in this field in 1872 and emphasized the significance of emotional communication for development and adaptation.

Peter Salovey and John Mayer first coined the term emotional intelligence in 1990 and used it in literary writing. Be that as it may, Darwin's initial work on the importance of emotional expression has reflected the basic principles of emotional intelligence survival in 1900. In 1920, Edward Thorndike portrayed the idea of social intelligence as the potential to get on with others through understanding each other's internal states, intentions, and traits. Most of these early experiments were intended to identify, characterize, and aim to measure socially responsible behavior.

After a year, David Wechsler came up with the concept of non-cognitive intelligence in 1940 asserting that it is vitally important to life's success; intelligence is indeed not finished until its non-cognitive facets are defined. John Mayer and Peter Salovey published their breakthrough article Emotional Intelligence in the journal Imagination, Cognition, and Personality in 1900. Since the book by Daniel Goleman, Emotional Intelligence: How It Could Matter More than IQ, the definition of EI became popular in 1995 and the distinction between trait & ability emotional intelligence was made in 2000 by Konstantinos V. Petrides.

There are numerous definitions of emotional intelligence. In the Salovey and Mayer's view; Emotional intelligence is the ability of individuals to identify everyone's emotions, to differentiate and properly mark different feelings, To direct one's thoughts and actions, using emotional knowledge, and manage and/or modify emotions to adjust with the environment (Colman, 2015). But according to Konstantinos V. Petrides, Trait EI is "a constellation of emotional self-perceptions located at the lower levels of personality."

EI researchers have developed three key models over the past two decades (John, 2000): they are

1. **Ability Model**: Peter Salovey and John Mayer developed the ability model, stressing the capacity of the person to perceive and then use emotional knowledge to navigate the social environment. The four-level design of Mayer and Salovey follows emotional intelligence as mental ability and through which a person turns out to be emotionally intelligent.
    a. **Perceiving Emotions:** The potential to sense and decoding emotions in faces, photos, and sounds. It comprises the capability to recognize oneself emotions.

   b. **Using Emotions -** The potential to utilize emotional responses to make it easier for numerous psychological activities, including thinking and solving problems.
   c. **Understanding Emotions:** The potential to realize the meaning of feelings and recognize complex emotional relationships.
   d. **Managing Emotions:** The potential to monitor the emotions of everyone else's. The emotionally intelligent person can, therefore, use and control feelings, including bad ones, to accomplish desired goals.
2. **Bar-On: Emotional Intelligence Mixed Model:** Bar-On's emotional intelligence paradigm deals with success and achievement potential as opposed to accomplishment or achievement itself and is perceived to be process-oriented instead of results-oriented (Bar-On R, 2006). It accentuations on (1) a category of emotional skills, comprising the potential to be conscious of, understand and express oneself, and the potential to be conscious of, recognize and communicate with others, (2) The potential to cope with intense feelings and the adaptability to modify and address psychological or emotional problems. Bar-On referenced that through learning, programming, and counseling. Over time, emotional intelligence grows and that it can very well be enhanced.
3. **Goleman: Emotional Intelligence Mixed Model:** Goleman's design details the development of four major EIs (Daniel, 1995):
   a. **Self-Awareness:** The potential to read and acknowledge one's emotional responses when making use of gut feelings to direct decision making.
   b. **Self-Management:** To regulate one's emotional responses and desires and to adapt to the changing scenarios.
   c. **Social Awareness:** The ability to experience, Interpretation, and responding to other emotions through the understanding of social platforms.
   d. **Relationship Management:** The potential for promoting, motivating, and improving others in managing Conflict.
4. **Trait Model:** Konstantinos V. Petrides created the trait EI model. It "includes behavioral dispositions and self-perceived abilities and is measured through self-report." Trait EI is "a constellation of emotional self-perceptions located at the lower levels of personality (Petrides, 2010)." Inlay terms, trait Emotional Intelligence, applies to the self-perception of an individual's emotional capacity. An alternative name is the trait of emotional self-efficacy.

DIFFERENT SCALES FOR MEASURING EMOTIONAL INTELLIGENCE

While various scales, Essentially self-reporting models, have shown up in the previous years, we have chosen those tests that look encouraging to measure emotional intelligence, for example, have exhibited sensible psychometric properties and demonstrated valuable in both research and applied settings.

Mayer Salovey Caruso Emotional Intelligence Test (MSCEIT)

The most prominent measure of ability EI is the MSCEIT, although more recently, a variety of alternatives were established. MSCEIT is an EI capacity-based evaluation, taking into account how individuals accomplish things related to emotion, and solving emotional issues. It is focused on the four-pillar system of the researchers, including the capacity (1) to interpret emotions (in oneself, people, artifacts, crafts, music, etc.); (2) to produce & then utilize emotions to promote thinking; (3) to recognize emotional knowledge; and (4) to control emotions in self among others. The MSCEIT has 141 items in total and could be attempted in 30 to 45 minutes.

Situational Test of Emotional Understanding (STEU) and Situational Test of Emotional Management (STEM)

The STEU and STEM (Allen, V. D, 2014) are new methods of ability Emotional Intelligence. These models, as their tags, show, more explicitly evaluate emotional understanding & management, both of which are two of the Mayer's and Salovey's model's four EI dimensions. The STEU includes 42 questions with multiple choices, including 14 identified with particular situations, 14 identified with individual general life, and 14 identified with the working environment, through which a total score is inferred through calculation. The absolute scores are between 0 and 1. There have been 44 questions on the STEM, 18 focusing on the content of anger, 14 on sadness, and 12 aimed at the content of fear. The explanation for these two answer formats is to differentiate between the results of the checking and effects of designing.

Emotional Quotient Inventory (EQ-i)

Bar-On idealized EI as 'a collection of non-cognitive skills, knowledge, and talents that limit the ability of the person to adapt to psychological burdens and stresses in the community (Bar-On, R, 2000).' The EQ components are premised on the Bar-On EI model consisting of 15 specific elements falling into five conceptual groups: intrapersonal, interpersonal, stress management, adaptability, and General Mood. There are 133 questions measuring each of the dimensions of the model with 7-9 items. Everything is presented as a self-declaration, graded varying from 1 (very occasionally accurate or not valid for me) to 5 (very often true for me or false for me) on a 5-point Likert scale.

Trait Emotional Intelligence Questionnaire (TEIQue)

Trait Emotional Intelligence is characterized in the low levels of hierarchies as a cluster of personal self-perceptions of personality. The paradigm concerns the self-perceptions of individual people about their emotional capacities, which is why it was additionally named as a trait of emotional self-efficacy. As of now, in version 1.50, the TEIQue contains many constructs and has been translated and accepted in different dialects. The 15 dimensions were simplified to a combination of international EI traits, and four factors are emotionality, self-control, well-being, and sociability.

Wong and Law Emotional Intelligence Scale (WEIS)

Centered on the applicable model of Salovey and Mayer, WEIS represented EI as something of a four-dimensional structure, comprising Self Emotional Assessment (SEA), Regulation of Emotion (ROE), Other Emotional Assessment (OEA), and Use of Emotion (UOE). The Scale of Emotional Intelligence Wong and Law is a self-report test composed of 16 elements and answering on an answer scale of 7 point Likert-type (Wong, 2002). SEA, OEA, ROE, and UOE are used to evaluate. By summarizing the reactions to all 16 products, a general EI rating can be produced.

Schutte Self Report Emotional Intelligence Test (SSEIT)

The SSEIT is a technique for evaluating emotional intelligence that utilizes the perception of emotions, the use of emotions, manages self-relevant emotions, and control the emotions of others as its four sub-scales (Bailie K, 2005). The SSEIT is formed from the EI framework by Salovey and Mayer. The model is closely linked to the EQ-I framework of Emotional Intelligence.

Genos Emotional Intelligence Inventory

The EI of Genos (Gignac, 2010) is commonly expressed as 'the potential through using emotionally relevant processes to adapt, shape, and select environments purposely.' The test was designed to identify, select, and progress workers. Seventy questions are made from these seven domains Emotional Expression, Emotional Self-Awareness, Other people's Emotional Awareness, Emotional Reasoning, Emotional Self-Control, Other people's Emotional Management, and Emotional Self-Management. These questions evaluated over a five-point Likert scale varying from Seldom to Almost Always, which generates a Total EI score.

EMOTIONAL INTELLIGENCE IN EVERYDAY LIFE

Emotional Intelligence has a great influence on one's work life and career. When it comes to the fields such as conflict management, relationship building, and maintaining successful partnership, EI is the sword and shield. Emotional Intelligence benefits us in certain ways.

1. **Well-Being and Emotional Health:** Anxiety and depression are by far the most common problems that drive people to psychotherapy. Therefore, the abilities correlated with emotional intelligence must help individuals cope with unsettling emotions effectively and encourage pleasurable emotions to facilitate personal development and well-being. It leads to a greater understanding of health habits.
2. **Social Functioning:** Emotional intelligence is theorized to encourage better social functioning by helping people recognize emotional states of the others, incorporating viewpoints of others, improving communication, and controlling social behavior. Increasing emotional intelligence can increase levels of human comprehension and accessibility in every environment.
3. **Academic Achievement:** Emotional intelligence is speculated to help prioritize thinking and allow someone to handle emotions in situations that cause anxiety, such as standardized testing. Emotional intelligence is being associated with greater academic achievement. Research also found that EI is linked to academic and professional achievement, which leads to human cognitive-based output beyond the level of general knowledge.
4. **Performance in the Work Environment:** The emotional intelligence hypothesis affects the success of employees communicating with peers, Conflict or stress management techniques, and overall job efficiency. Great management requires emotional qualities and behavioral traits and thus Emotional Intelligence is important.

THE TRUTHS BEHIND SOCIAL MEDIA

Several factors contribute to emotional intelligence. The most crucial factor is the social network. The exponential rise of social media platforms such as facebook, Twitter, Snapchat, etc. certainly triggered several huge changes in how people communicate and engage with each other. It has become an enormous part of our lives. Social media is powerful. It's got the strength and depth of shaping and breaking people. It provides a convenient way to share or express daily lives on a global platform. From sharing to checking your likes or comments constantly, posting filtered photos to make them more appealing, sharing information, promoting business; chatting, etc. we are always on the go with social media.

Facebook, YouTube, Twitter, etc. are the most popular social media sites and have been enlisted, refer Table 1. Facebook is the most popular social media site for personal networking that allows users to create profiles, add other friends, exchange messages, post status updates, and share videos.

Table 1. List of some famous social network platforms

Facebook	A network formed of a large number of users who create personal profiles, add other users as friends, and share content. Subsequently, users can also join user groups of common interest, grouped by common features.
Twitter	Twitter is a microblogging service that enables its users to send and read publicly accessible messages. Tweets are text-based messages that appear on the user profile account.
Linkedin	A social networking forum used mainly for professional networking purposes. Users keep a list of contact details, called connections, of people they have relationships with. A list of contacts will also be used to create a network that serves various companies and to locate employment, individuals, and business opportunities.
YouTube	A streaming video website that enables users to upload, share, and view videos. A wide range of user-generated video content is also shown including movies and TV clips. Most videos allow users to exchange comments.
Wikipedia	A shared encyclopedic initiative focused on the web; Its 18 million articles were written collaboratively by users all over the world, and roughly all articles are openly editable by any user.

But social media also have some disadvantages too like it has become a safe haven for bullying and trolls. It reduces empathy and thoughtfulness and leads to more relationship problems. People typically lie on social media about their lives generating distorted Self-Image to appear more popular and successful.

The fascination with uploading and sharing has grown to the point that there has been a cause for concern. It influences how someone thinks and how someone feels. People need some kind of satisfaction from strangers. Because of this, people have many problems, such as depression and lower self-esteem. Anxiety and depression are by far the most common problems that drive people to psychotherapy. Many case studies and examples are available which shows that there exists some relationship between emotional intelligence and physical health.

Figure 1. Users using social media to gain likes

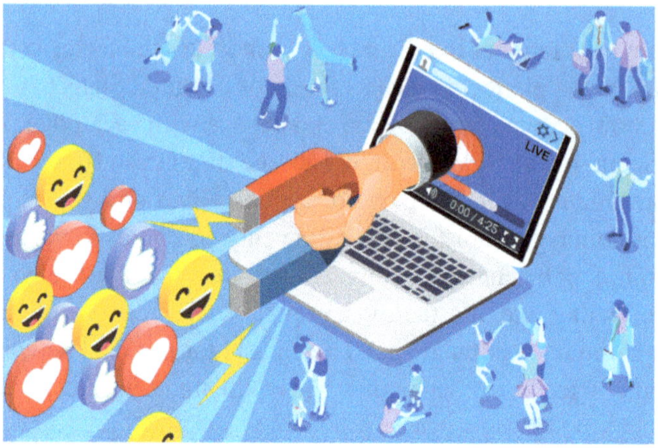

HEALTH CONCERNS ASSOCIATED WITH SOCIAL MEDIA

If someone is incapable of understanding, or controlling their feelings, they may also fail to develop close ties. This in turn will make them feel depressed and alone, exacerbating any mental health issues.

Now day's mental health problems such as depression, anxiety, panic attack are very much often seen in individuals. The main factor behind this is social pressure. People are trying so hard to cop up with social standards. Individuals need this kind of satisfaction from strangers. Even browsing makes people insecure about how they look and what's going on in their life. Envy and disappointment emotions are very prominent today, because of the beautiful bubble that social media has set up.

The urge to gain "likes" on social media can lead teenagers to take decisions that they'd never take, such as manipulating their image, participating in unhealthy behaviors, accepting dangerous social media competitions.

Though many teenagers know their peers are only sharing their big plays on digital networking, comparisons are very hard to resist. In social media everything from body appearance to working standards and alleged achievements and failures would be under a spotlight.

Excessive use of the social media often contributes to sleep deprivation. People check their social media last thing at night, first thing in the morning. That disrupts your sleep, which can seriously affect your mental health, too.

HOW SOCIAL MEDIA AFFECTS EMOTIONAL INTELLIGENCE AND HEALTH

There are several studies suggesting that emotional intelligence is compromised by social media and has also influenced wellbeing in some ways or other. The desire to look nice, to get more likes, views, comments, to demonstrate their ideal life has altered the user's viewpoint. This has also been seen that the modern society struggles from problems of depression and self-esteem induced by the Internet.

Facebook Depression

Facebook depression happens when users spend excessive time on social media sites, such as Facebook, Twitter, and start experiencing classic symptoms of depression. But it is specifically called Facebook depression because Facebook is the growing and most frequently used social network; it took its name from the trend in social media that triggered depression.

Figure 2. Facebook Depression

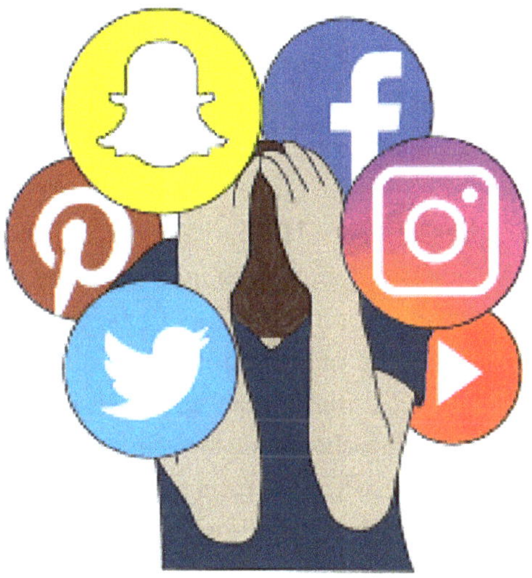

Kraut et al. conducted one of the first experiments in 1998 to demonstrate that internet use dramatically impacts intimate interactions and group life engagement. The authors found in this study that increased time spent online is correlated with a decrease in contact with family members that can also lead to a greater sense of depressive moods and suicidal thoughts.

In 2013 Kross released a study on the connection regarding use of Facebook and psychological well-being among adolescents. The research strategy concentrated on the participants' text messages for 2 weeks five days a day to assess their temperament, feelings of depression, social experiences, and social media use. The findings have shown that users can compromise the subjective sense of wellbeing and happiness with life. Needless to say, any such downturn will increase the symptoms and signs of depression.

One part of social life is to find recognition and continue to stay linked with peer groups. Additionally, the stress of the virtual environment, which constantly needs engagement, tends to create an aspect of self-awareness that can cause significant emotional and psychological distress. Individuals with emotional problem are at danger of victimization or often migrate to dangerous sites that encourage substance addiction, unhealthy sexual, violent behavior. Social media is becoming the go-to medium for all these regular conversations, allowing for the constant revival of the debates about these people's "problems," causing them to become obsessed with the "problem," and keeping them from moving forward in life. Such "problems" are typically minor concerns for the most part, or even being aware about demeanor; wondering regarding social approval, or contemplating whether affection is being reciprocated.

Social Network and Self Esteem

Some scholars describe the word "self-esteem" as "the aspect of the self-assessment-the degree to which one appreciates values, endorses, or likes oneself." Numerous mental conditions are associated with poor self-esteem, including depression, eating disorders, and addiction. One plausible justification for Facebook's pessimistic self-esteem connection is out across all social networking platforms where self-portrayal is the primary source across user engagement, and promotes narcissistic behavior. A study by Mehdizadeh identified results in which 100 York University Facebook users demonstrated a conscience-esteemed, self-reporting personality disorder. The studies have found that people with poorer self-esteem are more involved digitally when it comes to having more self-promotional posts on their social media site. These are all factors that can affect self-esteem positively or negatively.

Social Media Addiction

The psychological literature also addresses several findings pertaining to internet and social media addiction. Social media's addictive existence is demonstrated by the mental distress of frequent social media users who then tend to ignore other facets of their social life. For several papers, online social networking has so far been addressed as a possible issue of addiction. The Facebook Addiction Scale was created in 2012 by Andreassen, a rating scale that initially focused on 18 items, measuring compulsion symptoms as heterogeneity, behavioral disorder, forbearance, conflict, and recurrence. The authors tested the measure on a group of 423 students, along with other questionnaires. The analysis demonstrated fairly high reliability, and was reasonable to the student community.

Catfishing Through Social Media

As people spend so much time on social media networks they start withdrawing from their real-life connections. Due to this, as more of our attention and energy is poured into the theory of digital network, many important relationships with our relatives crumbled. Catfish a series based on a documentary film, Is a clear illustration to show the illusory side of social media connections. Using a false or stolen identity, "catfishing" is the process of online friendship with strangers. It is an intangible gesture that has wrecked other people's lives, marriages.

FOMO Effect

FOMO (Fear of Missing Out) is essentially heightened and persistent fear or discomfort of missing out on social activities or interactions perceived by others. Sadly, FOMO leads to a compulsive need to remain online linked to the lives of others. We become addicted to Facebook, Twitter, Instagram, etc. to an extent that it is all-important and all-consuming to check what others are doing or how they respond to our posts.

Table 2. The sample Population profiles (No of users are 444)

Item	Characteristics	Frequency	Ratio
Gender	Male	110	25%
	Female	334	75%
Daily Social media use time	Less than 2 h	51	17%
	2 – 4 h	223	50%
	More than 4 h	146	33%
Most popular social media platforms	WhatsApp	387	87%
	Instagram	342	77%
	YouTube	237	53%
	Twitter	103	23%
	Facebook	85	19%
	Google+	77	17%
	Snapchat	36	8%

STUDY WAS CONCEPTUALIZED SHOWING HOW SOCIAL MEDIA IMPACTS EMOTIONAL INTELLIGENCE

Study 1: Irfan Sural et al. (2019) presented that trait emotional intelligence is specifically correlated with the use of problematic social media and indirectly associated with motivations to show a successful side and pass time, to verify refer Table 3. A sample of 444 individuals aged ranged from 18 to 43 years having an active digital account was taken. The statistical analysis was done with the program SPSS 23, AMOS 23, and for route analysis, the maximum probability calculation was used. Table 2 shows the categorization of sample population profiles according to their gender, how much time they spend on social media and what are their most favorite social media platforms.

Table 3. TEI association with PSMU

Classification	Effect	Standardized Error	Total Effect (%)
Trait Emotional Intelligence è Problematic Social Media Use (total effect)	-.46***	.04	–
Trait Emotional Intelligence è Problematic Social Media Use (direct effect)	-.39***	.04	85
Trait Emotional Intelligence è Problematic Social Media Use (total indirect effect)	-.07**	.02	15
Trait Emotional Intelligence è Most Popular Self è Problematic Social Media Use (indirect effect)	-.03**	.01	6
Trait Emotional Intelligence è Pass Time è Problematic Social Media Use (indirect effect)	-.02**	.01	4

$^{**}p < .01$; $^{***}p < .001$

The proposed model was evaluated using path analysis. Results showed that the TEI was directly correlated with Problematic Social Media Use ($\beta = -0.39$, $p < 0{,}001$; 95%) and indirectly ($\beta = -0.07$, $p < 0.01$; 95%) through social media uses motives to communicate or portray a famous self and to pass time.

Study 2: A research conducted by Inwon Kang (2019), based on the FOMO as a method of understanding consumer compliance intake. The author finds that of the 187 people surveyed who completed the questionnaires, men with 52.4% was marginally greater than women with 47.6%. The participants below twenty recorded the maximum proportion of 66 persons with 35.3%, preceded by others in their twenties with 27.8% and thirties with 21.4%, and much more than forties with 15.5%. Refer Table 4.

Table 4. Specified test characteristics (No. of users are 187)

Item	Characteristics	Occurrence	Ratio (%)
Gender	Men	98	52.4
	women	89	47.6
Age	Below 20	66	35.3
	20-30	52	27.8
	30-40	40	21.4
	Above 40	29	15.4
Occupancy	Scholars	55	29.4
	Private workers	63	33.7
	Public workers	29	15.5
	Homemakers	15	8.0
	Freelancer	20	10.7
	Other	5	2.7

Study 3: Rajita Panditharadhyula et al. (2018) identified the effect of movies and social media on patterns of emotional intelligence over a random sample of 131 students (63 male and 68 female) ages between 16 – 18 years. Mangal Emotional Inventory tool was used to collect data in small groups. T-test, f- test, and univariate analysis was conducted on the obtained data leads to the results that biographical factors like gender, family type of the individual have a significant influence on the emotional intelligence and Facebook and Instagram have a higher influence on interpersonal management. The findings also show that individuals who do not use Facebook have higher intrapersonal awareness and interpersonal management of emotional intelligence than individuals who use Facebook, Refer Table 5.

Table 5. Individuals who use Facebook and who does not (N=131)

Domain of EI	Facebook	N	Mean	S.D.	T
Intra Personal Awareness	Don't use	61	16.3443	3.19314	2.116
	Use	70	15.1143	3.42431	
Inter-Personal Management	Don't use	61	16.4426	2.96943	1.933
	Use	70	15.4571	2.85741	

RELATIONSHIP BETWEEN EMOTIONAL INTELLIGENCE AND THE ELEMENTS OF PHYSICAL AND MENTAL WELLBEING

Many studies have been examined which proves the relationship between emotional intelligence and elements of physical and mental wellbeing. Martins et al. (2010) in his paper "A comprehensive meta-analysis of the relationship between Emotional Intelligence and health." suggests that high emotional intelligence is tied to enhance long-term health.

Freudenthaler et al. (2008) reported a negative relation of psychological symptoms with wellbeing, self-control, and sociability dimensions. Even though Mikolajczak et al. highlighted the positive association between general wellbeing and the four dimensions of the EI. Tsaousis and Nikolaou have evaluated the link between EI and lifestyle habits, reported a negative interaction with overall EI and smoking and alcohol, and reported a positive relationship with exercise.

The TMMS was applied by Limonero to demonstrate the connection among EI and university students' consumption of cigarettes and cannabis; found that Students who consumed tobacco were likely to have begun cigarettes or cannabis at a younger age and presented lower levels of the Repair dimension.

A study done by Enrique g. fernández-abascal (2015) investigated that the EI measurements are adequate to describe multiple health aspects and specific types of health patterns. A survey had been taken of 855 people, who completed two measures of EI as a measure of health patterns. The researcher concluded that analyzed aspects of EI are significant predictor of mental wellness (48.4%) than of physical wellness which is 15.6%. The information gleaned has important results to be able to outline the most strongly associated basic measurements of the EI. The aspects of the EI that strongly describe the element of physical health are the TEIQue's well-being, self-control, and sociability. Results revealed that nearly all of the measurements of the EI measured are positively linked to components of general wellbeing, except for attention that has a destructive connection.

Researchers also found that Gender acts as a wellness indicator, that man possessing greater standards than women in both the mental wellness component and the physical wellness dimension. While Age indicates less medical risk habits, as older people practice better prevention behaviors.

Also, according to the research done by Audrone Dumciene et al. (2018) the gender interaction has been studied as a possible measure of mental wellbeing and possible balance of emotional intelligence and wellness sustainability. That analysis comprised of samples of 1214 students among which 597 male and 617 female students were taken.

The study found that the average all measures of emotional intelligence had a strong and optimistic correlation with the aspects of the health, except for the aspects of motivation and appraisal; this had significant but adverse associations with risk taking of the drug.

CONCLUSION

This chapter examined the Incautious Usage of Social Media and its Impact on Emotional Intelligence and Health. This chapter gives a brief introduction to the emotional intelligence and the conceptualization and evaluation of this construct in detail describing how emotions can affect an individual's perspective. A variety of case studies has been discussed in this chapter shed light on social media, emotional intelligence, and healthy relationships. It serves a social role to be in tune with feelings, linking users to society around them. Emotional intelligence helps the individual to identify enemy mates, to assess the desire of another person in them, to regulate their nervous system, and to feel safe and happy. The chapter also discussed how the abilities correlate with emotional intelligence and help individuals cope with unsettling emotions effectively and encourage pleasurable emotions to facilitate personal development and well-being. Our research, therefore, leads to a greater understanding of health habits.

This research received no specific grant from any funding agency in the public, commercial, or not-for-profit sectors.

REFERENCES

AbdelKader, W., & Elnakeeb, M. (2017). The relationship between the use of media and emotional intelligence among youth nursing students. *Journal of Nursing and Health Science*, *6*(5), 63–77.

Alabi, O. F. (2013). A survey of Facebook addiction level among selected Nigerian university undergraduates. *New Media and Mass Communication, 10*, 70–80.

Allen, V. D., Weissman, A., Hellwig, S., MacCann, C., & Roberts, R. D. (2014). Development of the situational test of emotional understanding–brief (STEU-B) using item response theory. *Personality and Individual Differences*, *65*, 3–7. doi:10.1016/j.paid.2014.01.051

Bailie, K. (2005). *An exploration of the utility of a self-report emotional intelligence measure* (Doctoral dissertation). Stellenbosch: University of Stellenbosch.

Bar-On, R. (2006). The Bar-On model of emotional-social intelligence (ESI). *Psicothema*, *18*, 13–25. PMID:17295953

Bar-On, R., & Parker, J. D. A. (2000). *BarOn emotional quotient inventory: Youth version*. Multi-Health System, Incorporated.

Colman, A. M. (2015). *A dictionary of psychology*. Oxford Quick Reference.

Fernández-Abascal, E. G., & Martín-Díaz, M. D. (2015). Dimensions of emotional intelligence related to physical and mental health and to health behaviors. *Frontiers in Psychology*, *6*, 317. doi:10.3389/fpsyg.2015.00317 PMID:25859229

Freudenthaler, H. H., Neubauer, A. C., Gabler, P., Scherl, W. G., & Rindermann, H. (2008). Testing and validating the trait emotional intelligence questionnaire (TEIQue) in a German-speaking sample. *Personality and Individual Differences*, *45*(7), 673–678. doi:10.1016/j.paid.2008.07.014

García-Sancho, E., Salguero, J. M., & Fernández-Berrocal, P. (2014). Relationship between emotional intelligence and aggression: A systematic review. *Aggression and Violent Behavior*, *19*(5), 584–591. doi:10.1016/j.avb.2014.07.007

Gignac, G. E. (2010). Genos Emotional Intelligence Inventory. Technical Manual (2nd ed.). Sydney: Academic Press.

Goleman. (1995). *Emotional Intelligence: Why It Can Matter More Than IQ*. Bantam Books. https://en.wikipedia.org/wiki/David_Wechsler

GradesFixer. (2019). *A literature review of Emotional Intelligence*. Author.

Gugliandolo, M. C., Costa, S., Cuzzocrea, F., Larcan, R., & Petrides, K. V. (2015). Trait emotional intelligence and behavioral problems among adolescents: A cross-informant design. *Personality and Individual Differences*, *74*, 16–21. doi:10.1016/j.paid.2014.09.032

Hawi, N. S., & Samaha, M. (2017). The relations among social media addiction, self-esteem, and life satisfaction in university students. *Social Science Computer Review*, *35*(5), 576–586. doi:10.1177/0894439316660340

Howard Gardner. (n.d.). https://en.wikipedia.org/wiki/Howard_Gardner

Kang, I., Cui, H., & Son, J. (2019). Conformity consumption behavior and FoMO. *Sustainability*, *11*(17), 4734. doi:10.3390u11174734

Kuss, D. J., & Griffiths, M. D. (2017). Social networking sites and addiction: Ten lessons learned. *International Journal of Environmental Research and Public Health*, *14*(3), 311. doi:10.3390/ijerph14030311 PMID:28304359

Limonero, J. T., Tomás-Sábado, J., & Fernández-Castro, J. (2006). Perceived emotional intelligence and its relation to tobacco and cannabis use among university students. *Psicothema*, *18*, 95–100. PMID:17295964

Malinauskas, R., Dumciene, A., Sipaviciene, S., & Malinauskiene, V. (2018). *Relationship between emotional intelligence and health behaviours among university students: The predictive and moderating role of gender.* Academic Press.

Martins, A., Ramalho, N., & Morin, E. (2010). A comprehensive meta-analysis of the relationship between emotional intelligence and health. *Personality and Individual Differences*, *49*(6), 554–564. doi:10.1016/j.paid.2010.05.029

Mayer, J. D., & Salovey, P. (1993). *The intelligence of emotional intelligence.* Academic Press.

Mikolajczak, M., Luminet, O., & Menil, C. (2006). Predicting resistance to stress: Incremental validity of trait emotional intelligence over alexithymia and optimism. *Psicothema*, *18*, 79–88. PMID:17295962

Panditharadhyula, R., & Kumar, P. (2018). Impact of Biographical Variables and Social Networking Platforms on Emotional Intelligence among Adolescents. *International Journal of Scientific Research (Ahmedabad, India)*, *7*(5), 1320–1326.

Petrides, K. V. (2010). Trait emotional intelligence theory. *Industrial and Organizational Psychology: Perspectives on Science and Practice*, *3*(2), 136–139. doi:10.1111/j.1754-9434.2010.01213.x

Petrides, K. V. (2011). *Ability and trait emotional intelligence.* Academic Press.

Ryan, T., Chester, A., Reece, J., & Xenos, S. (2014). The uses and abuses of Facebook: A review of Facebook addiction. *Journal of Behavioral Addictions, 3*(3), 133–148. doi:10.1556/JBA.3.2014.016 PMID:25317337

Salovey, P., Mayer, J., & Caruso, D. (2004). Emotional intelligence: Theory, findings, and implications. *Psychological Inquiry, 15*(3), 197–215. doi:10.120715327965pli1503_02

Satici, S. A. (2018). Facebook addiction and subjective well-being: A study of the mediating role of shyness and loneliness. *International Journal of Mental Health and Addiction.*

Schutte, N. S., & Malouff, J. M. (2011). Emotional intelligence mediates the relationship between mindfulness and subjective well-being. *Personality and Individual Differences, 50*(7), 1116–1119. doi:10.1016/j.paid.2011.01.037

Shensa, A., Escobar-Viera, C. G., Sidani, J. E., Bowman, N. D., Marshal, M. P., & Primack, B. A. (2017). Problematic social media use and depressive symptoms among US young adults: A nationally-representative study. *Social Science & Medicine, 182*, 150–157. doi:10.1016/j.socscimed.2017.03.061 PMID:28446367

Sternberg, R. J. (Ed.). (2000). *Handbook of intelligence.* Cambridge University Press. doi:10.1017/CBO9780511807947

Süral, I., Griffiths, M. D., Kircaburun, K., & Emirtekin, E. (2019). Trait Emotional Intelligence and Problematic Social Media Use Among Adults: The Mediating Role of Social Media Use Motives. *International Journal of Mental Health and Addiction, 17*(2), 336–345. doi:10.100711469-018-0022-6

ThorndikeE. L. (n.d.). https://en.wikipedia.org/wiki/E._L._Thorndike

Tsaousis, I., & Nikolaou, I. (2005). Exploring the relationship of emotional intelligence with physical and psychological health functioning. *Stress and Health, 21*(2), 77–86. doi:10.1002mi.1042

Whaite, E. O., Shensa, A., Sidani, J. E., Colditz, J. B., & Primack, B. A. (2018). Social media use, personality characteristics, and social isolation among young adults in the United States. *Personality and Individual Differences, 124*, 45–50. doi:10.1016/j.paid.2017.10.030

Wong, C. S., & Law, K. S. (2002). The effects of leader and follower emotional intelligence on performance and attitude: An exploratory study. *The Leadership Quarterly, 13*(3), 243–274. doi:10.1016/S1048-9843(02)00099-1

Chapter 9
Epileptic Seizure Detection Using Machine Learning Techniques

Can Eyupoglu
https://orcid.org/0000-0002-6133-8617
Air Force Academy, National Defence University, Turkey

ABSTRACT

Epilepsy is a brain disorder that can be defined as a short-time and temporary occurrence of symptoms because of abnormal extreme or synchronous neuronal activity of the brain. Almost one percent of the world's population is struggling with epilepsy illness. The detection of epileptic seizures is mainly realized with reading the electroencephalogram (EEG) recordings by medical doctors due to the unpredictable and complex nature of the disease. This process takes much time and depends on the expert's experience. For this reason, automatic seizure detection using EEG recordings is necessary and of great importance for the comfort of medical doctors and patients. While detecting epileptic seizure automatically, machine learning techniques are used in the field of computer science. This chapter deals with the methods, approaches, models, and techniques which are utilized to detect epileptic seizures.

INTRODUCTION

There are various definitions for epilepsy and epileptic seizure in the literature. The International League Against Epilepsy (ILAE) and the International Bureau for Epilepsy (IBE) took a joint decision on the descriptions of epilepsy and epileptic seizure. In the sequel, they described these terms as "*a disorder of the brain characterized by an enduring predisposition to generate epileptic seizures and by the neurobiologic, cognitive, psychological, and social consequences of this condition*" for epilepsy and "*a transient occurrence of signs and/or symptoms due to abnormal excessive or synchronous neuronal activity in the brain*" for epileptic seizure. Besides, at least one epileptic seizure must occur to describe epilepsy (Fisher et al., 2005).

DOI: 10.4018/978-1-7998-6527-8.ch009

All over the world, epilepsy is one of the most widespread neurological illnesses and many people of different races, geographical areas, and ages suffer from this disease. Globally, almost 50 million people have epilepsy disease and approximately 80% of them live in low- and middle-income countries (WHO, 2019; WHO, 2020). As seen from Figure 1 indicating worldwide idiopathic epilepsy age-standardized prevalence per one hundred thousand population among males and females in 2016, idiopathic epilepsy is the most common in southern, western, and eastern sub-Saharan Africa, Andean and central Latin America, and central and southeast Asia (Feigin et al., 2019; WHO, 2019).

Figure 1. Worldwide idiopathic epilepsy prevalence per one hundred thousand population in 2016 *(Feigin et al., 2019; WHO, 2019)*

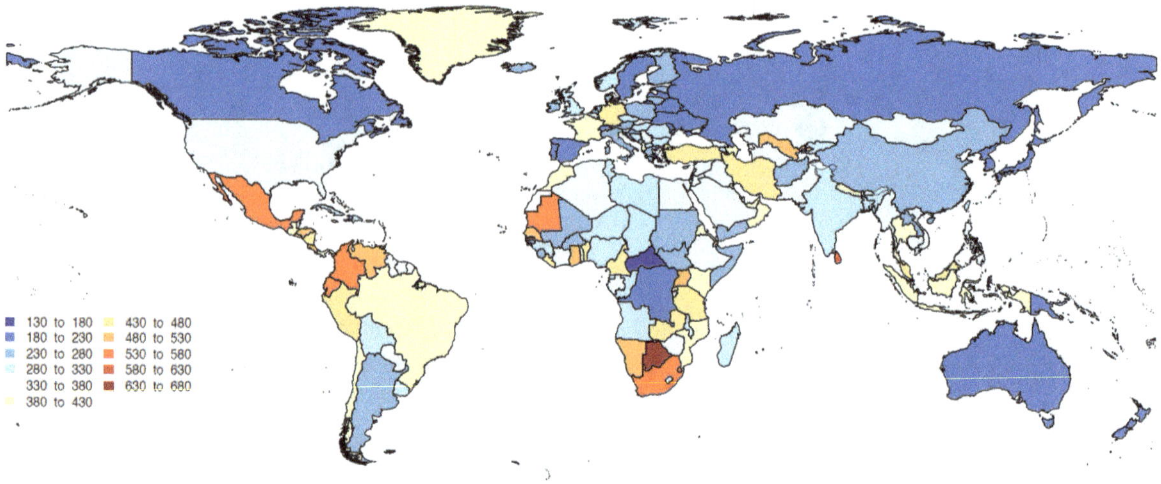

Timely diagnosis of the occurrence of epileptic seizures is one of the basic difficulties. The epileptic seizure detection process is fundamentally carried out by medical doctors with reading the electroencephalogram (EEG) recordings because of the unpredictable and complex nature of the illness, taking much time and depending on the experts' practice. Consequently, automated seizure detection using EEG signals is required and crucial for the comfort of medical specialists and patients (Yavuz, Kasapbaşı, Eyüpoğlu, & Yazıcı, 2018). Machine learning (ML) techniques are utilized while detecting epileptic seizure automatically. This chapter describes how ML methods are utilized to detect epileptic seizures and investigates the existing studies in the literature. Furthermore, the basic aim and contribution of this chapter are to inform the researchers who will work in this area.

The rest of the chapter is organized as follows. The second section expresses how epileptic seizures are detected and how epilepsy disease is diagnosed. In the third section, existing ML techniques utilized for epileptic seizure detection are investigated. Finally, the fourth section concludes the chapter.

DETECTING EPILEPTIC SEIZURES AND DIAGNOSING EPILEPSY

Epilepsy disease is described with repetitive seizures that are short episodes resulted from extreme electrical discharges in some brain cells. Various sections of the brain may become the place of these discharges. Moreover, frequency of seizures ranges from less than one per year to several per day. As a result of these seizures, different types of nonpermanent symptoms may occur, such as loss of the senses of hearing, sight and taste, and defects of movement, consciousness or other cognitive functions. Patients with epilepsy suffer from physical problems including injuries and fractures related to epileptic seizures, and psychological consequences regarding depression and anxiety (WHO, 2020).

In order to early detect the disease and manage a variety of etiologies, it is vital to analyze the causes of epilepsy. The causes of epilepsy disease are split into six types which are genetic, structural, immune, infectious, metabolic and unknown, as demonstrated in Table 1 (Scheffer et al., 2017; WHO, 2019).

Table 1. Causes of epilepsy disease

Causes	Description
Genetic	An assumed or common genetic mutation that epileptic seizures are major symptoms of defect.
Structural	Genetic abnormalities such as malformation in development of the cerebral cortex or the abnormalities that might be seen via structural neuroimaging, such as trauma, infection and stroke.
Immune	An immune problem that epileptic seizures are major symptoms and influences multiple organ systems.
Infectious	A common infection in which epileptic seizures are a basic symptom, such as tuberculosis, meningitis, cerebral malaria, HIV, encephalitis, neurocysticercosis and congenital infections like Zika virus.
Metabolic	An assumed or common metabolic problem in which epileptic seizures are a main symptom, such as uraemia, porphyria and pyridoxine-dependent seizures.
Unknown	The cause of the disease is unknown.

In the diagnosis process of this disease, a detailed analysis for the scalp EEG signals is required. EEG is an electrophysiological monitoring procedure in order to record brain electrical activities. Electrodes are placed all over the scalp during EEG recording process (Niedermeyer & da Silva, 2005). This process including electrodes and EEG signals is demonstrated in Figure 2. EEG is also utilized to make diagnosis of other neurological diseases such as stroke, brain damage, head injury, dementia, brain tumor, sleep disorder and brain inflammation (Siuly, Li, & Zhang, 2016). EEG signals being nonstationary and low frequency carry too much information regarding brain electrical activities and heavy computing load is necessary for processing them. Medical professionals visually examine EEG signal recordings for the diagnosis of epilepsy. Therefore, real-time processing is very difficult to perform (Yavuz et al., 2018).

Figure 2. EEG recording process
(Siuly, Li, & Zhang, 2016)

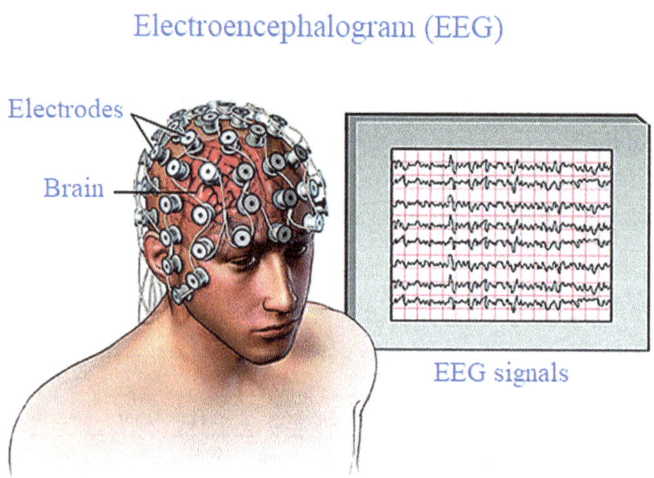

For preventing the possibilities of any missing signs about the disease, developing automatic epileptic seizure detection systems is very important. Thanks to these systems, timely diagnosis of epilepsy can be realized, and the treatment process of the patients can be started quickly. Extracting features from EEG recordings is the most significant part for epileptic seizure detection systems. For this reason, developing and implementing appropriate feature extraction technique for characterizing EEG signals and extracting the most beneficial information from these signals are the main challenge (Yavuz et al., 2018).

MACHINE LEARNING TECHNIQUES FOR EPILEPTIC SEIZURE DETECTION

Many studies have been done on epileptic seizure detection up to now. Various models, techniques and systems have been proposed to detect epileptic seizures. Most of these studies have used a public and well-recognized EEG time series data set comprising of 500 EEG recording samples (Andrzejak et al., 2001; University of Bonn Department of Epileptology, 2001). To explain the data set in more detail, it contains 5 sets which are symbolized as Z, O, N, F and S, each including 100 single channel segments. Besides, the duration of these segments is 23.6 seconds. Figure 3 shows some EEG instances for each set.

This section investigates and summarizes the studies using this data set. In the work of Srinivasan, Eswaran, and Sriraam (2007), an epileptic EEG identification approach depended on approximate entropy (ApEn) and artificial neural network (ANN) was presented. ApEn was used to extract features from the EEG recordings. Afterwards, probabilistic neural networks (PNN) and Elman network (EN) were utilized to detect epilepsy disease. The classification accuracy of 100% was acquired by means of the system.

Subasi (2007) proposed a mixture of expert systems (ME) model for detecting epileptic seizures. On account of decomposing the EEG recordings to the frequency sub-bands, discrete wavelet transform (DWT) was utilized and the extracted sub-band frequencies were utilized to feed the ME having two output which are epileptic and normal. Subsequently, expectation–maximization (EM) technique was applied to the model for efficient training. The proposed model obtained the accuracy of 94.5%.

In the study presented by Tzallas, Tsipouras, and Fotiadis (2007), principal component analysis (PCA), time-frequency analysis (TFA) and feed-forward neural network (FFNN) were used to detect seizures automatically. First, to compute the spectrum of the EEG signals, TFA was used and this spectrum was utilized for feature extraction. After feature extraction phase, PCA was applied to decrease the dimension of the features which are the input for FFNN. The best accuracy of the presented method was 100%.

In another study, Polat and Güneş (2007) proposed a two-stage hybrid system on the strength of decision tree (DT) for classification and fast Fourier transform (FFT) for feature extraction. FFT was applied to the EEG signals for the aim of feature extraction. Subsequently, the obtained features were employed qua an input for DT classifier. Finally, the proposed system classified the EEGs as normal or epileptic with the accuracy of 98.72%.

In the work of Bao, Lie, and Zhang (2008), an automatic epileptic identification system depending on various feature extraction parameters and PNN was introduced for helping medical doctors. FFT, relative intensity ratio (RIR), power spectral intensity (PSI), Higuchi fractal dimension (HFD), Petrosian fractal dimension (PFD), Hjorth parameters (HP), means and standard deviations were evaluated in the feature extraction step. 38 EEG features were extracted utilizing these calculations and the extracted features were used to feed PNN after normalization process. The overall classification accuracy of 99.5% was attained by the system.

Figure 3. EEG instances for each set
(Yavuz et al., 2018)

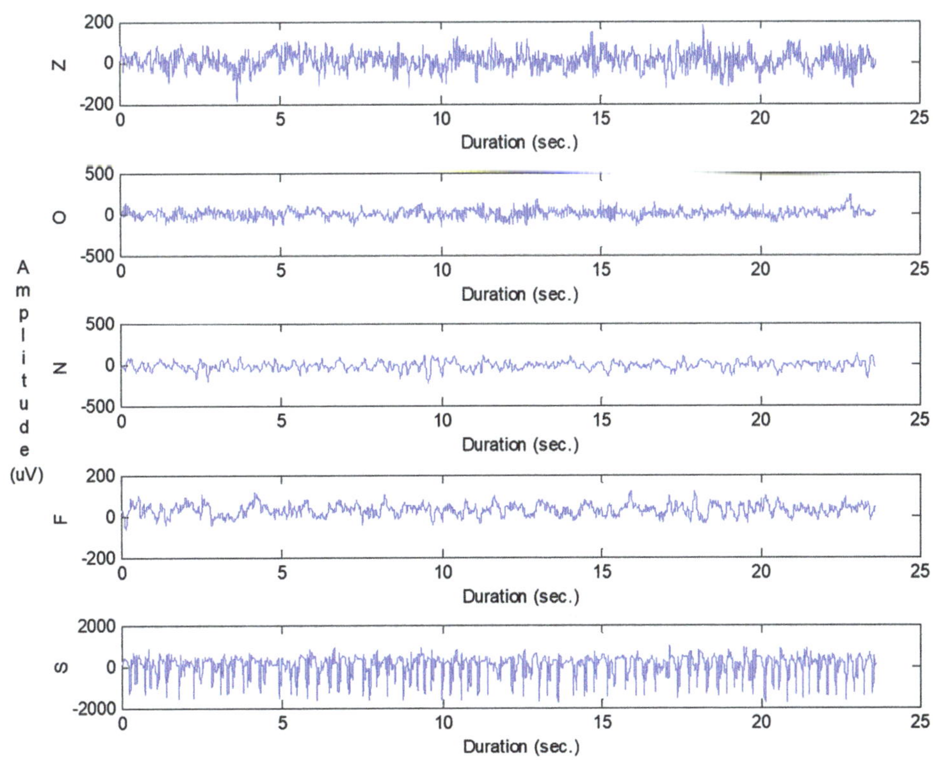

Ocak (2009) presented an automatic epileptic diagnosis scheme comprising of two phases. Fistly, ApEn was utilized for extracting features from the EEG signals and later DWT was applied to decompose the signals into frequency sub-bands as the second phase. The classification success of the presented scheme was 96%. In the same year, Chandaka, Chatterjee, and Munshi (2009) acquired the accuracy of 95.96% employing support vector machine (SVM) for classification and cross-correlation (CC) measure for feature extraction.

In the work of Guo, Rivero, Dorado, Rabunal, and Pazos (2010), multi-layer perceptron neural network (MLPNN) and DWT were utilized together to detect epileptic seizures. First, the decomposition of EEGs was performed with employing DWT. In the sequel, line length features were computed using every sub-band and a feature vector was created to feed MLPNN. In order to train MLPNN, Bayesian regularization back-propagation technique was chosen. Consequently, the proposed method classified the EEG signals into healthy or epileptic with the accuracy of 99.6%.

Murugavel and Ramakrishnan (2011) introduced an epileptic seizure identification approach exploiting ApEn, DWT and PNN. In the data transformation phase, DWT was applied to decompose the EEGs. Afterwards, ApEn was employed for the aim of feature extraction and sixty ApEn features were attained. Among these features, the best thirty features were chosen for faster processing. Lastly, the selected features were used to feed PNN. The accuracy rate of 100% was acquired with employing the method.

In the same year, Orhan, Hekim, and Ozer (2011) introduced an epileptic seizure classification model using DWT, *K*-means clustering algorithm and MLPNN. The proposed model obtained the best classification accuracy of 100%.

In the study presented by Song, Crowcroft, and Zhang (2012), a classification method based on extreme learning machine (ELM) and optimized sample entropy (O-SampEn) was proposed to designate epileptic seizures automatically. After feature extraction with O-SampEn, ELM was utilized for classifying the EEGs concerning the existence of epileptic or healthy. The accuracy of the presented method was 97.5%. In another study of the same year, Nicolaou and Georgiou (2012) introduced an epileptic seizure classification method utilizing SVM and permutation entropy (PE). The classification accuracy of the system was 93.55%.

Dehuri, Jagadev, and Cho (2013) proposed an ensemble approach for identification of epileptic seizures, which is based upon DWT and differential evolution-radial basis function neural networks (DE-RBFN). The proposed method utilized DWT for decomposing the EEGs to several sub-bands. After, the extracted features were utilized to feed the ensemble of DE-RBFN. The identification success of the presented ensemble method was as high as 100%. In the work of Zainuddin, Huong, and Pauline (2013), a seizure detection system employing DWT, type-2 fuzzy C-means (T2FCM) clustering and wavelet neural network (WNN) was presented and the system achieved the classification accuracy of 98.87%.

In another study conducted in 2014 (Kaya, Uyar, Tekin, & Yıldırım, 2014), a two-stage classification technique depending on one-dimensional local binary pattern (1D-LBP) and five classifiers was offered on behalf of classifying the EEG signals as epileptic or healthy. After feature extraction stage with 1D-LBP, various classifiers which are logistic regression (LR), functional tree (FT), BayesNet, SVM and ANN were applied to the extracted features. The best classification accuracy of 99.5% was attained with BayesNet.

In the study of Kumar, Dewal, and Anand (2014), three techniques, FFNN for classification, ApEn for feature extraction and DWT for EEG preprocessing, were used together to detect epileptic seizures. The proposed scheme achieved the classification accuracy of 100%. Das, Bhuiyan, and Alam (2014) presented a statistical approach using SVM, ANN and dual-tree complex wavelet transform (DT-CWT). The accuracy of the approach was 100%.

Kang, Chung, and Kim (2015) employed HP, FFT, autoregressive (AR) model, quadratic discriminant analysis (QDA) and MLPNN for effective epileptic seizure detection. The accuracy rate of the method was 99.78%. In the study of Sharma and Pachori (2015), an epileptic seizure identification method exploiting phase space representation (PSR), empirical mode decomposition (EMD), least squares support vector machine (LS-SVM) and intrinsic mode functions (IMF) was introduced and the method obtained the accuracy of 98.67%.

In the work by Tiwari, Pachori, Kanhangad, and Panigrahi (2016), an epilepsy diagnosis method depended on SVM and local binary pattern (LBP) was proposed. The accuracy rate of 99.31% was achieved. Tawfik, Youssef, and Kholief (2016) used weighted permutation entropy (WPE) and SVM together and then attained the classification accuracy of 93.75%.

In the study of Hassan, Siuly, and Zhang (2016), using bootstrap aggregating (bagging) and tunable-Q factor wavelet transform (TQWT), epileptic seizure classification was carried out. The accuracy of 100% was obtained by the presented method. In the same year, Bhardwaj, Tiwari, Krishna, and Varma (2016) employed utilized constructive genetic programming (CGP) and EMD. The best accuracy of 100% was acquired. In the work introduced by Das, Bhuiyan, and Alam (2016), DT-CWT and SVM were used and the accuracy rate of 100% was achieved.

In 2017, Mursalin, Zhang, Chen, and Chawla (2017) introduced an epileptic seizure classification technique utilizing DWT, random forest (RF) and improved correlation-based feature selection (ICFS). The technique obtained 100% detection success. In the work performed by Li, Chen, and Zhang (2017), an epilepsy diagnosis method was presented using neural network ensemble (NNE) and DWT-based envelope analysis (EA). The presented method attained the classification accuracy of 98.78%.

Satapathy, Dehuri, and Jagadev (2017) utilized artificial bee colony (ABC) algorithm, DWT and RBFN to determine epileptic seizures. The classification success of the study was 98.5%. In another study carried out in the same year (Jaiswal & Banka, 2017), two feature extraction methods, namely local neighbor descriptive pattern (LNDP) and one-dimensional local gradient pattern (1D-LGP), were proposed and the EEG signals were classified using nearest neighbor (NN), DT, ANN and SVM. This study achieved the accuracy of 99.82%.

Sharma, Pachori, and Acharya (2017) used analytic time-frequency flexible wavelet transform (ATF-FWT), HFD, and LS-SVM in order to identify epileptic seizures. According to experimental results, the proposed scheme obtained the accuracy of 100%.

In the work realized by Acharya, Oh, Hagiwara, Tan, and Adeli (2018), to automatically designate epileptic seizures, a computer-aided diagnosis (CAD) system exploiting deep convolutional neural network (CNN) with 13-layer was proposed. The proposed system attained the accuracy of 88.7%. In the same year, Ullah, Hussain, and Aboalsamh (2018) used a different type of CNN for diagnosis of epilepsy, namely pyramidal one-dimensional convolutional neural network (P-1D-CNN) and achieved the classification success of 100%.

In the study of Jaiswal and Banka (2018), 2 feature extraction methods which are one-dimensional local ternary pattern (1D-LTP) and local centroid pattern (LCP) were developed and various ML methods which are ANN, NN, DT and SVM were applied for classification. The best accuracy of 100% was obtained utilizing ANN.

Yavuz et al. (2018) proposed a system exploiting generalized regression neural network (GRNN) and cepstral analysis (CA) for diagnosis of epilepsy. The accuracy of the system was 99.6%. Siuly, Alcin,

Bajaj, Sengur, and Zhang (2018) presented an epileptic seizure identification approach based on LS-SVM and Hermite transform and achieved the accuracy of 99.67%.

In recent years, researchers have continued to utilize the EEG time series data (Andrzejak et al., 2001; University of Bonn Department of Epileptology, 2001). In the work presented by Lahmiri and Shmuel (2019), a CAD model was introduced exploiting generalized Hurst exponent (GHE) and k-nearest neighbors (k-NN). The classification success of the model was 100%. Thara, PremaSudha, and Xiong (2019) used deep neural network (DNN) for automatic epileptic seizure detection and achieved the classification accuracy of 97.21%. Akyol (2020) also employed DNN and obtained the accuracy of 97.17%.

In another study (Gao, Yan, Gao, Gao, & Zhang, 2020), ApEn, recurrence quantitative analysis (RQA) and CNN were applied, and the proposed approach attained the classification success of 99.26%. Amin, Yusoff, and Ahmad (2020) introduced a CAT system using Naïve Bayes (NB), DWT, arithmetic coding (AC), k-NN, SVM and MLPNN. The accuracy of the proposed system was 100% for all variations of the data set.

Hassan, Subasi, and Zhang (2020) introduced an approach to detect epileptic seizures using a type of EMD called as complete ensemble empirical mode decomposition with adaptive noise (CEEMDAN). In this study exploiting IMF, normal inverse Gaussian (NIG) and Adaptive Boosting (AdaBoost), the classification accuracy of 100% was achieved.

In the work of Rout and Biswal (2020), Hilbert transform (HT), variational mode decomposition (VMD) and error-minimized random vector functional link network (EMRVFLN) were used together for efficient epileptic seizure detection. The best accuracy of 100% was acquired by this approach.

In a recent study (Al-Hadeethi, Abdulla, Diykh, Deo, & Green, 2020), an epileptic seizure identification method was presented using AdaBoost LS-SVM and covariance matrix, and the accuracy rate of this method was 99%.

The aforementioned studies are compared with regard to the methods used and classification accuracy in Table 2. When all researches are examined, it is seen that neural network-based classifiers for classification and wavelet transform-based methods for feature extraction are mostly used techniques for epileptic seizure detection.

CONCLUSION

Worldwide, one of the most widespread neurological disorders is epilepsy. About %1 of the world's population is struggling with this disease. In order for epileptic seizure detection, medical specialists read the EEG recordings owing to the unpredictability and complexity of the disease. This process takes a lot of time and reading time varies with the expert's experience. Therefore, automatic detection of epileptic seizures is essential to comfort patients and medical experts. ML techniques are utilized during automatic epileptic seizure detection. In this chapter, the systems, techniques, methods, and models used for epilepsy diagnosis are investigated. When the existing studies in the literature are analyzed, it is seen that the most used techniques are neural network-based classifiers for classification and wavelet transform-based methods for feature extraction.

Table 2. Comparison of existing works regarding methods used and accuracy rate

Authors	Year	Methods	Classification Accuracy (%)
Srinivasan et al.	2007	ApEn – EN – PNN	100
Subasi	2007	DWT – EM – ME	94.5
Tzallas et al.	2007	TFA – PCA – FFNN	100
Polat and Güneş	2007	FFT – DT	98.72
Bao et al.	2008	FFT – PSI – RIR – PFD – HFD – HP – PNN	99.5
Ocak	2009	ApEn – DWT	96
Chandaka et al.	2009	CC – SVM	95.96
Guo et al.	2010	DWT – MLPNN	99.6
Murugavel and Ramakrishnan	2011	DWT – ApEn – PNN	100
Orhan et al.	2011	DWT – *K*-means – MLPNN	100
Song et al.	2012	O-SampEn – ELM	97.5
Nicolaou and Georgiou	2012	PE – SVM	93.55
Dehuri et al.	2013	DWT – DE-RBFN	100
Zainuddin et al.	2013	DWT – WNN – T2FCM	98.87
Kaya et al.	2014	1D-LBP – LR – FT – BayesNet – SVM – ANN	99.5
Kumar et al.	2014	DWT – ApEn – FFNN	100
Das et al.	2014	DT-CWT – ANN – SVM	100
Kang et al.	2015	HP – FFT – AR – QDA – MLPNN	99.78
Sharma and Pachori	2015	EMD – PSR – IMF – LS-SVM	98.67
Tiwari et al.	2016	LBP – SVM	99.31
Tawfik et al.	2016	WPE – SVM	93.75
Hassan et al.	2016	TQWT – Bagging	100
Bhardwaj et al.	2016	EMD – CGP	100
Das et al.	2016	DT-CWT – SVM	100
Mursalin et al.	2017	DWT – ICFS – RF	100
Li et al.	2017	DWT-based EA – NNE	98.78
Satapathy et al.	2017	DWT – ABC – RBFN	98.5
Jaiswal and Banka	2017	LNDP – 1D-LGP – NN – DT – ANN – SVM	99.82
Sharma et al.	2017	ATF-FWT – HFD – LS-SVM	100
Acharya et al.	2018	13-layer deep CNN	88.7
Ullah et al.	2018	P-1D-CNN	100
Jaiswal and Banka	2018	LCP – 1D-LTP – NN – ANN – SVM – DT	100
Yavuz et al.	2018	CA – GRNN	99.6
Siuly et al.	2018	LS-SVM – Hermite transform	99.67
Lahmiri and Shmuel	2019	GHE – k-NN	100
Thara et al.	2019	DNN	97.21
Akyol	2020	DNN	97.17
Gao et al.	2020	ApEn – RQA – CNN	99.26
Amin et al.	2020	DWT – AC – NB – k-NN – SVM – MLPNN	100
Hassan et al.	2020	CEEMDAN – IMF – NIG – AdaBoost	100
Rout and Biswal	2020	HT – VMD – EMRVFLN	100
Al-Hadeethi et al.	2020	AdaBoost LS-SVM – Covariance matrix	99

ACKNOWLEDGMENT

This research received no specific grant from any funding agency in the public, commercial, or not-for-profit sectors.

REFERENCES

Acharya, U. R., Oh, S. L., Hagiwara, Y., Tan, J. H., & Adeli, H. (2018). Deep convolutional neural network for the automated detection and diagnosis of seizure using EEG signals. *Computers in Biology and Medicine*, *100*, 270–278. doi:10.1016/j.compbiomed.2017.09.017 PMID:28974302

Akyol, K. (2020). Stacking ensemble based deep neural networks modeling for effective epileptic seizure detection. *Expert Systems with Applications*, *148*, 113239. doi:10.1016/j.eswa.2020.113239

Al-Hadeethi, H., Abdulla, S., Diykh, M., Deo, R. C., & Green, J. H. (2020). Adaptive boost LSSVM classification approach for time-series signal classification in epileptic seizure diagnosis applications. *Expert Systems with Applications*, *161*, 113676. doi:10.1016/j.eswa.2020.113676

Amin, H. U., Yusoff, M. Z., & Ahmad, R. F. (2020). A novel approach based on wavelet analysis and arithmetic coding for automated detection and diagnosis of epileptic seizure in EEG signals using machine learning techniques. *Biomedical Signal Processing and Control*, *56*, 101707. doi:10.1016/j.bspc.2019.101707

Andrzejak, R. G., Lehnertz, K., Mormann, F., Rieke, C., David, P., & Elger, C. E. (2001). Indications of nonlinear deterministic and finite-dimensional structures in time series of brain electrical activity: Dependence on recording region and brain state. *Physical Review. E*, *64*(6), 061907. doi:10.1103/PhysRevE.64.061907 PMID:11736210

Bao, F. S., Lie, D. Y. C., & Zhang, Y. (2008, November). A new approach to automated epileptic diagnosis using EEG and probabilistic neural network. In *2008 20th IEEE International Conference on Tools with Artificial Intelligence* (Vol. 2, pp. 482-486). IEEE. 10.1109/ICTAI.2008.99

Bhardwaj, A., Tiwari, A., Krishna, R., & Varma, V. (2016). A novel genetic programming approach for epileptic seizure detection. *Computer Methods and Programs in Biomedicine*, *124*, 2–18. doi:10.1016/j.cmpb.2015.10.001 PMID:26645791

Chandaka, S., Chatterjee, A., & Munshi, S. (2009). Cross-correlation aided support vector machine classifier for classification of EEG signals. *Expert Systems with Applications*, *36*(2), 1329–1336. doi:10.1016/j.eswa.2007.11.017

Das, A. B., Bhuiyan, M. I. H., & Alam, S. S. (2014, May). A statistical method for automatic detection of seizure and epilepsy in the dual tree complex wavelet transform domain. In *2014 International Conference on Informatics, Electronics & Vision (ICIEV)* (pp. 1-6). IEEE. 10.1109/ICIEV.2014.6850758

Das, A. B., Bhuiyan, M. I. H., & Alam, S. S. (2016). Classification of EEG signals using normal inverse Gaussian parameters in the dual-tree complex wavelet transform domain for seizure detection. *Signal, Image and Video Processing*, *10*(2), 259–266. doi:10.100711760-014-0736-2

Dehuri, S., Jagadev, A. K., & Cho, S. B. (2013). Epileptic seizure identification from electroencephalography signal using DE-RBFNs ensemble. *Procedia Computer Science*, *23*, 84–95. doi:10.1016/j.procs.2013.10.012

Feigin, V. L., Nichols, E., Alam, T., Bannick, M. S., Beghi, E., Blake, N., ... Fisher, J. L. (2019). Global, regional, and national burden of neurological disorders, 1990–2016: A systematic analysis for the Global Burden of Disease Study 2016. *Lancet Neurology*, *18*(5), 459–480. doi:10.1016/S1474-4422(18)30499-X PMID:30879893

Fisher, R. S., Boas, W. V. E., Blume, W., Elger, C., Genton, P., Lee, P., & Engel, J. Jr. (2005). Epileptic seizures and epilepsy: Definitions proposed by the International League Against Epilepsy (ILAE) and the International Bureau for Epilepsy (IBE). *Epilepsia*, *46*(4), 470–472. doi:10.1111/j.0013-9580.2005.66104.x PMID:15816939

Gao, X., Yan, X., Gao, P., Gao, X., & Zhang, S. (2020). Automatic detection of epileptic seizure based on approximate entropy, recurrence quantiðcation analysis and convolutional neural networks. *Artificial Intelligence in Medicine*, *102*, 101711. doi:10.1016/j.artmed.2019.101711 PMID:31980085

Guo, L., Rivero, D., Dorado, J., Rabunal, J. R., & Pazos, A. (2010). Automatic epileptic seizure detection in EEGs based on line length feature and artificial neural networks. *Journal of Neuroscience Methods*, *191*(1), 101–109. doi:10.1016/j.jneumeth.2010.05.020 PMID:20595035

Hassan, A. R., Siuly, S., & Zhang, Y. (2016). Epileptic seizure detection in EEG signals using tunable-Q factor wavelet transform and bootstrap aggregating. *Computer Methods and Programs in Biomedicine*, *137*, 247–259. doi:10.1016/j.cmpb.2016.09.008 PMID:28110729

Hassan, A. R., Subasi, A., & Zhang, Y. (2020). Epilepsy seizure detection using complete ensemble empirical mode decomposition with adaptive noise. *Knowledge-Based Systems*, *191*, 105333. doi:10.1016/j.knosys.2019.105333

Jaiswal, A. K., & Banka, H. (2017). Local pattern transformation based feature extraction techniques for classification of epileptic EEG signals. *Biomedical Signal Processing and Control*, *34*, 81–92. doi:10.1016/j.bspc.2017.01.005

Jaiswal, A. K., & Banka, H. (2018). Local transformed features for epileptic seizure detection in EEG signal. *Journal of Medical and Biological Engineering*, *38*(2), 222–235. doi:10.100740846-017-0286-5

Kang, J. H., Chung, Y. G., & Kim, S. P. (2015). An efficient detection of epileptic seizure by differentiation and spectral analysis of electroencephalograms. *Computers in Biology and Medicine*, *66*, 352–356. doi:10.1016/j.compbiomed.2015.04.034 PMID:25982199

Kaya, Y., Uyar, M., Tekin, R., & Yıldırım, S. (2014). 1D-local binary pattern based feature extraction for classification of epileptic EEG signals. *Applied Mathematics and Computation*, *243*, 209–219. doi:10.1016/j.amc.2014.05.128

Kumar, Y., Dewal, M. L., & Anand, R. S. (2014). Epileptic seizures detection in EEG using DWT-based ApEn and artificial neural network. *Signal, Image and Video Processing*, *8*(7), 1323–1334. doi:10.100711760-012-0362-9

Lahmiri, S., & Shmuel, A. (2019). Accurate classification of seizure and seizure-free intervals of intracranial EEG signals from epileptic patients. *IEEE Transactions on Instrumentation and Measurement*, *68*(3), 791–796. doi:10.1109/TIM.2018.2855518

Li, M., Chen, W., & Zhang, T. (2017). Classification of epilepsy EEG signals using DWT-based envelope analysis and neural network ensemble. *Biomedical Signal Processing and Control*, *31*, 357–365. doi:10.1016/j.bspc.2016.09.008

Mursalin, M., Zhang, Y., Chen, Y., & Chawla, N. V. (2017). Automated epileptic seizure detection using improved correlation-based feature selection with random forest classifier. *Neurocomputing*, *241*, 204–214. doi:10.1016/j.neucom.2017.02.053

Murugavel, A. M., & Ramakrishnan, S. (2011). Wavelet domain approximate entropy-based epileptic seizure detection. *The 5th International Conference on Information Technology.*

Nicolaou, N., & Georgiou, J. (2012). Detection of epileptic electroencephalogram based on permutation entropy and support vector machines. *Expert Systems with Applications*, *39*(1), 202–209. doi:10.1016/j.eswa.2011.07.008

Niedermeyer, E., & da Silva, F. L. (Eds.). (2005). *Electroencephalography: basic principles, clinical applications, and related fields*. Lippincott Williams & Wilkins.

Ocak, H. (2009). Automatic detection of epileptic seizures in EEG using discrete wavelet transform and approximate entropy. *Expert Systems with Applications*, *36*(2), 2027–2036. doi:10.1016/j.eswa.2007.12.065

Orhan, U., Hekim, M., & Ozer, M. (2011). EEG signals classification using the K-means clustering and a multilayer perceptron neural network model. *Expert Systems with Applications*, *38*(10), 13475–13481. doi:10.1016/j.eswa.2011.04.149

Polat, K., & Güneş, S. (2007). Classification of epileptiform EEG using a hybrid system based on decision tree classifier and fast Fourier transform. *Applied Mathematics and Computation*, *187*(2), 1017–1026. doi:10.1016/j.amc.2006.09.022

Rout, S. K., & Biswal, P. K. (2020). An efficient error-minimized random vector functional link network for epileptic seizure classification using VMD. *Biomedical Signal Processing and Control*, *57*, 101787. doi:10.1016/j.bspc.2019.101787

Satapathy, S. K., Dehuri, S., & Jagadev, A. K. (2017). ABC optimized RBF network for classification of EEG signal for epileptic seizure identification. *Egyptian Informatics Journal*, *18*(1), 55–66. doi:10.1016/j.eij.2016.05.001

Scheffer, I. E., Berkovic, S., Capovilla, G., Connolly, M. B., French, J., Guilhoto, L., ... Nordli, D. R. (2017). ILAE classification of the epilepsies: Position paper of the ILAE Commission for Classification and Terminology. *Epilepsia*, *58*(4), 512–521. doi:10.1111/epi.13709 PMID:28276062

Sharma, M., Pachori, R. B., & Acharya, U. R. (2017). A new approach to characterize epileptic seizures using analytic time-frequency flexible wavelet transform and fractal dimension. *Pattern Recognition Letters*, *94*, 172–179. doi:10.1016/j.patrec.2017.03.023

Sharma, R., & Pachori, R. B. (2015). Classification of epileptic seizures in EEG signals based on phase space representation of intrinsic mode functions. *Expert Systems with Applications*, *42*(3), 1106–1117. doi:10.1016/j.eswa.2014.08.030

Siuly, S., Alcin, O. F., Bajaj, V., Sengur, A., & Zhang, Y. (2018). Exploring Hermite transformation in brain signal analysis for the detection of epileptic seizure. *IET Science, Measurement & Technology*, *13*(1), 35–41. doi:10.1049/iet-smt.2018.5358

Siuly, S., Li, Y., & Zhang, Y. (2016). Electroencephalogram (EEG) and Its Background. In *EEG Signal Analysis and Classification* (pp. 3–21). Springer. doi:10.1007/978-3-319-47653-7_1

Song, Y., Crowcroft, J., & Zhang, J. (2012). Automatic epileptic seizure detection in EEGs based on optimized sample entropy and extreme learning machine. *Journal of Neuroscience Methods*, *210*(2), 132–146. doi:10.1016/j.jneumeth.2012.07.003 PMID:22824535

Srinivasan, V., Eswaran, C., & Sriraam, N. (2007). Approximate entropy-based epileptic EEG detection using artificial neural networks. *IEEE Transactions on Information Technology in Biomedicine*, *11*(3), 288–295. doi:10.1109/TITB.2006.884369 PMID:17521078

Subasi, A. (2007). EEG signal classification using wavelet feature extraction and a mixture of expert model. *Expert Systems with Applications*, *32*(4), 1084–1093. doi:10.1016/j.eswa.2006.02.005

Tawfik, N. S., Youssef, S. M., & Kholief, M. (2016). A hybrid automated detection of epileptic seizures in EEG records. *Computers & Electrical Engineering*, *53*, 177–190. doi:10.1016/j.compeleceng.2015.09.001

Thara, D. K., PremaSudha, B. G., & Xiong, F. (2019). Auto-detection of epileptic seizure events using deep neural network with different feature scaling techniques. *Pattern Recognition Letters*, *128*, 544–550. doi:10.1016/j.patrec.2019.10.029

Tiwari, A. K., Pachori, R. B., Kanhangad, V., & Panigrahi, B. K. (2016). Automated diagnosis of epilepsy using key-point-based local binary pattern of EEG signals. *IEEE Journal of Biomedical and Health Informatics*, *21*(4), 888–896. doi:10.1109/JBHI.2016.2589971 PMID:27416609

Tzallas, A. T., Tsipouras, M. G., & Fotiadis, D. I. (2007). Automatic seizure detection based on time-frequency analysis and artificial neural networks. *Computational Intelligence and Neuroscience*, *2007*, 80510. doi:10.1155/2007/80510 PMID:18301712

Ullah, I., Hussain, M., & Aboalsamh, H. (2018). An automated system for epilepsy detection using EEG brain signals based on deep learning approach. *Expert Systems with Applications*, *107*, 61–71. doi:10.1016/j.eswa.2018.04.021

University of Bonn Department of Epileptology. (2001). *EEG time series data* [Data file]. Available from http://epileptologie-bonn.de/cms/front_content.php?idcat=193&lang=3&changelang=3

World Health Organization (WHO). (2019). *Epilepsy: a public health imperative*. World Health Organization.

World Health Organization (WHO). (2020). *Epilepsy*. Retrieved from https://www.who.int/news-room/fact-sheets/detail/epilepsy

Yavuz, E., Kasapbaşı, M. C., Eyüpoğlu, C., & Yazıcı, R. (2018). An epileptic seizure detection system based on cepstral analysis and generalized regression neural network. *Biocybernetics and Biomedical Engineering*, *38*(2), 201–216. doi:10.1016/j.bbe.2018.01.002

Zainuddin, Z., Huong, L. K., & Pauline, O. (2013). Reliable epileptic seizure detection using an improved wavelet neural network. *The Australasian Medical Journal*, *6*(5), 308–314. doi:10.4066/AMJ.2013.1640 PMID:23745153

KEY TERMS AND DEFINITIONS

Electroencephalogram (EEG): An electrophysiological monitoring procedure in order to record brain electrical activities.

Epilepsy: A brain disorder that can be defined as a short-time and temporary occurrence of symptoms because of abnormal extreme or synchronous brain neuronal activities.

Epileptic Seizure: A temporary emergence of symptoms on account of abnormal extreme or synchronous brain neuronal activities.

Machine Learning: An area of techniques and algorithms that learn from data and perform a particular task.

Chapter 10
Public Health Surveillance System:
Infectious Diseases

Manish Kumar Dwivedi
Indira Gandhi National Tribal University, India

Suvashish Kumar Pandey
https://orcid.org/0000-0001-6524-475X
School of Bio-Sciences and Technology, VIT University, India

Prashant Kumar Singh
https://orcid.org/0000-0002-8117-4592
Indira Gandhi National Tribal University, India

ABSTRACT

To guard people against some grave infectious disease, the surveillance system is a key performance measure of global public health threats and vulnerability. The diseases surveillance system helps in public health monitor, control, and prevent infectious diseases. Infectious diseases remain major causes of death. It's important to monitor and surveillance worldwide for developing a framework for risk assessment and health regulation. Surveillance systems help us in understanding the factors driving infectious disease and developing new technological aptitudes with modeling, pathogen determination, characterization, diagnostics, and communications. This chapter discussed surveillance system working, progress toward global public healthy society considering perspectives for the future and improvement of infectious disease surveillance without limited and fragmented capabilities, and making even global coverage.

INTRODUCTION

Infectious diseases have been a huge health burden in the global history of mankind. New emerging disease such as Corona virus disease (COVID-19), Ebola, H5N1 and H7N9 avian influenza viruses,

DOI: 10.4018/978-1-7998-6527-8.ch010

and the Middle East respiratory syndrome corona virus along with emergence of drug resistance in pathogens causing infectious disease like tuberculosis and malaria are the major causes for morbidity and mortality worldwide (Fauci, A.S., 2001). A competent surveillance system is a powerful tool that can play a dynamic role in controlling and monitoring the outbreak of infectious diseases. The results of the surveillance system result in the establishment of new public health policies that may be useful in protecting public health. The surveillance system is a basic tool in understanding the burden of a disease over time, detect changes in disease outbreaks, determine risk factors for the disease and populations at greatest risk, guide immediate public health actions for individual patients or the community and thus formulate policies for the effective control measures for preventing the infectious diseases and other epidemics. The surveillance method for the controlling of diseases was first time applied by William Farr and Wales from the General Registrar's Office of England and Wales in the mid-1800s where they collected morbidity data from few communities in other countries (Thacker, S. B., 2000; Brachman, 2009). In 1878, the Public Health Service of the United States collected the morbidity data due to plague, yellow fever, cholera, and smallpox (Langmuir, A. D., 1963; Thacker, S. B., & Berkelman, R. L., 1988). In this period, surveillance system covered communicable diseases, non-communicable diseases, bioterrorism trials, immunizations, and other health care delivery (Thacker, S. B., 2000; Brachman, 2009). In 1961, all of the data related to the morbidity of infectious diseases was moved to the communicable disease center currently known as the Centers for Disease Control and Prevention (CDC), Atlanta, Georgia.

In recent years, the surveillance system is comprehensive on viral outbreaks with focus on Human Immunodeficiency Virus and Acquired Immune Deficiency Syndrome (HIV/AIDS), West Nile virus infection, avian influenza, severe acute respiratory syndrome (SARS), and current spread of COVID-19 worldwide. At present, 59 diseases are reported weekly to the CDC and seven other diseases are informed exclusively (monthly or yearly). Three diseases namely yellow fever, plague, and cholera are subject to the International Health Regulations adopted by the World Health Assembly (1951). These mechanisms provide security against the international spread of epidemic diseases with a minimum interference with world traffic. Each country should inform World Health Organization (WHO) within the first 24 hours of diagnosis of the first suspected case on its territory and all following cases and deaths are to be reported to WHO. In case of infectious diseases with high fatality rates (such as meningococcal disease), most countries require rapid reports of the first occurrences of suspect cases. For diseases, such as pneumonia or AIDS, weekly, monthly, or quarterly case reports are required. The reporting requirements for infectious diseases are nationally or sub-nationally determined. For example leishmaniasis needs to be notified in high risk countries but not in all. Similarly, reporting of HIV is required in some states in the United States of America but not in others. The WHO maintains surveillance for Yellow fever, Plague, Cholera, African trypanosomiasis, Meningococcal disease, Dengue, Influenza, HIV/AIDS, Leishmaniasis and Leishmania/HIV co-infection. WHO helps several countries in the world to maintain their National disease surveillance programs and report cases differently according to the type and frequency of the disease. Detection and reporting of all infectious diseases is of prime importance since new emerging strains have the potential to cause new epidemics and pandemics leading to huge economic loss. For example England is a small country with a population of approximately 66.87 million individuals. The infectious diseases account for 7% of deaths and annual costs of £30bn (Health Protection Agency, 2020). The disease epidemic can economically weaken any country as evident by the 2003 SARS outbreak that were not only limited to Asian countries but were also seen worldwide. The economic cost (direct and indirect) of SARS are assessed at US$80 billion (Knobler, S., et al., 2004). The discussion in the current chapter is based on the risks associated with the endemic diseases and how the health problems must be defined in terms of etiology, distribution, and mechanism of infection. The major information that is collected during disease outbreaks include features such as identifying the pathogen involved, associated symptoms, population infected, and the morbidity and mortality rates. Without surveillance system, the health officials cannot predict the intensity and spread patterns of the disease that would lead to waste of precious resources. The surveillance data helps in understanding the pathogen involved helps scientists design health policies that can successfully intervene in containing and eradication the infectious diseases.

BACKGROUND

As per the WHO around 5.72 billion people are at the risk of many infectious diseases that are responsible for the death of more than 17 million people annually, including about 9 million deaths in young children. A microscopic technique has developed in the second half of the 19th century and has been used for the detection of diseases. The progressive results from this innovation allowed new concepts to improve the study of spread and contributing factors of infectious diseases among the quantified population. Epidemiology is the branch of science that studies the patterns, causes, and effects of Infectious diseases on health in population under study. Public health policies and decisions are based on the evidence based outcomes of such studies that identify risk factors for disease and targets for preventive medicine (Ziegler, 2015; World Health Organization, 2018). The term of infectious agents is referred to the all microorganisms or macro-organisms such as bacteria, viruses, protozoa, parasites, and fungi collectively called pathogens that are capable of producing an infection called infectious diseases (Barreto, 2006). Infectious disease were considered the greatest severe health problem worldwide until the beginning of the 20th century as they are difficult to control and evolve resistance against drugs and then chronic degenerative and cancerous disease originated to lead this situation in established countries. Plagues, Cholera and Malaria used to overwhelm important extents of the residents of the European capitals shifting investments by all private investors treating these and ignoring all poor men's disease (Ziegler, 2015; WHO publications, 1993; Evans, R.J., 1995).

For virtuous public health it is essential to concurrently practice plan, implement, and evaluate the ongoing or existing, analysis, and systematic collection method of health-related statistics. It is faithfully included with distribution of these data to those in authority for prevention, control, and generates interferences that increase the health of the objective residents. The word surveillance is imitative from the French roots, sur (over) and veiller (to watch over) (Choi, 2012). It is also defined as the nearby and incessant supervision, or control of one or more individuals (Brachman, 2009). The key goal is to be responsible for evidence that can be used for health action by public health staffs, administration representative and to guide public health policy and program's serious constituents of a well-functioning public health system. Broad-spectrum values of public health surveillance are used in programs to control, and prevent the spread of infectious disease amongst the population. Public health surveillance systems are allowed for surveillance, and are central for practicing of contemporary public health. The system includes data collection, investigation and elucidation of data, characterization of the burden, prioritization of public health actions, distribution of adverse health events, control measures and recognition of initial health situations that may have an important effect on people health (Brownson & Petitti, 2006).

The Greek physician Hippocrates, known as the father of medicine was the first epidemiologist who studied the effects of environmental influences and the occurrence of disease. He believed that sickness of the human body is caused by an imbalance of the four Humors (air, fire, water and earth "atoms"). The distinction between "epidemic" and "endemic" was explained by Hippocrates. The diseases that are "visited upon" a population are epidemic and that "reside within" a population are endemic. Through various milestones of public health actions, awareness development of health surveillance came into existence and different diseases lead to different interventions. Public health surveillance is used to evaluation the public health status by departments of health, ministries of finance, NGOs, and contributors. It is useful for both measuring interventions and effects of interval (Galley, 1995).

Globally International Classification of Diseases (ICD) is used as provides a common language for reporting and monitoring diseases allowing the countries to compare and share data in a consistent and standard way. Similar statistics facilitates the collection and storage of data for analysis and evidence-based decision-making. ICD serves as the diagnostic classification standard for all clinical and research purposes defining the diseases, disorders, injuries and other related health conditions. The benefits of ICD usage are easy storage, retrieval and analysis of health information, sharing and comparing health information and data comparisons in the same location across different time periods. The global data is compiled, examined and reported by WHO in their "World Health Statistics" publications (McNabb, 2004).

Figure 1. Flow chart of working surveillance system

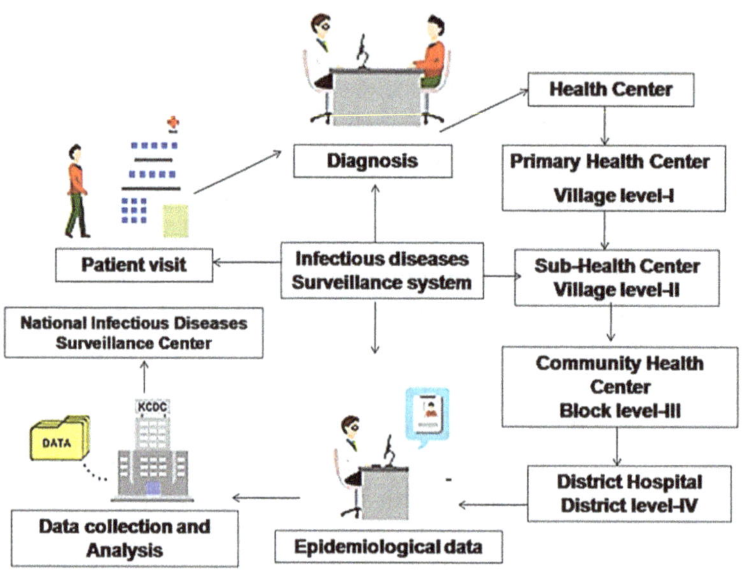

SURVEILLANCE SYSTEM

Public health surveillance system is the ongoing systematic collection, analysis, and interpretation of health data, essential to the planning, implementation, and evaluation of public health practice, closely integrated to the dissemination of these data to those who need to know and linked to prevention and control. The system is beneficial in measuring the need for interventions and studying the effects of interventions. The outcome of the surveillance data empowers the decision makers to design evidence based health policies and manage the health system more effectively (Figure 1). In developing countries like India that have very big population, surveillance systems are a very hard thing to create and are often non-existent. The main reasons are restricted accessible assets, shortage of experienced staff, disorganization, and deprived structure for data collection. The health system in India is very fragmented both administratively and thematically which limits and deter the prevention and control of infectious diseases whenever there is an outbreak. Robust public health infrastructure surveillance systems in countries such as India are required that will permit data to be more precisely documented and evaluated to resolve the national of health problems. It can help in improving health advancement plans, assist in policy implementation and justified use of the resources (Haveman-Nies, et al., 2017; Birkhead & Maylahn, 2010; Woodruff, 2006; Nsubuga, P., et al, 2006). The basic terms and definitions related to health surveillance system are being listed below:

Basic Terms and Definitions

1. **Incidence**: Refers to the number of individuals who develop a specific disease or experience a specific health-related event during a particular time period.
2. **Prevalence**: Existing number of cases in the population at a certain time period or a specific time point. It is usually expressed as a percentage of the population.
3. **Mortality rate:** The number of deaths in a given area or period, or from a particular cause.
4. **Years of Potential Life Lost (YPLL)**: An estimate of the average years a person would have lived if he / she had not died prematurely. It is, therefore, a measure of premature mortality.
5. **Disability-Adjusted Life Year (DALY)**: DALYs for a disease or health condition are calculated as the sum of the Years of Life Lost (YLL) due to premature mortality in the population and the Years Lost due to Disability (YLD) for people living with the health condition or its consequences.
6. **Adjusted rates**: Statistically modified rates to disregard the effect of positive types in people surveillance data. Such as, due to higher communicable infectious diseases caused higher death rates in the city, thus mortality data might be location-adjusted to account for the demographic difference when matching it with data from another city.
7. **Crude rates:** A crude rate is the number of new cases (or deaths) occurring in a specified population per year, usually expressed as the number of cases per 100,000 population at risk.
8. **Case-Fatality Rate (CFR):** It is the proportion of deaths from a certain disease compared to the total number of people diagnosed with the disease during a particular period of time.
9. **Cluster:** When a patient with disease is closely tangled with place and time of outbreaks, birth defects, cancers, and other serious diseases.
10. **Endemic:** The typical rise in prevalence or frequency of a certain disease in a group of people.
11. **Epidemic**: Epidemic occurs when an agent and susceptible hosts are present in adequate numbers, and the agent can be effectively conveyed from a source to the susceptible hosts.
12. **Pandemic**: An epidemic arises over a number of cities, country or regions and affecting a huge group of the people.
13. **Health indicator**: It's a capacity that shows the wellbeing state of individuals in a region. For example, the mortality rate death rate, etc.
14. **Validity**: A degree that the accuracy of measures of procedures what it's significant to measure.
15. **Vital Statistics**: Systematic information registered by local health authorities about population births, marriages, divorces, and deaths.
16. **Sensitivity**: The ability to identify true and positive cases with a low rate of false negatives.

17. **Specificity**: The capability of a test to identify eliminate which are not true cases, or people without the disease with highly specific tests having a low rate of false positives.
18. **Routine Health Information System:** Regular reporting around diseases and programs are accomplished by public health officials, hospitals, and diagnostic laboratories.
19. **Health Information and Management System:** A system of routine report collection almost administrative public health logistic, financial, clinical and other involved processes that can be used for surveillance.
20. **Active Surveillance:** Employing health officials and other staff members for contact health care providers or the population representatives for data collection about health conditions providing more accurate and timed information. This method is an expensive surveillance system.
21. **Passive Surveillance:** A system of report submission from clinics, public health units, laboratories including other sources covering large areas giving critical information about community health and also helps in constant monitoring. Data collection from different institutions makes data controlling difficult and providing data with data quality and timeliness.
22. **Categorical Surveillance:** The active or passive surveillance system focusing on one or more diseases of interest in an intervention program.
23. **Integrated Surveillance:** Combination of both passive and active systems for gathering data about several diseases of interest to more than a few intervention programs using a single infrastructure.
24. **Syndromic Surveillance:** A data collection system based completely on clinical infrastructures with clinical or laboratory diagnosis combining an active or passive system implemented by developing country during an epidemic.
25. **Behavioral Risk Factor Surveillance System (BRFSS):** An active system of repetitive surveys as a measure of behaviors that are acknowledged for causing disease or injury.

Categories of Surveillance Approaches

Surveillance systems are aimed and designed to meet top administrations requirements for dedicated, consistent, timely collection of evidence that can be presented efficiently. These needs are diverge and dependent on geographical location, population size and nation medical policies, thus several diverse strategies have been established that have been explained below (Birkhead & Maylahn, 2010).

1. **Sentinel Surveillance:** When the passive system fails to obtain high-quality data on the high probability of growth in several cases of the disease in question, then informed staff recognizes and inform on stated diseases using laboratory facilities (Arita, I, et al., 2004). Data collected can be used to detect outbreaks, indicate trends, monitor existing diseases in regions, suggest alternative and effective surveillance systems as it is not effective in identifying a rare disease or outside the selected area (Birkhead, G. S., & Maylahn, C. M., 2000). Although a passive system collects data from multiple health workers and facilities. For example, hospitals are huge network used to gather high-quality data on different diseases, for example offensive bacterial disease caused by *Hemophilus influenzae* type b, *pneumococcus* or *meningococcus* (World health statistics, 2005).
2. **Periodic Population-Based Surveys:** A consistent data collection on regular interval through survey produced by representatives of nationally and globally with different demographic, rates, ratios, probabilities and social indicators with the help of trained enumerators using standard instruments, scientifically designed questionnaires with administrative guidelines to minimize statistical

errors, non-sampling errors made through calculation and humans respectively (Thacker, S. B., & Berkelman, R. L., 1988). A comparable time series surveillance data gives information about health, population size with resources existing in a specific demographic location with medical infrastructure. Some background inequalities are also revealed through time to time survey between sub-population, a socioeconomic group existing in that region. The survey datasets also link and characterize health outcomes, estimates independent effects on various determents on ill health and mortality findings with other non-medical determinants communicability of diseases, treatment, and precautious approach by people network coverage by services. Validation of data is also an important step that suggests fertility, motility of regional and global statistical data collection system (Wang, et al., 2019; Birkhead & Maylahn, 2010).

3. **Laboratory-Based Surveillance:** This method forms a spectrum that evolves with the economic development of a country and depends on more resources and infrastructure. This type of surveillance requires enough resources, facilities, and trained personnel. A dedicated and centrally regulated public health reference laboratory is must for quality control purposes. A systematic sampling scheme and referral mechanism is being followed in this type of system. The information is regularly shared amongst the microbiology laboratories and epidemiologists so that the information can be used to its full potential. Molecular detection methods have expanded the power of laboratory-based surveillance methods for the detection of outbreaks in the background of sporadic cases by distinguishing the molecular "fingerprint" of an outbreak strain. Standardized protocols for several pathogens have been developed along with advancement in gene-based detection technologies (Herikstad, H., et al., 2000).
4. **Integrated Disease Surveillance and Response (IDSR):** IDSR is an approach used for linking epidemiologic and laboratory data in Infectious disease surveillance systems at all levels of the health system, with emphasis on integrating surveillance with response. It indicates established and existing links between health facility, community, national levels, district, use of resources for disease control and prevention. Major steps in IDSR implementation are sensitization of key health authorities and stakeholders, carrying out situational analysis, formulating a strategic IDSR plan, creating well training and motivated individuals, developing national IDSR technical guidelines, planning and implementation, monitoring and evaluating (WHO 2000b; International Health Regulations 2005, 2008).
5. **Injury Surveillance:** Injuries are the most important public health problems that kill more than five million people globally per year. They are the main cause of disabilities especially for low-income groups that are even less likely to make full recovery (Peden, M., et al., 2002). The surveillance for injury includes monitoring the incidence, causes and circumstances of fatal and nonfatal injuries. Injuries are classified by the intention of the act into two groups: unintentional injuries and violence-related injuries. Guidelines have been developed for establishing injury surveillance systems by WHO and the Pan American Health Organization (Holder, Peden, & Krug 2001; Concha-Eastman & Villveces 2001)

Violence Prevention Department has provided guidelines for both investigators and medical practitioners in the field, on how to categorize and code data on injuries according to agreed international standards (Sharma, et al., 2000; Villaveces, et al., 2010).

6. **Complex Emergency Surveillance:** Complex Emergency Surveillance is used during the acute phase of the emergency. Community exposed diseases in highly populated area are major cause to the high mortality and morbidity leading to an outbreak. Poor nations with large population are more susceptible to epidemic-prone outbreaks, therefore precautious approach should be taken for the calculation of indicators and determinants estimating, improving current research regarding complex emergencies epidemiologic indicators used for these typical situations (Salama, et al., 2004; Burkle, 1999). While planning a disaster surveillance system, the key elements to be included are establishing objectives, developing case definitions, determining data sources, developing simple data collection instruments, field testing the methods, developing and testing the analysis strategy, developing a dissemination plan for the report or results, and assessing the usefulness of the system. The requirements of the surveillance system need to be varied during the pre-impact, impact, and post-impact phases (Binder & Sanderson 1987). The following framework of activities should be included in disaster surveillance:
    a. Pre-disaster activities (hazard mapping, provision of guidelines, and training for medical and rescue teams)
    b. Regular monitoring and surveillance for priority health problems in affected populations.
    c. Prospective surveillance of affected populations focusing on the natural history of exposure and health effects and long-term effects of stress disorders among survivors.
7. **Surveillance for Biologic Terrorism:** A significant rise in biological agents for disseminating purpose to harm public health and the socioeconomic environment is known as bioterrorism (Buehler, J. W., et al., 2004). Positively, till date intentional bioterrorism has not been reported being potentially most lethal and weapons of mass destruction (WMDs). Its risk assessment involves constant monitoring surveillance over nations, laboratories further preparedness, de-containment and prevention with casualties management. Giving these developments, nations and authorities should consider that new ways of networking of data and data sharing of surveillance should be made (Grundmann, 2014). Biological terrorism surveillance is conducted mainly to detect outbreak and its management. Surveillance must be capable for early detection of an act of biologic terrorism and it should be able to characterize it in the same way as that of naturally occurring outbreaks of infectious diseases. Timely detection can be achieved by the following:
    a. Timely and complete receipt, review, investigation of disease case reports, prompt recognition and reporting to or consultation with health departments by physicians, health care facilities, and laboratories.
    b. Use of analytical tools for early recognition of indicative patterns of a possible outbreak.
    c. Acquiring data that is not routinely observed (increased demand in procurement of health care products, absences from offices/ school, increased patients visits to diagnostic centers).

Surveillance System: Establishment and Maintenance

Health administrators who have undertaken to utilize public health surveillance system as a health management tool must be aware of the fact political support along with human and financial resources are regularly needed for successful implementation. A health surveillance system to be successful requires qualified, well trained and enthusiastic health workers that need continuous supervision. The surveillance system is not constant and must evolve with time adapting to changes in the population and the physical and social environment. There are major six steps that are linked continuously and are required for establishing a successful surveillance system (Thacker & Stroup, 1998):

Table 1. Establishment and Maintenance

1	2	3	4	5	6
Goal Establishment	Design case definitions	Hire qualified personnel	Acquirement of tools & clearances for collection, analysis and dissemination of data and information.	Surveillance system implementation	Evaluation of surveillance activities

Analysis of Surveillance Data

The information gathered by surveillance system is analyzed by time, place, and person. The data should be reviewed regularly by competent technical staff and the authorities to ensure its validity and to retrieve important information from it. Surveillance data such as name, age, gender, symptoms, diagnostics test, pathogen identification, etc are collected scientifically. The data should be converted to tables and graphs for easy understanding, presentation and timely dissemination to the policy makers. Effective intervention programs should be designed based on critical information gathered from the surveillance system. The huge surveillance data has led to evolution of field of public health informatics that deals with collection, classification, storage, retrieval, analysis, and presentation of large amounts of health data, offering the potential for development of integrated public health surveillance systems. Such integrated system will benefit the understanding of epidemiology of diseases by incorporating a systematic approach to standards for data content. One such international standard computer program used globally for the analysis of surveillance data is Epi Info. The graphs generated by the programs are known Epi Curve that helps researchers in investigating the spread patterns, incubation period, and probable outcome the disease may take. Case data plotted on the map are called spot map that helps in detection patterns and clusters of disease and display geographic population at risk. For instance, 1000 cases occurred in a big city, even though 3 cases may have in a small rural town. A huge difference occurred due to the variant in exposures in differences in population size. The people affected in the population were detected by using spot maps. British physician John Snow used spot map for the study of Cholera outbreak in London and has been named as the "Father of Modern Epidemiology" (Buckeridge, D. L., 2007; Brownson, R. C., et al., 2009; Shaban-Nejad, A., et al., 2016; Vachon, D., 2005; Choi, 2012).

Regular interval analysis is done for detecting changes, to ensure their legitimacy, to identify new information using simple computer-generated tables and graphs through statistical programming for summarizing and interpretation of data generated through the strategical survey (Groseclose, S. L., & Buckeridge, D. L., 2017). Timely distribution of statistical results to policymakers and program implementing representatives and authorities helps in critical reasoning.

Health Problem and Programing

Data generated by the surveillance system helps public health administrators comprehend strategic policies for identifying the emerging infectious diseases (Heymann, D. L., 2004) and to understand the degree of changes in the distribution of well-known diseases. During data collection the information is collected on identical kind of pathogen involved, symptoms, the mortality and morbidity rates. Without suitable strategic surveillance, we would be wasting our precious time and resources with blind goals. Data generated through surveillance systems is compiled and analyzed by health officials to design a portrait of the present public depending on current data. New programs are shaped and implemented, after which continuous surveillance is implemented so that the public resources and manpower are utilized effectively. To measures the health events of specific geographic areas, the surveillance systems generate data that helps to identify novel facts about disease distribution patterns and factors responsible for its occurrence and distribution. The results enlightens representatives and administrations who can make more knowledgeable assessments about where, when, how to use resources and time. Without these data, the verdict would be imprudent and inefficient. Based on the statistics, funders and representatives gather their confidence in decision as efficient surveillance system generates information for crucial resource allocation (Groseclose & Buckeridge, 2017). Surveillance system together with information to measure the kin significance's of the disease are:

- Prevalence / Incidence
- Mortality rate.
- Yield loss.
- Preventability of disease.
- Premature mortality (YPLL).
- Severity (case fatality rate).
- Costs in medical care.

Schistosomiasis is a good example where surveillance and data collection played a major role for applied disease control program (Heymann, D., 2006). In one outbreak, schistosomiasis was caused by parasitic worm in the Sichuan province of China (Yang W., et al., 2017). Peoples were infected with schistosomiasis when contacted infected water with Schistosoma worm that entered the body through the skin. The parasite affected approx. 200 million people worldwide with symptoms such as liver enlargement, bladder cancer, stomach pain, fever and chills. Sichuan region has been successful in controlling Schistosomiasis with the help of a surveillance program to stop the transmission. Pesticides were used to kill the snail hosts involved in the life cycle of the parasites. The significance of surveillance systems and gathering of data in previous programs is necessity for the assessment making of mass drug administration and focuses on pathogenic control efforts in a particular situation as needed. It also gathers data about the success of past programs and policies for the regions to speak out "controlled" or "eradicated" of the pathogen at the time. Shortcomings in the surveillance system are mainly accountable for the ultimate failure of containment of disease in many countries.

Implementation of Advance Public Health Surveillance System

Public health administrators focus, timely, systematically comprehensive information for providing evidence in judgments making for improving health and sanitation of the population in their jurisdictional region. A major presentation of improving and existing public health is done through surveillance information for evidence-based decisions. The role of field epidemiologists is important in providing suggestions and partnering in an enhanced universal surveillance system. It also helps in defiance of gravity of funds, sharing raw data information, resources, and supporting public health policies and programs. Listed below are some agencies, initiatives, and companies that work on improving public health surveillance system throughout the globe.

1. **Global Health Security Initiative (GHSI):** GHSI is part of a surveillance system which emphasizes on chemicals and pathogens used for biological weaponry. GHSI also works on developing vaccine, antibiotics and rapid tests kit. It also works with WHO and builds communication between national and international labs and public health organizations (http://www.ghsi.ca/english/members.asp).
2. **Association of Public Health Laboratories (APHL):** APHL is involved in an improved laboratory practice globally. It is working to strengthen laboratory infrastructures in the United States and in other countries of the world. (https://www.aphl.org/AboutAPHL/Pages/default.aspx).
3. **The Global Fund:** It is working with a collaboration of government/public and private sector. The objectives of the global funds reduced infection/death caused by malaria, HIV/AIDS, and TB. (https://www.theglobalfund.org/en/about/whoweare/).
4. **Global Laboratory Initiative (GLI):** The objectives of the GLI expand the surveillance system by the enhancement in the diagnosis system and treatment of tuberculosis in the emerging countries. Therefore, low quantity of Tuberculosis patient identified in emerging country (http://www.stoptb.org/wg/gli/).
5. **US Global Health Initiative (GHI):** GHI is working with several national and international partners such as PEPFAR, defense organizations, and CDC. It is also working with the private sector and NGOs for Worldwide health improvement. The aim of the GHI is to improve the surveillance systems for infectious and non infectious diseases.
6. **Seeding Labs:** It provides laboratory materials to the lower-income countries for upgrading their facilities. It is a non-profitable organization that is helping the scientific community by helping in upgrading of their research infrastructure in the emerging countries.
7. **Foundation for Innovative New Diagnostics (FIND):** FIND aims to develop low cost diagnostic tests. FIND is working with academic and research Institutes, Universities, private organizations that are working for the development of diagnostic tools. The research interests are specifically dedicated to malaria, tuberculosis, leishmaniasis, and trypanosomiasis (http://www.finddiagnostics.org/about/).

Application of Surveillance System

The main component of the surveillance system is outbreak investigation and detection systems. Subtle surveillance systems help in the detection of abnormal health events taking place at the surveillance area, and alert authorities like regional health departments, CDC, WHO for examination and involvement wherever required. WHO and CDC are responsible for aid to the nations that are under an ongoing epidemic. There is strict protocol stated by CDC for out broke control surveillance that is followed by the specific countries (World Health Organization, 2018).

1. **Preparation for Fieldwork:** An investigator should collect all relevant information reported at the outbreak site. He or she should be organized for the work ahead and brings all materials such as lab apparatus for sample collection, and all wellbeing apparatus including bodysuit as necessary for protection. Whether a field investigation has to be done or not, the investigator should be well prepared before leaving for the field. There are two broad categories of the preparations that include scientific and investigative issues and management and operational issues. Complete scientific preparations for both categories of issues are required to facilitate a smooth field experience.
2. **Establish the Existence of an Outbreak:** Whenever the number of cases increases than expected in a particular area and among a specific community over a period of time, the disease is categorized as an outbreak or an epidemic. These cases are thought to have a common occurrence and are related to each another in some way. Epidemiologist defines outbreak as an epidemic limited to localized increase in the incidence of disease. A cluster is an aggregation of cases in a given area over a particular period regardless of the actual number of cases. The major task of the field investigator is to verify that a cluster of cases is indeed an outbreak. Many of the clusters turn out to be true outbreaks with a common cause; some are sporadic and unrelated cases of the same disease while other cases may be similar but unrelated diseases. The observed results are compared to the expected outcome. The expected number is the number calculated from the previous few weeks or months, or from a similar time period during the previous few years. A final survey of the community should be conducted to establish the background or historical level of disease. It is not necessary that if the current number of reported cases is more than that the expected number, an outbreak has occurred. The case number may be on higher side due to reporting procedures, case definition, increased awareness, or sophisticated diagnostic procedures. A newly recruited employee may report more cases as compared to the senior employees. Some number may be attributed to the false positives reported by laboratories. The decision to further investigate the disease does not depend on the observed number of cases. Many a times, the health agencies may take note of the small number of observed cases. The major factors responsible for launch of a field investigation are severity of disease, the spread potential, available control measures, political considerations, public relations, available resources, and other factors.
3. **Verification of the Diagnosis Process:** The verification of the diagnosis is the prime process that is linked to the verification of the existence of an outbreak. Diagnosis verification is important for the proper identification of the disease and to rule out the reporting of false positive laboratory results. The laboratory tests must be reviewed by reference laboratories, DNA or other chemical or biological fingerprinting, or polymerase chain reaction. The investigators must visit the patients for personal interaction that gives a better understanding of the clinical features and helps to design the appropriate preventive measures. The conversation also helps in drawing hypotheses about possible disease etiology and spread patterns. The clinical features must be summarized using frequency distributions that are useful in characterizing the spectrum of illness, verifying the diagnosis, and developing case definitions.
4. **Create Case Definition:** A case definition is a standard set of criteria for deciding whether an individual should be classified as having the health condition of interest. A case definition includes clinical criteria that are restricted by time, place, and person. The clinical criteria are to be simple

in nature such as measurement of fever, loose bowel movements per day and / or muscle pain that are severe enough to limit the patient's routine activities. The criteria must be applied consistently to all persons under investigation. The important factor that needs to be remembered is that the case definition should not include the risk factor the investigator is interested in evaluating. Different categories of a case definition may be defined such as confirmed, probable, and possible or suspect, that allow for uncertainty. A case definition is a tool for classifying whether a person as contracted or not contracted the disease of interest.

Step 5: Find cases systematically and record information. Before reporting the outbreaks to the attention of health authorities, public health workers must scrutinize all the cases to determine the true geographic extent of the problem and the effected populations. In some outbreaks the health official may aware the general public by sharing information through local media. The official can also collect information using a questionnaire or by collecting laboratory specimens to verify the number of asymptomatic cases. Information may be obtained from the patients for other infected persons. Specifically constructed data collection form can be used to gather the outbreak data. The following information should be necessarily obtained while collecting the data:

- Identifying information (name, address, and contact number)
- Demographic information (Age, sex, race, occupation)
- Clinical information
- Risk factor information
- Reporter information (physician, clinic, hospital, or laboratory).

Step 6: Perform Descriptive Epidemiology: The process, in which the outbreak is characterized by time, place, and person, is called descriptive epidemiology. It helps in data summarizing by key demographic variables and provides a comprehensive characterization of the outbreak. The population at risk can be identified by this method. The result gives insights on the etiology, source, and modes of transmission. The result helps to begin intervention and prevention measures and to enable the investigator to identify and correct errors and missing values.

Step 7: Hypotheses Development: The hypothesis is generated at the time of first information that may address the source of the agent, the mode of transmission, and the exposures that caused the disease. The generated hypotheses should be testable that need to be evaluated. Apart from infected patients the local health department staffs are also key person from whom important information may be gathered. If the epidemiology does not fit the natural pattern, then other points may be thought off like bioterrorism.

Step 8: Evaluate Hypotheses Epidemiologically: When a hypothesis about the possible outbreak has been developed, it must be evaluated to test the plausibility of that hypothesis. During field investigation the hypotheses are evaluated using a combination of environmental evidence, laboratory science, and epidemiology either by comparing the hypotheses with the established facts or by using analytic epidemiology to quantify relationships and assess the role of chance.

Step 9: Reconsider, Refine, and Re-Evaluate Hypotheses: When the hypotheses cannot be evaluated with the help of analytic epidemiology, than the hypotheses may be re-evaluated. Even when the association between an exposure and disease has been established by an analytic study, the hypothesis may need to be testified. Many a times, more specific control group are required for testing a hypothesis. The investigators may utilize the outbreak to study the different clinical parameters in the patients for upto some years after infection leading to the understanding of the disease and thus designing better control and prevention strategies.

Step 10: Compare and reconcile with laboratory and environmental studies: The results of an epidemiological survey can associate vehicles and direct appropriate public health action. It is always the laboratory results that confirm the findings. Environmental studies frequently explain the cause of an occurrence of an outbreak. The epidemiologic, environmental and laboratory findings during an investigation may be complementary to each another and may lead plausible conclusion regarding an outbreak under investigation.

Step 11: Implementation of Control and Prevention Measures: The main objective of the outbreak investigations is to control the outbreak and further prevent the spread of the infection. Protection of the public health is the prime responsibility of the government and the health departments. Appropriate control measures should be implemented at earliest. The confidentiality of the patients should be maintained at all points of investigation during collection, management and sharing of data. The control measures are targeted against one or more segments of transmission (agent, source, mode of transmission, portal of entry, or host). Controlling or eliminating the causative agent at source is the most authentic intervention for the control of the outbreak. Isolation, cohortion, decontamination, sterilization, sanitization, vaccination, filtration, vector control, insecticidal sprays are some of the routinely applied methods.

Step 12: Surveillance Maintenance: When the preventive measures have been initiated it is must to monitor them. Active surveillance should be done to monitor the situation and determine the effectiveness of the preventive and control measures being undertaken. It should be determined whether the outbreak has spread outside its original area or the area where the interventions were targeted. In case of spread outside the area, effective control and prevention measures are to be implemented in the new areas of spread.

Step 13: Communicate Findings: Detailed analysis of the outcome and its effective communication to the health administrators and politicians is critical. The results may be summarized in the form of a report and effectively communicated to the peers. This can be done either by orally briefing to the local authorities and persons responsible for implementing control and prevention measures. The findings must be presented in a scientifically objective fashion so that appropriate decisions may be taken. Additionally, a written scientific report may be submitted that will provide a blueprint for timely action. The report can also be used as a reference documents for future similar outbreaks.

Example of a Disease Investigation

Coronavirus diseases–2019 (COVID-19): In many countries COVID-19 outbreak spread rapidly starting in the month of creating epidemic. The COVID-19 title was at first released by WHO on January 12, 2020. An international committee was proposed to name SARS-CoV-2 of new coronavirus on February 11, 2020 (Rong et al., 2020). The Emergency Committee of the WHO declared an outbreak in Wuhan, China on January 30, 2020, which was considered to be community health emergency of global nature (Rodríguez et al., 2020). The WHO declared the novel coronavirus (COVID-19) outbreak a global pandemic on March 11, 2020. The number of cases outside China increased 13 fold over the past 2 weeks and the number of countries with cases increased threefold. WHO also reported that this is the first pandemic caused by a coronavirus. WHO suggested countries to detect, test, treat, isolate, trace, and mobilize their people in the response, those with a handful of cases can prevent those cases becoming clusters, and those clusters becoming community transmission. It is of utmost importance that all countries strike a fine balance between health protection and minimizing economic and social disruption altogether with respecting human rights. The four areas to give importance are to (i) be prepared and be ready, (ii) detect, protect and treat, (iii) reduce transmission and (iv) innovate and learn. Most of the countries tried to contain the spread of the virus but in most of the countries the virus could not be controlled, it is thriving on delay, denial, and division.

The world is fighting hard to find a cure for the disease; over 5000 patients in more than 20 countries have joined WHO's Solidarity Trial, which continues to answer questions about which treatments are most effective. Several donor contributions is helping the WHO to fund more than 108 COVID-19 national plans through the WHO Partners Platform. Through this generous funding, the WHO's COVID-19 Supply Chain System had procured 140 million items of personal protective equipment, 4.5 million laboratory test kits, and 5 million sample collection kits that will be distributed to the nations in need.

WHO is continuously working with expert in the field, more networks are being created around the world. WHO has published more than 130 guiding documents on various aspects of preparedness and response that are useful in knowledge updating and measures to contain and prevent the spread of the virus? WHO is providing constant online and in-person training, technical sessions and remote support? WHO has helped nations to develop their own guidance and strategic national plans? WHO are global and regional platforms, country offices, and collaborative initiatives such as the Global Outbreak Alert and Response network is helping the nations in implementing these plans at the ground level. However, the virus is still spreading quickly with potential to collapse the most versatile health systems. The pandemic continues to accelerate and at the current rate, cases are doubling around every six weeks. As per the latest situation report (August 2, 2020) from WHO, more than 17660523 confirmed cases, 680894 death and spread to 215 countries worldwide has been documented. In India 1750723 confirmed cases, 37364 deaths and 54735 new cases reported till August 2, 2020 (WHO, 2020).

Countries today need authoritative real-time information on the evolving epidemiology and risks, time bound access to essential supplies, medicines and equipment and training of their health care workers as per the latest technical guidelines and best practices. All the countries are required to establish research and innovation priorities, scale-up research and development, and ensure that earliest development of candidate therapeutics, vaccines, and diagnostics is done. WHO has identified nine areas that need prioritization that includes 1) Country-level coordination, planning and monitoring, 2) risk communication and community engagement, 3) surveillance, rapid-response teams, and case investigation, 4) points of entry, 5) national laboratories, 6) infection prevention and control, 7) case management, 8) operations support and logistics and 9) maintaining essential health services and systems. Interrupting the spread of COVID-19 requires identifying and testing all suspected individuals so that confirmed cases are effectively isolated and provided appropriate health care. The persons who have been in close contacts of all confirmed patients are to be rapidly identified for quarantine and appearance of any symptoms for the 14-day incubation period of the virus. For this to achieve, the countries require to increase their COVID-19 testing capacity so that the cases from general population may be identified quickly. WHO has a mandate that all countries should have access to diagnostic testing as part of surveillance strategies designed by WHO. With the help of WHO 99% of countries and territories were able to conduct COVID-19 testing and had established access to an international laboratories within 72 hours. Apart from contact tracing surveillance more strategies are being used because of difference and difficulty in reporting methods, data collection through person to person contact. Some Asian countries are now using digital surveillance; countries like South Korea and India are using CCTV footage, geo-mapping location, cellular network pings, bank account transactions to track the suspected cases. China and Taiwan tracked down travel history using visa and flight-based databases and tagged people with reported health conditions. After identifying the people with COVID-19 positive they are put on quarantine and under surveillance to stop infecting other people and reduce health risk globally (World Health Organization, 2020).

FUTURE OF SURVEILLANCE

Public health agencies, ministries, and international donors and organizations are trying to modify the current surveillance system to a meaningful data collection and analysis system that can provide reliable data to local health status and provide real-time warnings for the destructive disease outbreaks. This requires developing critical surveillance systems with a coherent, integrated approach by commitment from all stake holders. Recent advances in the information technology, informatics and artificial intelligence can radically help in achieving this vision. Technological tools can facilitate the data collection, analysis, and use of surveillance data. With the use of artificial intelligence the data can be analyzed and automatic electronic message can be sent to the responsible public health personnel. Use of cell phones, wireless internet access, advances in geographic information system might also transform the capacities of the local health centers.

CONCLUSION

Public health surveillance is an essential tool for the health administrators, health and finance ministries, and donors. The results of the surveillance system help all the stake holders to take decisions to effectively and efficiently allocate resources and manage public health interventions. The public health surveillance systems should be designed in a scientific way that helps to address the critical concerns associated with the public health practice (Thacker, Berkelman, & Stroup 1989). The surveillance requirement of the countries differs and is based on the population size, geography, environment and economy. The need of the developing world is different from those of the developed countries. We are currently in a time when we are dealing with several deadly viruses like SARS, Ebola, avian influenza and COVID-19 virus. There is undeniable need to collaborate globally for research and development efforts in to find a therapeutic or prophylactic cure for such pathogenic microorganisms. There is a urgent need for collaboration among health practitioners, scientific community, nations, and international organizations in order to understand the epidemiology of the emerging infectious diseases so as to address the global needs of public health surveillance systems.

REFERENCES

Arita, I., Nakane, M., Kojima, K., Yoshihara, N., Nakano, T., & El-Gohary, A. (2004). Role of a sentinel surveillance system in the context of global surveillance of infectious disease. *The Lancet. Infectious Diseases*, *4*(3), 171–177. doi:10.1016/S1473-3099(04)00942-9 PMID:14998504

Barreto, M. L. (2006). Comentário: Tecnologias Em saúde E o sempre tenue equilíbrio entre riscos E benefícios. *Revista de Saude Publica*, *40*(3), 397–399. doi:10.1590/S0034-89102006000300005 PMID:16810361

Birkhead, G. S., & Maylahn, C. M. (2000). State and Local Public Health Surveillance. In Principles and Practices of Public Health Surveillance. Oxford University Press.

Birkhead, G. S., & Maylahn, C. M. (2010). State and local public health surveillance in the United States. *Principles & Practice of Public Health Surveillance*, 381-398. . doi:10.1093/acprof:oso/9780195372922.003.0018

Brachman, P. S. (2009). Public health surveillance. *Bacterial Infections of Humans*, 51-67. doi:10.1007/978-0-387-09843-2_2

Brownson, R. C., Fielding, J. E., & Maylahn, C. M. (2009). Evidence-based public health: A fundamental concept for public health practice. *Annual Review of Public Health*, *30*(1), 175–201. doi:10.1146/annurev.publhealth.031308.100134 PMID:19296775

Brownson, R. C., & Petitti, D. B. (2006). *Applied epidemiology: Theory to practice*. Oxford University Press. doi:10.1093/acprof:oso/9780195187410.001.0001

Buckeridge, D. L. (2007). Outbreak detection through automated surveillance: A review of the determinants of detection. *Journal of Biomedical Informatics*, *40*(4), 370–379. doi:10.1016/j.jbi.2006.09.003 PMID:17095301

Buehler, J. W., Hopkins, R. S., Overhage, J. M., Sosin, D. M., & Tong, V. (2004). Framework for Evaluating Public Health Surveillance Systems for Early Detection of Outbreaks: Recommendations from CDC Working Group. *MMWR. Recommendations and Reports*, *53*(RR-5), 1–11. PMID:15129191

Burkle, F. M. (1999). Fortnightly review: Lessons learnt and future expectations of complex emergencies. *BMJ (Clinical Research Ed.)*, *319*(7207), 422–426. doi:10.1136/bmj.319.7207.422 PMID:10445925

Centers for Disease Control and Prevention (CDC). (n.d.). *Encyclopedia of Public Health*. doi:10.1007/978-1-4020-5614-7_343

Choi, B. C. (2012). The past, present, and future of public health surveillance. *Scientifica*, *2012*, 1–26. doi:10.6064/2012/875253 PMID:24278752

Collins, C., Xu, J., & Tang, S. (2012). Schistosomiasis control and the health system in P.R. China. *Infectious Diseases of Poverty*, *1*(1), 8. doi:10.1186/2049-9957-1-8 PMID:23849320

Fauci, A. S. (2001). *Infectious diseases: considerations for the 21st century*. Clin Infect.

Galley, C. (1995). Terence ranger and Paul slack, EDS., epidemics and ideas. Essays on the historical perception of Pestilence. (Cambridge: Cambridge university press, 1992.) pages ix + 346. £35.00. *Continuity and Change*, *10*(2), 301–303. doi:10.1017/S0268416000002708

Groseclose, S. L., & Buckeridge, D. L. (2017). Public health surveillance systems: Recent advances in their use and evaluation. *Annual Review of Public Health*, *38*(1), 57–79. doi:10.1146/annurev-publhealth-031816-044348 PMID:27992726

Grundmann, O. (2014). The current state of bioterrorist attack surveillance and preparedness in the US. *Risk Management and Healthcare Policy*, *177*, 177. Advance online publication. doi:10.2147/RMHP.S56047 PMID:25328421

Haveman-Nies, A., Jansen, M., Oers, J. A., & Veer, P. V. (2017). *Epidemiology in public health practice*. Academic Press.

Health Protection Agency. (n.d.). *Health protection in the 21st century*. Available from: http://www.hpa.org.uk/ publications/2005/burden disease/default.htm

Herikstad, H., Motarjemi, Y., & Tauxe, R. V. (2002). Salmonella Surveillance: A Global Survey of Public Health Serotyping. *Epidemiology and Infection*, *129*(1), 1–8. doi:10.1017/S0950268802006842 PMID:12211575

Heymann, D. (2006). *Control, elimination, eradication and the re-emergence of infectious diseases: getting the message right.* Retrieved from Bulletin of the World Health Organization. https://www.who.int/bulletin/volumes/84/2/editorial10206html/en/

Heymann, D. L. (2004). *Control of Communicable Diseases Manual*. American Public Health Association.

International Health Regulations. (2008). (2nd ed.). Geneva: World Health Organization. https://www.who.int/ihr/publications/9789241596664/en

Knobler, S., Mahmoud, A., Lemon, S., Mack, A., Sivitz, L., & Oberholtzer, K. (2004). Workshop summary. In *Learning from SARS: Preparing for the Next Disease Outbreak* (p. 11). National Academies Press.

Langmuir, A. D. (1963). The surveillance of communicable diseases of national importance. *The New England Journal of Medicine*, *268*(4), 182–192. doi:10.1056/NEJM196301242680405 PMID:13928666

McNabb, K. (2004). Operations | Nursery operations. Encyclopedia of Forest Sciences, 649-657. doi:10.1016/b0-12-145160-7/00001-6

Niesters, H. G., Rossen, J. W., Van der Avoort, H., Baas, D., Benschop, K., Claas, E. C., Kroneman, A., Van Maarseveen, N., Pas, S., Van Pelt, W., Rahamat-Langendoen, J. C., Schuurman, R., Vennema, H., Verhoef, L., Wolthers, K., & Koopmans, M. (2013). Laboratory-based surveillance in the molecular era: The TYPENED model, a joint data-sharing platform for clinical and public health laboratories. *Eurosurveillance*, *18*(4). Advance online publication. doi:10.2807/ese.18.04.20387-en PMID:23369392

Nsubuga, P., White, M. E., Thacker, S. B., Anderson, M. A., Blount, S. B., Broome, C. V., Chiller, T. M., Espitia, V., Imtiaz, R., Sosin, D., Stroup, D. F., Tauxe, R. V., Vijayaraghavan, M., & Trostle, M. (2006). *Public Health Surveillance: A Tool for Targeting and Monitoring Interventions. Disease Control Priorities in Developing Countries* (2nd ed.). Oxford University Press.

Peden, M., McGee, K., & Sharma, G. (2002). *The Injury Chartbook: A Graphical Overview of the Global Burden of Injuries*. World Health Organization.

Ranger, T., & Slack, P. (Eds.), *Epidemics and ideas: essays on the historical perception of pestilences* (pp. 149–173). Cambridge University Press. doi:10.1017/CBO9780511563645

Rodríguez, M., Alfonso, P., MacGregor, J., Kanagarajah, K., Patel, S., & Schlagenhauf, D. (2020). Going global – Travel and the 2019 novel coronavirus. *Travel Medicine and Infectious Disease*, *33*. Advance online publication. doi:10.1016/j.tmaid.2020.101578 PMID:32044389

Rong, G. Y., Cao, Q. D., Hong, Z. S., Tan, Y. Y., Chen, S. D., Jin, H. J., Tan, K. S., Wang, D. Y., & Yan, Y. (2020). The origin, transmission and clinical therapies on coronavirus disease 2019 (COVID-19) outbreak – an update on the Status. *Military Medical Research*, *7*(1), 11. doi:10.118640779-020-00240-0 PMID:32169119

Salama, P., Spiegel, P., Talley, L., & Waldman, R. (2004). Lessons learned from complex emergencies over past decade. *Lancet*, *364*(9447), 1801–1813. doi:10.1016/S0140-6736(04)17405-9 PMID:15541455

Shaban-Nejad, A., Lavigne, M., Okhmatovskaia, A., & Buckeridge, D. L. (2016). (in press). PopHR: A knowledge-based platform to support integration, analysis and visualization of population health data. *Annals of the New York Academy of Sciences*. PMID:27750378

Sharma, G., Krug, E., & Lozano, R. (2000). Injury: A leading cause of the burden of disease. *Injury Control and Safety Promotion*, *7*(4), 261–267. doi:10.1076/icsp.7.4.261.7399

Snijder, E. J., Van der Meer, Y., Zevenhoven-Dobbe, J., Onderwater, J. J., Van der Meulen, J., Koerten, H. K., & Mommaas, A. M. (2006). Ultrastructure and origin of membrane vesicles associated with the severe acute respiratory syndrome coronavirus replication complex. *Journal of Virology*, *80*(12), 5927–5940. doi:10.1128/JVI.02501-05 PMID:16731931

Thacker, S. B. (2000). Historical development. In S. M. Teutsch & R. E. Churchill (Eds.), *Principles and Practice of Public Health Surveillance* (2nd ed., pp. 1–16). Oxford University Press.

Thacker, S. B., & Berkelman, R. L. (1988). Public Health Surveillance in the United States. *Epidemiologic Reviews*, *10*(1), 164–190. doi:10.1093/oxfordjournals.epirev.a036021 PMID:3066626

Thacker, S. B., & Stroup, D. F. (1998). Foreword. *Deciphering Global Epidemics*, *xix-xx*, xix xx. Advance online publication. doi:10.1017/CBO9780511549489.001

Vachon, D. (2005). Father of modern epidemiology. *Old News*, *16*(8), 8–10.

Villaveces, A., Peck, M., & Price, G. (2010). Process evaluation of emergency department use of an electronic data collection tool that incorporates the international classification of external causes of injury (ICECI) into the US national burn repository. *Injury Prevention*, *16*(Supplement 1), A73–A73. doi:10.1136/ip.2010.029215.266

Wang, W., Pullum, T., & Kishor, S. (2019). The demographic and health surveys (DHS). Encyclopedia of Gerontology and Population Aging, 1-5. doi:10.1007/978-3-319-69892-2_969-1

WHO publications. (1993). Article. *International Journal of Epidemiology*, *22*(6), 1212–1212. doi:10.1093/ije/22.6.1212

Woodruff, B. A. (2006). Interpreting mortality data in humanitarian emergencies. *Lancet*, *367*(9504), 9–10. doi:10.1016/S0140-6736(05)67637-4 PMID:16399135

World Health Organization. (2018). *Global tuberculosis report 2018*. WHO.

World Health Organization. (n.d.). *Infection prevention and control during health care when COVID-19 is suspected.* https://www.who.int/publications-detail/infection-prevention-and-control-during-health-care-when-novel-coronavirus-(ncov)infection-is-suspected-20200125

World Health Organization (WHO). (2020). *Coronavirus disease (COVID-19) Pandemic*. https://www.who.int/emergencies/diseases/novel-coronavirus-2019

World Health Statistics 2005. (2005). WHO.

Yang, W., Li, Z., Lan, Y., Ma, J., Jin, L., Lai, S., Liao, Y., Lv, W., Sun, Q., Wang, J. (2017). China Infectious Diseases Automated-Alert and Response System (CIDARS). *Early Warning for Infectious Disease Outbreak*, 131-161. . doi:10.1016/B978-0-12-812343-0.00007-2

Ziegler, M. (2015). *The Black Death and the future of the plague*. Pandemic Disease in the Medieval World. doi:10.2307/j.ctvmd83jc.14

Chapter 11
Applications of Nanoparticles in Various Fields

Vijeta Singh
Amity University, India

Sunishtha Singh Yadav
Amity University, India

Vandana Chauhan
Amity University, India

Shikha Shukla
Ranveer Ranjanay Post Graduate College, India

Krishan Kumar Vishnolia
University of Lübeck, Germany

ABSTRACT

Nanoparticles (NPs) are tiny particles having dimensions ranging from 1 nm to 100 nm. Nanoparticles are field of profound scientific interest, on account of diverse conceivable applications in various fields such as electronic, optical, agriculture, biomedical, etc. Many of the interesting properties of nanoparticles are intimately linked on shape and size of nanomaterials. In nanoparticles, percentage of surface atoms are high; nanoparticles show properties dependent on shape which are utilized in catalysis, optics, data storage, etc. Further, the physical properties of nanoparticles such as melting point, density, optical properties, electrical conductivity, chemical stability, etc. make them suitable candidates to be utilized in several fields. Many of the nanoparticles have been widely studied and many applications explored for example gold and silver nanoparticles, while research is being carried out to investigate the probable applications in several other fields. This review provides the readers a summary of the applications of various nanoparticles.

DOI: 10.4018/978-1-7998-6527-8.ch011

INTRODUCTION

Nanotechnology is well known, highly significant field of science which concern with the synthesis of nanoparticles of several chemical compositions, shapes, sizes and their uses for human welfare (Vineet and Sudesh, 2009). Nanoparticles have higher surface to volume ratio that transmit them different properties and hence make them feasible to be utilized in exclusive applications. In order to obtain nanoparticles for application, specific nano size of nanoparticle is attained through controlled synthesis (Fratoddi et al. 2017). Nanoparticles can either be hydrophilic or hydrophobic and this functionalization arbitrates their application. Nanoparticles consist of three layers (i) The first layer is characterized with various miniature particles, surfactants, metallic ions and polymers: the surface layer, (ii) the second layer distinct in configuration of chemicals from the origin segment, the shell layer, and (iii) central part of nanoparticles i.e. the core (Shin et al., 2016). Due to the remarkable properties, nanoparticles are of considerable interest for investigation in different fields. The nanoparticles can be utilized for various purposes in different fields such as medicine (Min-Dianey et al. 2018), agriculture (Rastogi et al. 2019), environmental remediation (Ghoto et al. 2019, Singh and Verma 2018), electronics (Tamilvanan et al. 2014), energy storage (Manj et al. 2018) etc (Figure 1). In the present chapter, we explain the several applications of nanoparticles as well as provide the future aspects of the applications of various nanoparticles.

Figure 1.

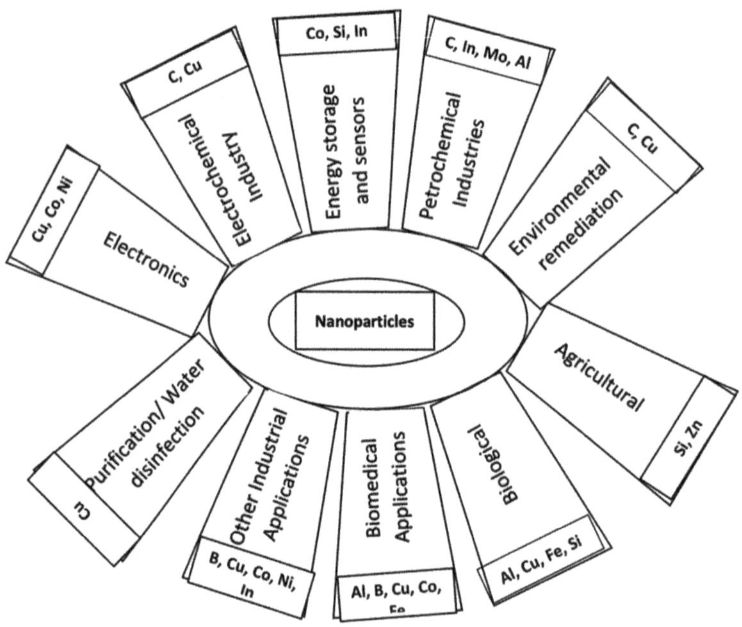

ALUMINUM NANOPARTICLES

Aluminum (Al) nanoparticles such as Al oxide (Al_2O_3) nanoparticles are the category of oxides of metal nanoparticles known to show varied biomedical utilities known to show varied biomedical utilities due to the extraordinary constitutional and physiochemical characteristics, for instance resistance to stresses against mechanical, chemical, wear besides their desirable optical traits and permeable ample surface area. The effortless handling, and small preparation cost are the other rationales for comprehensive usance of Al nanoparticles. The principle biomedical applications of Al nanoparticles are:

- **Antimicrobial Properties:** Al nanoparticles have extensive surface area as a result they exhibit substantial anti-microbial action. Antimicrobial effect of Al nanoparticles was verified by Sadiq. M. et al. (2009) against Escherchia coli (E. coli).
- **Cancer Therapy:** The nanotubes of Al oxide nanoparticles consisting of Thapsigarin, was administered along with an inhibitor of autophagy, viz. 3-methyladenine, so as to intent signaling of autophagy in both the normal as well as cancerous cells in human beings (Evdokiou et al. 2015).
- **Biosensing:** Al oxides nanoparticles are being contemplated as modern tools for apprehension of various molecules. The nanoparticles of Al oxides are being utilized to detect Bovine Serum Albumin (BSA) (Ito et al. 2017).
- **Drug Delivery:** Al nanoparticles such as mesoporous Al oxides are being utilized for enhanced oral administration of hypertension medication Telmisartan as a low water-soluble amalgam (Borbane et al. 2015).
- **Effective for Treatment of Other Diseases:** Alpha Al nanoparticles have been conjoined with intestinal peptide which is vasoactive so as to cure the asthma due to allergy in the model of mouse. The alpha Al nanoparticles were utilized for the stabilization of vasoactive peptides of intestine against degradation by enzymes in the pulmonary system of mouse model affected with asthma. It exhibited substantial activity against asthma in comparison to the non-conjoined beclomethasone and the vasoactive peptides of intestine (Shamsadin et al. 2016).
- **Stabilization and Preservation of Biomolecules**: Al nanoparticles could be used as nanoplatform to mend the protein molecules folding. Al nanoparticles interreact in electrostatic fashion with the remolded proteins which are negatively charged and hence avert their mis-folding and aggregation (Volodina et al. 2017).
- **Immunotherapy:** Al nanoparticles are found to exhibit the ability to induce autophagy. Induction of autophagy is the principle objective of vaccines for next generation and immunotherapy, this is due to the main aspect of autophagy in the introduction of the antigens to the T-lymphocytes. Aluminum nanoparticles conjugated to cysteine peptidase A as well as B were utilized as vaccination for leishmania so as to activate the process of autophagy in macrophage cells. The conjugated form of Al nanoparticles demonstrated the expeditious internalization via macrophages infected with leishmania consequent to administrating Al nanoparticles (Beyzay et al. 2017).

Other applications of Al nanoparticles:

- **Al Nanoparticles as Propellants:** Al nanoparticles of various sizes are being used for the production of compound for rocket propellent. Al nanoparticles have found application in various fields such as military as coolant and fuel for rocket, heat resistant layer of aircraft, corrosion, automobiles.
- **Al Nanoparticles as Energetic Materials:** Al nanoparticles are extensively used for military purposes as energetic materials. They are used in explosives to enhance the temperature of the reaction and elevate the energies of the bubbles in weapons used under the water. Aluminum

nanoparticles have application as constituents of explosives and propellants for rockets (Piercey and Klapotkes 2010).

- **Boron:** Boron is categorized as a metalloid and has an atomic number of 5. It is a fundamental trace element for plants. Due to boron electronic structure and its capacity to frame covalent bonds with carbon, boron is generally utilized in synthetic chemistry. Boron has intense scope of utilizations in chemistry, material science, energy research, and life sciences.

Materials made of boron have a differing scope of utilizations in regions, for example, Boron nitride as semiconductors (Zhou et al. 2018), insulating layer (Bekish et al. 2010), large density liquors (Millot et al. 2002), malignant growth therapy (Singh et al. 2019).

The expansion of substances added with boron enhance the friction coefficient that develops the conductance of anti-wear upon use as lubricant oil. Boron nanomaterial's have an assortment of fascinating properties that are reasonable for such decent variety. The large surface volume ratio of nanoparticles made of boron combined with the huge energy content of boron make these nanoparticles appealing to be used as fuel added substances for fuels as hydrocarbon for air-breathing pressure frameworks. The strong electrical and thermal stabilities contrasted with metallic nanowires, makes 1-D nanostructures of boron, for example, wires, rods, belts or tubes of boron nanoparticles favorable materials for application in Nano electronic gadgets as electric conducting interconnects. Nanoparticles mainly based on boron are currently being utilized in Boron Neutron Capture Therapy (BNCT) as a source of Boron. Nanowires of boron have potentiality to be employed in the field of electronics by assembling them to be modified as electric wires of nanoscale. The homogenous conductivity, mechanical aspect, thermal as well as chemical stability are prominent components for the functions firmly identified with the nanowire structure along with morphology.

- **Carbon:** Carbon is special amid the elements as it has the ability to articulate steadily secured chains enclosed via hydrogen atoms. Such hydrocarbons, which are typically used as the sources of non-renewable energy for example coal, gaseous petrol and oil are commonly made use as energizes. A small yet significant part is exploited in petrochemical industries as a source of feedstock conveying solvents, paints, plastics, polymers etc. (Alsaba et al. 2020).

The later disclosure of carbon nanotubes, different fullerenes and atom thin sheets of graphene have changed equipment improvements in the gadgets business and in nanotechnology by and large, while the utilization of nano diamonds, nano-onions, peapods, nanofibers, nano rings etc. are well known, the on-going functions mostly center around the operation of fullerenes and carbon nanotubes.

Carbon nanotubes (CNTs) as well as fullerenes serve as the most significant categories of nanoparticles based on carbon element. They have extensive advantage in industries and have widespread business due to the exclusive properties as great quality, high affinity to electrons, structure, flexibility and electrical conductivity (Astefanei et al. 2015). Because of their novel mechanical, physical, chemical attributes, these carbon nanotubes have significant applications in pristine form along with nano composites for some commercial operations, acting as fillers (Saeed and Khan 2014), in bioremediation as effective adsorbents of gas (Ngoy et al. 2014), as well as they are utilized for various organic media along with inorganic catalysts as a support medium (Mabena et al. 2011).

- **Copper Nanoparticles:** Copper nanoparticles find applications in various areas owing to their characteristic traits. Some of the important applications of copper nanoparticles are:
- **Antimicrobial activity of Copper Nanoparticles (CuNPs):** Copper nanoparticles antimicrobial activity is widely studied. As a result of antimicrobial effect of CuNPs, they are being used in the field of medicine and dentistry.
- **CuNPS in Medicine:** CuNPs are effective in treating common microbial infections especially bacterial infections in respiratory, circulatory and digestive systems. CuNPs have shown Imaging functions and increased antithrombic response. Drugs incorporated with CuNPs are utilized to damage cancerous and tumorous cells (Halevas and Pantazaki 2018).
- **CuNPs in Dentistry:** CuNPs fusion to orthopedic dental adhesive shows significant bactericidal response to S. aureus, S. mutans, and E. coli; increased adhesive properties without affecting the shear bond strength by incorporating as nanofillers. CuNPs are utilized for B. subtilis as they have affinity for surface active bacterial species (Ruparclia et al. 2008).
- **Cu nanoparticles in Antimicrobial Textile and Finishing Treatments:** CuNPs act on cotton fabric after altering its surface, they work either as fillers or cross-linking components, thereby strengthening the fabric and dye bond and improve the bond quality (Chattopadhyay and Patel 2010).
- **CuNPS in Electronic Applications:** CuNPs has vital applications in conductive printing. They can replace expensive silver nano inks in conductive printing. Recently, a technique has been developed which can develop a material consisting of CuNPs, can replace expensive silver and gold nanoparticles in electronics, and can be used to fabricate electronic components based on environment friendly production techniques (Tamilvanan et al. 2014). Thus, CuNPs finds important application in printed electronics. Further, CuNPs have potential to build a lead-free stable solder to be used for high stress environments and space missions.
- **Cu Nanoparticles in Biological and Biosensing Applications:** CuNPs can be employed in biosensing and biological operations. Preparation of CuNPs via nanosphere lithography method can be utilized in some applications in place of costly silver and gold nanoparticles (Goel et al. 2013).
- **Cu Nanoparticles in Electrochemical Capacitors:** Multilayer nanosheets of coper oxide exhibits hydrophilic character and the electrodes of copper oxide show high capacitance and hence they are reasonable material to be utilized in electrochemical capacitors (Wu et al. 2015).
- **Cu Nanoparticles in Pesticide Detection/ Environmental Remediation:** CuNPs coated as colorimetric probe on cetyltrimethyl ammonium bromide (CTAB) can be used for sensing Zineb, Ziram, Maneb and dithiocarbamates (DTCs) in the environment or as well as in beverages. Chitosan-copper nanocomposites can be utilized for the extraction of organophosphorous pesticides from the soil (Ghoto et al. 2019).
- **Cu Nanoparticles as Potent Anticancer Agents:** CuNPs have potential to alter surface properties as they can conjugate with biomolecules and hence can be used as components to cleave DNA and cogent therapeutics for cancer. They can also control growth of cancer cells by working in molecular doping techniques and as nano-formulations in drug delivery methods. Nanomaterials such as Chitosan-copper nanocomposites are being used in environmental remediation and biological applications. These nanomaterials can promote shrinkage and blebbing of cancer cells, lower the cell-cell interaction and cell density compared with untreated cells (Halevas and Pantazaki 2018).
- **Cu Nanoparticles as Water Disinfectant:** Microbial contamination of water is a noteworthy danger to human well-being and therefore number of methods to disinfect water have developed

rapidly as microbes become resistant to earlier antimicrobial components. A novel and effective technique is the use of CuNPs to disinfect wastewater (Ruparelia et al. 2008).

- **Cu nanoparticles as Catalyst:** CuNPs application in dye reduction, reduction of nitrobenzene etc. CuNPs work as heterogenous catalyst in several chemical transformations. CuNPs catalyzed reactions are small in catalyst loading, yield better, recyclable catalyst, cost effective, less reaction times and hence have more advantage compared with the conventional reactions catalyzed with metals (Ojha et al. 2017).
- **Cu Nanoparticles as Additives:** CuNPs when added to oil increase gasoline engine performance by improving the anti-wear and reduction in friction. The carbon-coated CuNPs addition to poly-alphaolefin reduced the wear and improved the capacity of the base oil in terms of load-import (Borda et al. 2018). Thus, these CuNPs can be utilized as additives in industry.
- **Cobalt Nanoparticles:** Cobalt is a chemical compound and symbolized as Co with atomic number 27. Cobalt is silver-white in colour with a somewhat blue tinge. It is a hard, ferromagnetic, weak element. Cobaltite, smaltite, and erythrite are the ores of cobalt. It is also obtained as a by-product from lead, nickel, silver, copper and iron mining.

Among the metallic Nanoparticles, Co is one among the potent elements and is of incredible interest over quite a while for scientists from different scientific fields for various relevance. Commonly, Co nanoparticles have magnificent attractive, reactant and electrical traits, that have scientific and mechanical use for different areas, inclusive of use as magnetic fluids and sensors (Dutz et al. 2020), record-keeping media, catalysis and so forth. As of late, Co NPs were additionally seen as appealing for electromagnetic wave retention applications, for example, the advancement of wireless communication. In particular, the Co NPs likewise have a natural favorable position in biomedical related ðelds like drug delivery (Ansari et al. 2017).

- **Iron (Fe) Nanoparticles:** There are distinctive properties of iron chemical compound nanoparticles (IONPs) that are useful in many biomedical applications such as, medicine, imaging tool, magnetic separator, drug delivery, cell proliferation regulator and tissue repair. The higher mixture stability, biocompatibility, and persistence magnetic properties of IONPs make them ideal for medical specialty applications (Huang et al. 2009).

There are few recent developments in the technology aiming towards the development of novel protein mimetics, nanozymes exhibiting biological enzyme, peroxidase, catalase, and superoxide dismutase-like activities (Karim et al. 2018). There are intrinsic biological enzyme-like properties possessed by Nanozymes. Nanozymes are nanomaterials which provide many benefits over natural enzymes such as high stability and activity at broad range of pH and temperatures. Nanozymes can be subjected to straightforward manipulation and multiple applications on one platform. The iron chemical compound nanoparticles (IONPs) have been exploited in medical applications and biotechnological advances such as resonance imaging, cell separation and detection, tissue repair, magnetic physiological condition and drug delivery.

Due to their outstanding properties, like super para magnetism, small size and risk of receiving a biocompatible coating. Also, to reduce drug resistance to standard antibiotics, antibiotic carrier nano-systems have been developed which could be an alternative to traditional antibiotics. These IONPs coupled with metal are used as carriers of antibiotic drug (El Zowalaty et al 2015). It was also demonstrated that a physical mixture of antibiotics showed a speedy unharness (20 min) in phosphate-buffered saline, whereas the nano based antibiotic system showed its full unharness was completed solely in 350 min, indicating the power of IONs to act in controlled release systems. Also new generation of environmental improvement technologies have been proposed by Nanoscale iron particles which might provide cost-efficient solutions to number of difficult environmental cleanup issues. Nanoscale iron particles have known to have massive surface areas and high surface reactivity. It is also important to point out that they have monumental flexibility for various applications. Analysis has shown that the high effectiveness of nanoscale iron particles towards the transformation and detoxification of common environmental contaminants, like chlorinated organic solvents, organochlorine pesticides, and PCBs.

The magnetic nanoparticles have some important physical and chemical characteristics that make them ideal for wide range of medical specialty applications, distinction agents in resonance imagining (MRI) (Wilczewska et al. 2012), cell separation and detection (Lin et al. 2017), treatment for physiological condition (Zhang et al. 2016) and drug delivery (Saikia et al. 2016). Especially, IONPs are biocompatible and environmentally safe (Lu et al. 2007), therefore presenting distinctive characteristics for clinical applications. However, once IONPs (Fe3O4 (magnetite) or -Fe2O3 (maghemite)) reach smaller sizes (about 10–20 nm for iron oxide), they acquire super paramagnetic properties and these particles reach a stronger performance for many of the above-mentioned applications (Lu et al. 2007.) Due to their strong magnetic properties, iron chemical compound NPs were initially used in biology in the magnetic separation of biological merchandise and cells furthermore as magnetic steering of particle systems for site-specific drug delivery (Estelrich et al. 2015).

The bio distribution of the NPs is determined by the surface chemistry, size, and charge of magnetic particles which influence activities within the clinical applications. The recent decades use of magnetic carriers and particles are augmenting due to their important role in medicine and treatment modalities (Mahdavi et al. 2013). Magnetic NPs have also attracted abundant role as a labeling material in life sciences and numerous alternatives in dominant fields of the experimental world.

- **Indium Nanoparticles:** The unusual material properties of indium its strong effective resonances which can be further extended up to the ultraviolet. When combined with low cost, this extended response, along with easy synthesis process, allow a range of applications of indium and makes it highly promising material of the era (Meshgi et al. 2016).
- **Semiconductor Application:** The most versatile use of Indium is in the semiconductor industry, like solders made through low-melting-point (soft-metal high-vacuum seals).
- **Conductive Coating Application:** The transparent conductive coatings of on glass is made of Indium nanoparticles called indium tin oxide (ITO).
- **Solar Cell Application:** The nano-powder or nanoparticles of Indium can be utilized for production of electronic devices and different materials such as solar cells. Based on this, researchers from the Lund University in Sweden came up with solar cell produced from indium phosphide nanowires, a novel type in January 2013. These nanowires match the electrical output of conventional thin-film solar cells and occupy only a fraction of the space (Wallentin et al. 2013).
- **LCD Panels Application:** These are also used in LCD panels and it is also mixed with welding alloy so that the melting point of the alloy shall be lowered down.
- **Combustion Application:** The nano-powder or nanoparticles of indium are also used in rocket fuel as combustion improver.

Researchers are looking at ways to further exploit the nanoparticles' potential magnetic, bioscience, biomedical, optical, electrical, optical and properties.

- **Molybdenum Nanopowder / Nanoparticles:** Molybdenum is not found as free metal naturally on earth, instead it exists in several oxidation states. Around 14% of the Molybdenum production of the world have industrial applications and are generally utilized either as catalysts, pigments or have elevated pressure and elevated temperature applications (Fakhri and Nejad 2016).
- **Lubricant & Coating Application:** Mo nanoparticles/nanopowder give very good result in situations where a lubricant is needed to withstand high temperatures. Molybdenum nanoparticles/nanopowder are well-known as a coating of choice in high-friction, heavy load Environments, due to the extreme lubrication they offer.
- **Anti-corrosive Application:** Molybdenum nanoparticles/nanopowder are used in steel as anti-corrosive additives, vacuum valves & hard alloys.
- **Sintering Additives Application:** In the manufacture of high-pressure vacuum tubes, heat tubes, X-Ray tubes Molybdenum Nanoparticles/Nanopowder can be useful.
- **Cutting Tools Application:** Molybdenum nanoparticles/nanopowder offer a simple, effective way to apply such coatings with extreme precision.
- **Nickel Nanopowder / Nanoparticles Application:** Several uses of nickel nanoparticles has been addressed like conductor, addictive, electromagnetic shield catalyst etc. Furthermore, the nanopowders of nickel can be handled as ethanol suspensions or in other solvents.
- **Catalyst for Combustion:** Research has already suggested the viability in a host of combustive applications of nickel nano-powder as a catalyst for combustion of liquid or solid propellants. The upcoming investigation suggests further possibilities and horizons for use of nickel in fuel production, even after ignored energetics due to its relatively low energy density. The extra ordinary behavior of nickel has been revisited as research into nano-powder resurges.
- **Application as Additive:** Due to the unusual properties' nano-powder of nickel it's one of the most common and popular additives in the manufacturing of several different materials which includes different varieties of ceramics and lubricants. Moreover, it provides sintering of another materials aid as an additive.
- **Applications in Electronics:** The most common application of nano-powder/nanomaterials of nickel is in different domains of electronics. Nickel has also been used in the manufacturing or as a component for electrode terminations, capacitors, metal base electrodes, electromagnetic shielding, pastes, conductive coatings, ferrofluids etc.
- **Uranium Purification Process:** Different research works have evidenced that nickel interacts with uranium and it's a viable and effective material which helps in the purification of uranium. Though further research is needed but the initial data proves the significance of nickel in various industrial applications and certain projects on environment (Crane et al. 2015).
- **Application as an Electrode:** These days the modified electrodes of nickel nanoparticles are utilized as an ultra-sensitive electrochemical insulin and urea detection.

Silicon Nanoparticles

- **Energy Storage and Sensors:** Silicon nanoparticles (SiNPs) possess characteristics such as stability, large surface area, magnificent electrical and optical properties and biocompatibility. SiNPs are porous and hence these mesoporous nanoparticles are suitable in bioscience as well as energy storage applications. SiNPs enhance the electrochemical characteristics in Lithium-ion batteries when replaced with Silicon anodes. These are showing good results in gas sensors and biosensors (Manj et al. 2018).

- **Biological Applications:** SiNPs, due to non-toxic, biocompatible and other unique properties find bio-applications as diagnostics, nanocarriers, and for cancer treatment (Min-Dianey et al. 2018).
- **Drug Delivery:** Mesoporous Silica Nanoparticles (MSNs) when modified can be utilized as multifunctional system for delivery of drugs. MSNs have structure, which is multi-functional, porous, less cytotoxic etc. MSNs can carry various sizes of molecules of drug as their morphologies and pores can be adjusted. MSNs can also enhance the solubility of compounds and hence make them bioavailable and their surfaces can be modified with various functional groups (Watermann and Brieger 2017). Therefore, MSNs delivery system has significant potential for tumor diagnosis and cancer treatment.
- **Regeneration of Tissues:** MSNs can generate nanosized apatite of carbon upon reacting with the physiological environment of the bone and hence by utilizing silanol groups on their surface MSNs have applications in tissue engineering of bones (Rosenholm et al. 2016).
- **Bioimaging:** Due to characteristic properties of MSNs they can support an imaging substance for development of targeted bioimaging. The properties of MSNs are thus suitable for high speed, long-term, real time bioimaging with laser irradiation (Cha and Kim 2019).
- **Energetic Material Applications:** Silicon quantum dots can be fabricated and modified which have the capacity to maintain properties of porous silicon which make it feasible for highly energetic material reaction to manifest (Adams et al. 2018). Hence, they can be utilized for applications of energetic material.
- **Applications in Agriculture:** SiNPs can be utilized as pesticides, delivery agent for herbicides and fertilizers, target specific delivery of proteins, nucleotides, and chemicals in plants, as a component of nanozeolite for increasing water-holding capacity and as nanosensors. Hence, SiNPs have prospects to reform agriculture (Rastogi et al. 2019).
- **Enhancement of Solar Cells:** Scientists have improved the performance of perovskite solar cells by using SiNPs which can absorb broad wavelength of light, without interaction with other battery elements. Such Perovskite solar cells are cost effective as SiNPs are inexpensive and easily produced (Furasova et al. 2018).
- **Adsorption and Separation of Protein:** MSNs are potential to act as protein carriers for in vivo and in vitro delivery. Further, they are optimal candidates for adsorption and separation of specific protein molecules. This is due to the physiochemical property, low cost, adjustable size of pores, structure, possibility of distinct surface functionalization (Lui and Xu 2019). Thus, they are useful for bio- separation, immunoassays, enzyme immobilization and biosensors.
- **Zinc Nanoparticles:** Zinc nanoparticles have widespread applications in various fields. Some of the uses of zinc nanoparticles are list below:
- **Zinc (Zn) Nanoparticles Medicinal Uses:** In rats zinc nanoparticles are found to regulate in vitro synaptic transmission and to alter the spatial cognition ability by increasing longstanding potentiation. It has been known that Zn Oxide nanoparticles revelation has the potential to cause genotoxicity via oxidative stress and lipid peroxidation. As a result of the targeting possibility Zinc Oxide nanoparticles can find therapeutic applications for the autoimmune related diseases and cancer treatment (Hanley et al. 2008).

Table 1.

Nanoparticles	Applications	References
Aluminum	Biomedical (antimicrobial, cancer therapy, biosensing, drug delivery, treatment of diseases, immunotherapy	Hassanpour et al. 2018
	Preservation and stabilization of biomolecules	Volodina et al. 2017
	Propellants and energetic materials	Piercey and Klapotkes 2010
Boron	Semiconductors, Insulating layer, Large density liquors	Zhou et al. 2018
	Malignant growth therapy	Singh et al. 2019
Carbon	Petrochemical Industries, Electrochemical conductivity, Fillers	Alsaba et al. 2020, Astefani et al. 2015
	Bioremediations	Ngoy et al. 2014
Copper	Medicine (anticancer agents) and Dentistry Biological and biosensing	Ruparelia et al. 2018 Goel et al. 2013
	Antimicrobial textiles	Chattopadhyay and Patel 2010
	Electronic applications Electrochemical capacitors	Tamilvanan et al. 2014 Wu et al. 2015
	Catalysts, additives	Borda et al. 2018
	Water disinfectant	Ruparelia et al. 2018
	Environmental remediation	Ghoto et al. 2019
Cobalt	Magnetic fluids and sensors, Record-keeping media, Catalysis, Electromagnetic wave retention applications	Dutz et al. 2020
	Drug delivery	Ansari et al. 2017
Iron	Biomedical applications Protein mimetics	Karim et al. 2018
Indium	Semiconductor, conductive coating, solar cell, LDC panels, combustion applications	Wallentin et al. 2013
Molybdenum	Lubricant and coating, anti-corrosive sintering and cutting applications	Fakhri and Nejad 2016
Nickel	Combustion, additives, electronics, purification, electrode	Crane et al. 2015
Silicon	Energy storage and sensors	Manj et al. 2018
	Biological	Watermann and Brieger 2017
	Agricultural	Rastogi et al. 2018
Zinc	Medical uses	Hanley et al. 2008
	Agricultural applications	Prasad et al. 2012

- **Agricultural Applications of Zn Nanoparticles:** Zinc oxide nanoparticles have the capability to enhance the growth and yield of crop plants. Zinc oxide at various concentrations were used as treatment to enhance germination of seed, growth of plant, vigor of seedlings. Zinc oxide nanoparticles were noticed to be efficient to enhance root and stem growth of Peanut plants (Prasad et al. 2012). The zinc oxide nanoparticles solution can be used as fertilizer. Such nano fertilizer performs significant part in the agriculture. Another benefit of nanoparticles is they can be applied in very less quantity.
- **Skin Penetration:** Zinc oxide nanoparticles are specially used in sunscreens as they have inherent capacity to permeate UVA and UVB radiation. Because of this exceptional trait Zinc oxide

nanoparticles-based sunscreens provide extensive protection compared to other sunscreen agents. However, these nanoparticles have the potential via skin surface and to enter feasible cells causing the probable toxic effect expended by them (Mohammed et al. 2019).

CONCLUSION

Evidences are very clear that the nanoparticles have applications in several fields (Table 1). The various nanoparticles have been explored for drug delivery, antimicrobial properties, imaging, biosensing etc. in biomedical field. Similarly, various nanoparticles have potential to be used effectively to solve problems related to environmental field such as for bioremediation, agriculture, water purification as well as manufacturing of clean and efficient energy. However, for metallic nanoparticles to be further used more effectively in various aspects such as therapeutic treatment, it is important to study the in vivo toxicity and effects associated with long-term exposure. Further, more studies are needed to establish safe design, use, and dispose products including metal nanoparticles without novel hazard to human beings or the surroundings.

REFERENCES

Adams, S. K., Piekiel, N. W., Ervin, M. H., & Morris, C. J. (2018). Silicon quantum dots for energetic material applications. *Applied Physics Letters*, *112*(23), 233108. doi:10.1063/1.5022587

Alsaba, M. T., Al Dushaishi, M. F., & Abbas, A. K. (2020). A comprehensive review of nanoparticles application in the oil and gas industry. *Journal of Petroleum Exploration and Production Technology*, *10*(4), 1389–1300. doi:10.100713202-019-00825-z

Ansari, S. M., Bhoi, R. D., Pai, K. R., Sen, D., Mazumder, D., Ghosh, K., Kolekar, Y. D., & Ramana, C. V. (2017). Cobalt nanoparticles for biomedical applications: Facile synthesis, physiochemical characterization, cytotoxicity behavior and biocompatibility. *Applied Surface Science*, *414*, 171–187. doi:10.1016/j.apsusc.2017.03.002

Astefanei, A., Nunez, O., & Galceran, M. (2015). Characterization and Determination of Fullerenes: A Critical Review. *ChemInform*, *46*(33), 19–21. doi:10.1002/chin.201533304

Bekish, Y. N., Poznyak, S. K., Tsybulskaya, L. S., & Gaevskaya, T. V. (2010). Electrodeposited Ni–B alloy coatings: Structure, corrosion resistance and mechanical properties. *Electrochimica Acta*, *55*(7), 2223–2231. doi:10.1016/j.electacta.2009.11.069

Beyzay, F., Hosseini, A. Z., & Soudi, S. (2017). Alpha alumina nanoparticle conjugation to cysteine peptidase A and B: An efficient method for autophagy induction. *Avicenna Journal of Medical Biotechnology*, *9*(2), 71–81.

Bogart, L.K., Morozov, I.G., Parkin, I.V., & Kuznetcov, M.V. (2018). Fe Mössbauer study of NiFe2O4 nanoparticles produced by the levitation-jet aerosol technique. *Journal of Materials Science: Materials in Electronics, 29*(10). 1007/s10854-018-9569

Borbane, S. A., Pande, V. V., Vibhute, S. K., Kendre, P. N., & Dange, V. U. (2015). Design and Fabrication of ordered meso-porous alumina scaffold for drug delivery of poorly water-soluble drug. *Austin Therapeutics*, *2*(1), 1015.

Borda, F.L.G., Oliveria, S.J.R., Lazaro, L.M.S.M., & Leiroz, A.J.K. (2018). *Experimental investigation of the tribological behavior of lubricants with additive containing copper nanoparticles*. Academic Press.

Cha, B. G., & Kim, J. (2019). Functional mesoporous silica nanoparticles for bio-imaging applications. *Wiley Interdisciplinary Reviews. Nanomedicine and Nanobiotechnology*, *11*(1), 1–22. doi:10.1002/wnan.1515

Chattopadhyay, D. P., & Patel, B. H. (2010). Effect of Nanosized Colloidal Copper on Cotton Fabric. *Journal of Engineered Fibers and Fabrics*, *5*(3), 1–6. doi:10.1177/155892501000500301

Crane, R. A., Pullin, H., Macfarlane, J., Silion, M., Popescu, I. C., Andersen, M., Calen, V., & Scott, T. B. (2015). Field Application of Iron and Iron-Nickel Nanoparticles for the Ex Situ Remediation of a Uranium-Bearing Mine Water Effluent. *Journal of Environmental Engineering*, *141*(8), 8. doi:10.1061/(ASCE)EE.1943-7870.0000936

Dorn, V., Chopa, A., & Radivoy, G. (2016). Mild bottom-up synthesis of indium (0) nanoparticles: Characterization and application in the allylation of carbonyl compounds. *RSC Advances*, *6*(28), 23798–23803. doi:10.1039/C5RA27928C

Dutz, S., Buske, N., Landers, J., Grafe, C., Wende, H., & Clement, J. H. (2020). Biocompatible Magnetic Fluids of Co-Doped Iron Oxide Nanoparticles with Tunable Magnetic Properties. *Nanomaterials (Basel, Switzerland)*, *10*(6), 1019. doi:10.3390/nano10061019

El Zowalaty, M. E., Hussein-Al-Ali, S. H., Husseiny, M. I., Geilich, B. M., Webster, T. J., & Hussein, M. Z. (2015). The ability of streptomycin-loaded chitosan-coated magnetic nanocomposites to possess antimicrobial and antituberculosis activities. *International Journal of Nanomedicine*, *10*, 3269–3274. doi:10.2147/IJN.S74469

Estelrich, J., Escribano, E., Queralt, J., & Busquets, M. A. (2015). Iron oxide nanoparticles for magnetically guided and magnetically responsive drug delivery. *International Journal of Molecular Sciences*, *16*(4), 8070–8101. doi:10.3390/ijms16048070

Fakhri, A., & Nejad, A. P. (2016). Antimicrobial, antioxidant and cytotoxic effect of Molybdenum trioxide nanoparticles and application of this for degradation of ketamine under different light illumination. *Journal of Photochemistry and Photobiology*, *159*, 211–217. doi:10.1016/j.jphotobiol.2016.04.002

Fazio, E., Speciale, A., Spadaro, S., Bonsignore, M., Cimino, F., Cristani, M., Trombetta, D., Saija, A., & Neri, F. (2018). Evaluation of biological response induced by molybdenum oxide nanocolloids on in vitro cultured NIH/3T3 fibroblast cells by micro-Raman spectroscopy. *Colloids and Surfaces. B, Biointerfaces*, *1*(170), 233–241. doi:10.1016/j.colsurfb.2018.06.028

Fratoddi, I., Matassa, R., Fontana, L., Venditti, I., Familiari, G., Battocchio, C., Magnono, E., Nappini, S., Leahu, G., Belardini, A., & … . (2017). Electronic Properties of a Functionalized Noble Metal Nanoparticles Covalent Network. *The Journal of Physical Chemistry C*, *121*(33), 18110–18119. doi:10.1021/acs.jpcc.7b07176

Furasova, A. D., Zakhiodov, A. A., Di Carlo, A., & Makarov, S. V. (2018). Resonant Silicon Nanoparticles for Enhanced Light Harvesting in Halide Pervskite Solar Cells. *Journal of Physics: Conference Series*, *1092*(012038).

Ghoto, S. A., Khuhawar, M. Y., Jahangir, T. M., & Mangi, J. D. (2019). Applications of copper nanoparticles for colorimetric detection of dithiocarbamate pesticides. *Journal of Nanostructure in Chemistry*, *1*(2), 1–17. doi:10.100740097-019-0299-4

Goel, S., Chen, F., & Cai, W. (2013). Synthesis and biomedical applications of copper sulfide nanoparticles: From sensors to theranostics. *Small*, *10*(4), 631–645. doi:10.1002mll.201301174

Halevas, E. G., & Pantazaki, A. A. (2018). Copper Nanoparticles as Therapeutic Anticancer Agents. *Nanomedicine and Nanotechnology Journal*, *2*(1), 119.

Hanley, C., Layne, J., Punnoose, A., Reddy, K. M., Coombs, I., Coombs, A., Feris, K., & Wingett, D. (2008). Preferential killing of cancer cells and activated human T cells using ZnO nanoparticles. *Nanotechnology*, *19*(29), 295103. doi:10.1088/0957-4484/19/29/295103

Hassanpour, P., Panahi, Y., Ebrahimi-Kalan, A., Akbarzadeh, A., Davaran, S., Nasibova, A. N., Khalilov, R., & Kavetskyy, T. (2018). Biomedical applications of aluminium oxide nanoparticles. *Micro & Nano Letters*, *13*(9), 1227–1231. doi:10.1049/mnl.2018.5070

Huang, D. M., Hsiao, J. K., Chen, Y. C., Chien, L. Y., Yao, M., Chen, Y. K., Ko, B. S., Hsu, S. C., Tai, L. A., Cheng, H. Y., Wang, S. W., Yang, C. S., & Chen, Y. C. (2009). The promotion of human mesenchymal stem cell proliferation by superparamagnetic iron oxide nanoparticles. *Biomaterials*, *30*(22), 3645–3651. doi:10.1016/j.biomaterials.2009.03.032

Ito, T., Matsuda, Y., Jinba, T., Asai, N., Shimizu, T., & Shingubara, S. (2017). Fabrication and Characterization of nonoporous lattice biosensor using anodic aluminum oxide substrate. *Japan Society of Applied Physics*, *56*, 6S1.

Karim, M. N., Anderson, S. R., Singh, S., Ramanathan, R., & Bansal, V. (2018). Nanostructured silver fabric as a free-standing NanoZyme for colorimetric detection of glucose in urine. *Biosensors & Bioelectronics*, *110*, 8–15. doi:10.1016/j.bios.2018.03.025

Kuznetcov, M. V., Morozov, Y. G., & Belousova, O. V. (2012). Levitation jet synthesis of nickel ferrite nanoparticles. *Inorganic Materials*, *48*(10), 1044–1051. doi:10.1134/S0020168512100020

Lin, R., Li, Y., MacDonald, T., Wu, H., Provenzale, J., Peng, X., Huang, J., Wang, L., Wang, A. Y., Yang, J., & Mao, H. (2017). Improving sensitivity and specificity of capturing and detecting targeted cancer cells with anti-biofouling polymer coated magnetic iron oxide nanoparticles. *Colloids and Surfaces. B, Biointerfaces*, *150*, 261–270. doi:10.1016/j.colsurfb.2016.10.026

Lu, A. H., Salabas, E. L., & Schüth, F. (2007). Magnetic nanoparticles: Synthesis, protection, functionalization, and application. *Angewandte Chemie International Edition in English*, *46*(8), 1222–1244. doi:10.1002/anie.200602866

Lui, H-J., & Xu, P. (2019). Smart Mesoporous Silicon Nanoparticles for Protein Delivery. *Nanomaterials*, *9*(511), 1-23.

Mabena, L. F., Sinha, R. S., Mhlanga, S. D., & Coville, N. J. (2011). Nitrogen-doped carbon nanotubes as a metal catalyst support. *Applied Nanoscience*, *1*(2), 67–77. doi:10.100713204-011-0013-4

Mahdavi, M., Ahmad, M. B., Haron, M. J., Namvar, F., Nadi, B., Rahman, M., & Amin, J. (2013). Synthesis, surface modification and characterization of biocompatible magnetic iron oxide nanoparticles for biomedical applications. *Molecules (Basel, Switzerland)*, *18*(7), 7533–7548. doi:10.3390/molecules18077533

Manj, R. Z. A., Chen, X., Rehman, W. U., Zhu, G., Luo, W., & Yang, J. (2018). Big Potential from Silicon-Based Porous Nanomaterials: In Field of Energy Storage and Sensors. *Frontiers in Chemistry*, *6*, 539. doi:10.3389/fchem.2018.00539

Meshgi, M. A., Kriechbaum, M., Biswas, S., Holmes, J. D., & Marschner, C. (2016). Synthesis of indium nanoparticles at ambient temperature; simultaneous phase transfer and ripening. *Journal of Nanoparticle Research*, *18*(12), 363. doi:10.100711051-016-3683-8

Millot, F., Rifflet, J. C., Sarou-Kanian, V., & Wille, G. (2002). High-Temperature Properties of Liquid Boron form Contactless Techniques. *International Journal of Thermophysics*, *23*(5), 1185–1195. doi:10.1023/A:1019836102776

Min-Dianey, K. A. A., Zhang, H. C., Brohi, A. A., Yu, H., & Xia, X. (2018). Optical spectrea of composite silver-porous silicon (Ag-pSi) nanostructure based periodical lattice. *Superlattices and Microstructures*, *115*, 168–176. doi:10.1016/j.spmi.2018.01.028

Mohammed, Y. H., Holmes, A., Haridass, I. N., Sanchez, W. Y., Studier, H., Grice, J. E., Benson, H. A. E., & Roberts, M. S. (2019). Support for the safe use of zinc oxide nanoparticles sunscreens: Lack of Skin Penetration or Cellular Toxicity After Repeated Application in Volunteers. *The Journal of Investigative Dermatology*, *139*(2), 308–315. doi:10.1016/j.jid.2018.08.024

Ngoy, J. M., Wagner, N., Riboldi, L., & Bolland, O. (2014). A CO_2 capture technology using multi-walled carbon nanotubes with polyaspartamide surfactant. *Energy Procedia*, *63*, 2230–2248. doi:10.1016/j.egypro.2014.11.242

Nguyen, N. S., Gautam, D., & Hee, Y. H. (2016). Nickel/cobalt oxide-decorated 3D graphene nanocomposite electrode for enhanced electrochemical detection of urea. *Biosensors & Bioelectronics*, *77*, 372–377. doi:10.1016/j.bios.2015.09.046

Ojha, N. K., Zyryanov, G. V., Majee, A., Charushin, V. N., Chupakhin, O. N., & Santra, S. (2017). Copper nanoparticles as inexpensive and efficient catalyst: A valuable contribution in organic synthesis. *Coordination Chemistry Reviews*, *353*, 1–57. doi:10.1016/j.ccr.2017.10.004

Piercey, D. G., & Klapoetke, T. M. (2010). Nanoscale Aluminium Metal Oxide (Thermite) Reactions for Application in Energetic Materials. *Central European Journal of Energetic Materials*, *7*(2), 115–129.

Prasad, T. N. V. K. V., Sudhakar, P., Sreenivasulu, Y., Latha, P., Munaswamy, V., Reddy, K. R., Sreeprasad, T. S., Sajanlal, P. R., & Pradeep, T. (2012). Effect of nanoscale Zinc Oxide Particles on the Germination, Growth and Yield of Peanut. *Journal of Plant Nutrition*, *35*(6), 905–927. doi:10.1080/01904167.2012.663443

Rastogi, A., Tripathi, D.K., Yadav, S., Chauhan, D.K., Ghorbanpour, M.Z.M., El-Sheery, N.I., & Brestic, M. (2019). Applications of silicon nanoparticles in agriculture. *Biotech, 9*(90), 1-11.

Rosenholm, J. M., Zhang, J., Linden, M., & Sahlgren, C. (2016). Mesoporous silica nanoparticles in tissue engineering- a prospective. *Nanomedicine (London), 11*(4), 391–402. doi:10.2217/nnm.15.212

Ruparelia, J. P., Chatterjee, A. K., Duttagupta, S. P., & Mukherji, S. (2008). Strain specificity in antimicrobial activity of silver and copper nanoparticles. *Acta Biomaterialia, 4*(3), 707–716. doi:10.1016/j.actbio.2007.11.006

Sadiq, M., Chowdhury, B., Chandrasekaran, N., & Mukherjee, A. (2009). Antimicrobial sensitivity of Escherichia coli to alumina nanoparticles. *Nanomedicine; Nanotechnology, Biology, and Medicine, 5*(3), 282–286. doi:10.1016/j.nano.2009.01.002

Saeed, K., & Khan, I. (2014). Preparation and properties of single-walled carbon nanotubes/poly (butylene terephthalate) Nano composites. *Iranian Polymer Journal, 23*(1), 53–58. doi:10.100713726-013-0199-2

Saikia, C., Das, M. K., Ramteke, A., & Maji, T. K. (2016). Effect of crosslinker on drug delivery properties of curcumin loaded starch coated iron oxide nanoparticles. *International Journal of Biological Macromolecules, 93*, 1121–1132. doi:10.1016/j.ijbiomac.2016.09.043

Shamsadin, S., Pourpak, Z., Folkerts, G., Garssen, J., Moin, M., Adcock, I. M., Movassaghi, M., Ardestani, M. S., Moazzeni, S. M., & Mortaz, E. (2016). Conjugated alpha-alumina nanoparticle with vasoactive intestinal peptide as a nono-drug in treatment of allergic asthma in mice. *European Journal of Pharmacology, 791*, 811–820. doi:10.1016/j.ejphar.2016.10.014

Shin, W. G., Calder, S., Ugurlu, O., & Girshick, S. L. (2011). Production and characterization of boron nanoparticles synthesized with a thermal plasma system. *Journal of Nanoparticle Research, 13*(12), 7187–7191. doi:10.100711051-011-0633-3

Singh, A., Kim, B. K., Mackeyev, Y., Rohani, P., Mahajan, S. D., Swihart, M. T., Krishan, S., & Prasad, P. N. (2019). Boron-Nanoparticles loaded folic acid functionalized liposomes to achieve optimum boron concentration for boron Neutron capture Therapy of Cancer. *Journal of Biomedical Nanotechnology, 15*(8), 1714–1723. doi:10.1166/jbn.2019.2800

Singh, V., & Verma, K. (2018). Metals from cell to environment: connecting metallomics with other omics. *Open Journal of Plant Science, 3*(1), 1-14

Tamilvanan, A., Balamurugan, K., Ponappa, K., & Madhan, K. B. (2014). Copper Nanoparticles: Synthesis Strategies, Properties and Multifunctional Application. *International Journal of Nanoscience, 13*(2), 143001–143022. doi:10.1142/S0219581X14300016

Thomas, E., Rathore, I., & Tarafdar, J. (2017). Bioinspired Production of Molybdenum Nanoparticles and Its Effect on Chickpea (Cicer arietinum L). *Journal of Bionanoscience., 11*(2), 1–7. doi:10.1166/jbns.2017.1425

Vineet, K., & Sudesh, K. Y. (2009). Plant mediated synthesis of silver and gold nanoparticles and their applications. *Journal of Chemical Technology and Biotechnology (Oxford, Oxfordshire), 84*(2), 151–157. doi:10.1002/jctb.2023

Volodina, K. V., Anvir, D., & Vinogradov, V. V. (2017). Alumina nanoparticle-assisted enzyme refolding: A versatile methodology for proteins renaturation. *Scientific Reports*, *7*(1), 1458. doi:10.103841598-017-01436-6

Wallentin, J., Anttu, N., Asoli, D., Huffman, M., Aberg, I., Magnusson, M.H., Siefer, G., Fudd-Kailuweit, P., Dimroth, F., Witzigmann, B., Xu, H.Q., Samuelson, L., Deppert, K., & Borgstrom, M.T. (2013). In P Nanowire Array Solar Cells Achieving 13.8% Efficiency by Exceeding the Ray Optics Limit. *Science*.

Watermann, A., & Brieger, J. (2017). Mesoporous Silica Nanoparticles as Drug Delivery Vehicles in Cancer. *Nanomaterials (Basel, Switzerland)*, *7*(7), 189. doi:10.3390/nano7070189

Wilczewska, A. Z., Niemirowicz, K., Markiewicz, K. H., & Car, H. (2012). Nanoparticles as drug delivery systems. *Pharmacological Reports*, *64*(5), 1020–1037. doi:10.1016/S1734-1140(12)70901-5

Wu, Q., Wang, X., Liao, C., Wei, Q., & Wang, Q. (2015). Microgel coating of magnetic nanoparticles via enzyme-mediated free-radical polymerization for colorimetric detection of glucose. *Nanoscale*, *7*(40), 16578–16582. doi:10.1039/C5NR05716G

Wu, R., Wang, D. P., Kumar, V., Zhou, K., Adrian, W. K. L., Lee, P. S., & Lou, J. (2015). MOFs-derived copper sulfides embedded within porous carbon octahedra for electrochemical capacitor applications. *Chemical Communications*, *15*(51), 3109–3112. doi:10.1039/C4CC09065A

Yanan, Y., Meisong, G., Mengwei, Y., Weitong, L., & Jingbo, H. (2016). Nickel nanoparticle-modified electrode for ultra-sensitive electrochemical detection of insulin. *Biosensors & Bioelectronics*, *77*, 215–219. doi:10.1016/j.bios.2015.09.036

Zhang, X. W., Zou, Y. J., Yan, H., Wang, B., Chen, G. H., & Wong, S. P. (2000). Electrical properties and annealing effects on the stress of RF-sputtered c-BN films. *Materials Letters*, *45*(2), 1110–1115. doi:10.1016/S0167-577X(00)00086-0

Zhang, Z. Q., & Song, S. C. (2016). Thermosensitive/superparamagnetic iron oxide nanoparticle-loaded nano capsule hydrogels for multiple cancer hyperthermia. *Biomaterials*, *106*, 13–23. doi:10.1016/j.biomaterials.2016.08.015

Zhou, C., Lai, C., Zhang, C., Zeng, G., Huang, D., Cheng, M., Hu, L., Xiong, W., Chen, M., Wang, J., Yang, Y., & Jiang, L. (2018). Semiconductor /boron nitride composites: Synthesis, properties, and photocatalysis applications. *Applied Catalysis B: Environmental*, *238*, 6–18. doi:10.1016/j.apcatb.2018.07.011

Chapter 12
Internet of Things (IoT) in Healthcare

Shashwat Pathak
Amity School of Engineering and Technology, Amity University, India

Shreyans Pathak
Jaypee Institute of Information Technology, India

ABSTRACT

The recent decade has seen considerable changes in the way the technology interacts with human lives and almost all the aspects of life be it personal or professional has been touched by technology. Many smart devices have also started playing a vital role in many fields and domains and the internet of things (IoT) has been the harbinger of the advent of IoT devices. IoT devices have proven to be monumental in imparting 'smartness' in the otherwise static machines. The ability of the devices to interact and transfer the data to the internet and ultimately to the end-user has revolutionized the technological world and has brought many seemingly disparate fields in the technological purview. Out of the many fields where IoT has started gaining momentum, one of the most important ones is the healthcare sector. Many wearable smart devices have been developed over time capable to transmit real-time data to hospitals and doctors. It is essential for tracking the progress of the critically ill patients and has opened the horizon for attending patients remotely using these smart devices.

INTRODUCTION

One of the most basic and yet essential services which need to be at the disposal of any human being is access to healthcare. Thanks to the improvements in the medical sciences in recent times we are currently living in an era where life expectancy has hit the best possible values in most of the countries. Providing the best possible healthcare and the best professionals in the business is the need of the hour for many of the developing countries and the rise of the technology is heralding a new era for both healthcare and technology as well. One of the recent additions to technological advancement is the advent of the Internet of Things. With the Internet of Things, many handheld or wearable devices can help to provide data

DOI: 10.4018/978-1-7998-6527-8.ch012

to the end-users, which in the case of healthcare would be the medical professionals or in some cases the ability to diagnose and interact with the patients without having any geographical limitations. The scope of the Internet of Things is wide and is on a rise and many seemingly disparate fields have come in the purview of the Internet of Things and many more fields are expected to incorporate the Internet of Things in their business in the coming future.

BACKGROUND

Internet of things, colloquially termed as IoT is a general term given to any device or artifact having the capability to collect and transmit the information via any source, generally, the internet or a broader definition of an IoT device is any device that is connected with the internet. Such devices are also termed as 'smart' devices as we can infer important information from the data provided. The initial IoT devices were the consumer devices like vending machines which could transmit the current status of the items to the users on a real-time basis and now with wider and easier access to the internet even more devices are now equipped with internet which can transfer data to the end-users whenever required. As mentioned earlier as well, the areas in which IoT can play a considerable role are expanding and one of the most important areas in which it covers is Healthcare. Healthcare domain has always been adapting the latest trends in science and technology and in current times with the advent in latest trends in technology, it is imperative for the healthcare domain to keep up with the latest developments in the field of science and technology and incorporate developments that ease and facilitate the tracking and monitoring of the patients on a real time basis, and IoT has just done that. With the provision of having the real time confrontation with the patient data, the healthcare professionals can have a better understanding of the patient's health aspects and another way in which it is beneficial is that it comes in pretty handy for the patients who are immobile due to some reason or have difficulty in travelling to the healthcare centers on a regular basis. Thus by having this virtual vigilance the patients and the professionals both will have considerable benefits in many different ways. Although setting up the infrastructure for effective transmission of data is quite essential here, which must be taken care of as we can not expect delays or lag in communication while the data is in transit. We can utilize the existing vast cloud computing architecture here for efficient data transfer, we will look into this in the upcoming sections (Erl et al., 2014).

IOT CONSTITUENTS

IoT comprises both hardware and software components and it is the combined work of these two core components which make the IoT devices function the way they do. Apart from these two main components, we can also integrate some of the existing technologies for our benefit in the IoT devices (Panigrahi et al., 2018). The main two components, hardware and software are mentioned briefly below

Hardware Components for IoT

The hardware components which are mostly used in the IoT applications employ a plethora of sensors as they are the primary source of collecting information from their surroundings. The major hardware components used in IoT are mentioned below

- **Sensors** As mentioned earlier as well sensors are the central to the success of the IoT devices as in the case of healthcare, mostly the sensors are embedded in the devices which are in close contact with the human body and can record and transmit data on a real time or in some cases they might not be put inside any specific device but are attached with the surface directly
- **Wearable Devices** These are the most common form of IoT devices and this has seen a surge in the recent years. These wearable devices are either in the form of smartwatches or bands which can easily be worn and these IoT devices are connected with a parent app where the users can see all the stats about their activities. Such devices have been in use in the fields of athletics, where the teams working on athletes used these wearable devices to monitor various parameters like heart rate, blood pressure etc and in the healthcare domain as well these kind of devices are quite handy and provide accurate data on real time (Vora, Tanwar, Tyagi et al, 2019). This is particularly helpful when the patient needs urgent care and such devices can really prove to be life saving

Software Components of IoT

The software components of the IoT comprise of the applications or software which can process the raw information provided by the sensors and then can elicit meaningful information and send the same to the concerned. The application might need to perform some pre-processing of the data followed by processing of the data and then finding relations and patterns in the data, something which is the domain of data mining and machine learning. The final data is then displayed on the front end to the end user.

Potential Technologies for IoT

Various technologies and protocols have been integrated for utilizing their potential in the IoT domain and some of the most common technologies are listed down below (David et al., 2017)

- **NFC:** NFC which is also called Near Field Communication, is a technology using which devices can share data when placed in close proximity with each other. This technology is being used in many mobile phones now-a-days for transferring data and the same way the IoT devices can also transfer data on a NFC enabled device very quickly and this can prove to be quite beneficial when we have a huge amount of data to transfer.
- **RFID:** Radio Frequency Identification System or RFID is another technology where radio waves are used for identifying distinct objects. This has found it's usage in many of the vehicles wherein the toll booths are equipped with the RFID identifiers and they can differentiate between the vehicles using their unique RFID tags
- **WiFi Direct:** Wifi Direct which is also known as WiFi P2P, is another protocol which is used for connecting various devices using WiFi only but without any access point and the connected devices can transfer data and which again can prove to be useful for IoT devices placed in close proximity with each other.

This is not an exhaustive list as many other technologies like Bluetooth, Zigwave etc can also be used for providing quick and fast data transfer speeds and this very much is dependent on how we are aiming to use the IoT devices.

IOT AND HEALTHCARE

Healthcare has incorporated technology for quite a long period of time. The rudimentary methods of tests and assessment of a patient's well being have been replaced with the advanced scanning and imaging techniques which allow the medical professionals to get a clear overview of the patient's health using non-intrusive methods which are not only cost-effective but also time-saving. The recent times have seen a growth in many wearable devices, the most common example is that of the fitness bands which monitor the steps, sleep patterns, etc, similarly many other wearable devices with embedded sensors have also been developed which can collect the data from the patient and can transfer the data to the concerned medical professionals in no time. Such devices are nothing but just the IoT devices which have already begun to redefine the healthcare of the modern century. The doctors can assess the progress of the patients by utilizing the real-time data of the patients and can provide their feedback without geographical distance being a constraint. The real benefit of IoT devices is for the patients who due to any reason are immobile or can not manage to visit the doctors in person. This inclusion of IoT and technology in the healthcare domain also constitutes what has been termed as 'Healthcare 4.0' (Tanwar et al., 2019a). This is not restricted just till virtual visits as now the doctors can even operate from a distant location using the robotic operating systems in place. This really has the potential to revolutionize the whole Healthcare Industry. However, the challenges in implementing a fool proof and reliable infrastructure are no less daunting. The flawless data transfer with minimal to almost no data loss is the goal of implementing such systems in place and this calls for resilient data processing to ensure that critical data operations are performed with minimal lag and as mentioned earlier as well, we can make use of the cloud computing architecture for efficiently transferring the data with minimal loss to any part of the globe. We will look into the same in the next section.

IOT AND CLOUD COMPUTING

As we have been stressing, cloud computing can have major implications for the success of IoT in healthcare as the data is of paramount importance here and to ensure that the data gets transmitted properly and in time is even more essential. Over the course of time, the cloud computing paradigm has taken over as the most preferred way of accessing and managing data due to a plethora of reasons - it is convenient, accessible, has round the clock availability and most important of all, it requires minimal to none of the intervention of the users as the platform being offered is maintained by the providers themselves. Having said that, the need for cloud is underscored by the fact that the IoT devices, in order to share the data with the concerned, need connectivity and since it potentially generates a huge amount of data and so managing and channeling the data becomes necessary. The cloud infrastructure is quite flexible and quite recently we have seen emergence of something called as Fog computing, which is nothing but a logical extension of the existing cloud computing architecture, in which we create virtual localized nodes of servers which act much like a load balancer for the main cloud server as some of the computational logic is performed on those nodes themselves prior to sending the data to the main cloud server which essentially takes some of the pressure off the main cloud server and at the same time adds to the overall efficiency of the system. Thus as the healthcare IoT devices are in constant internet connectivity and produce lots of data, it is important to have efficient data management tools at our disposal and cloud computing is quite perfect for our requirements. We will quickly go through the cloud computing paradigm to get an idea of how the cloud architecture is organized and how we can reap the benefits by utilizing them in an efficient manner (Kavis, 2014).

CLOUD COMPUTING OVERVIEW

Cloud computing has been around for a while now with the global footprint increasing over the course of time.

There are various ways to define cloud computing but the simple definition is that it is a system which is present at a remote location providing the infrastructure to the clients on a need basis. There are different types of services which the clients might require and cloud service providers provide the same on a pay-per-use basis. Another inherent benefit for the clients is that they need not consume their precious time in the intricacies of setting up the environment for usage as this has already been taken care of by the cloud service provider and this takes off quite a load from the clients and they can focus on other important things related to the product or solution they intend to deploy (Erl et al., 2014).

The cloud computing system is concerned with providing 'services' to the clients, we can consider public transport system as an analogy for the same, where the passengers board on the trains, pay for the tickets and reach their destination thus terminating the service usage, on a similar note the cloud computing also provides services, which we will enlist below; which users can seek and use. The main features that cloud computing offers are listed down below:

- The services are fully accessible over the internet, that is anyone with an active internet connection can use the services without any special requirements (Erl, 2015).
- Another added benefit offered by cloud computing is that it is available all the time which is handy for the clients as they can choose their convenient time for accessing the services without any dependency on the service providers active hours as the services are available round the clock
- The users can 'plug and play' with the features, in other words the users can add or remove services as and when needed as per their requirement.
- It can also prove to be cost effective for the clients as they need not invest their energy or resources on getting the prerequisites done, as the service provider has got much of this covered already.

Now the main categories or models in which we can divide the cloud services are deployment and service models. The main functionalities that these models provide is that in the service model the focus of the providers is to provide a resource as a service and in the deployment model, the deployment model guides the way in which these resources should be provided to the clients as a service. We will quickly go through these in the next section.

Types of Deployment Models

So, the deployment model defines the way in which the services have to be provided to the clients, some of the most common deployment types in existence are briefly described below

Public Cloud

Figure 1. Public cloud

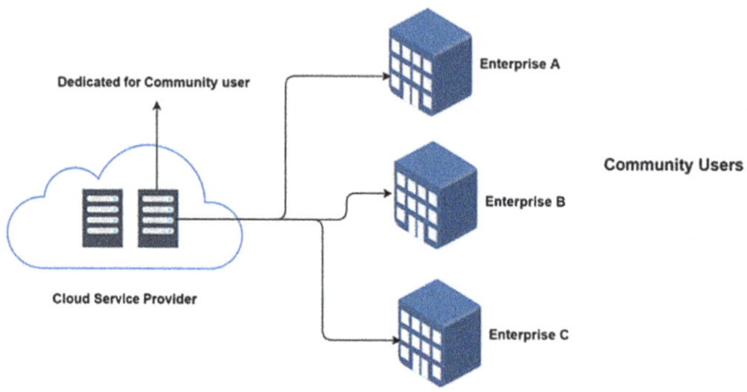

This is one of the most common types of cloud architecture, they are extensively being used and we on a daily basis use them as well, many websites and applications are deployed on the public cloud accessible to anyone with an active internet connection. For instance, the online document and image storage services open to the public also make use of the public cloud and we knowingly or unknowingly use the same almost daily. The key points about the public cloud model are listed down below

- As this service is open to all, all we need is an internet connection to get access to all of the services and no special hardware is required for accessing the service.
- This model can be used when the applications are intended to reach to a wider user based as in contrast to be used by individual clients, for which we have different deployment models
- The services provided by the public cloud are quite reliable and robust as the services would be used by a lot of people
- Although for general purposes the public cloud caters the requirements extensively, it is not recommended when the services that would be getting used are of critical importance, in that case the private model serves us best.

Private Cloud

Figure 2. Private cloud

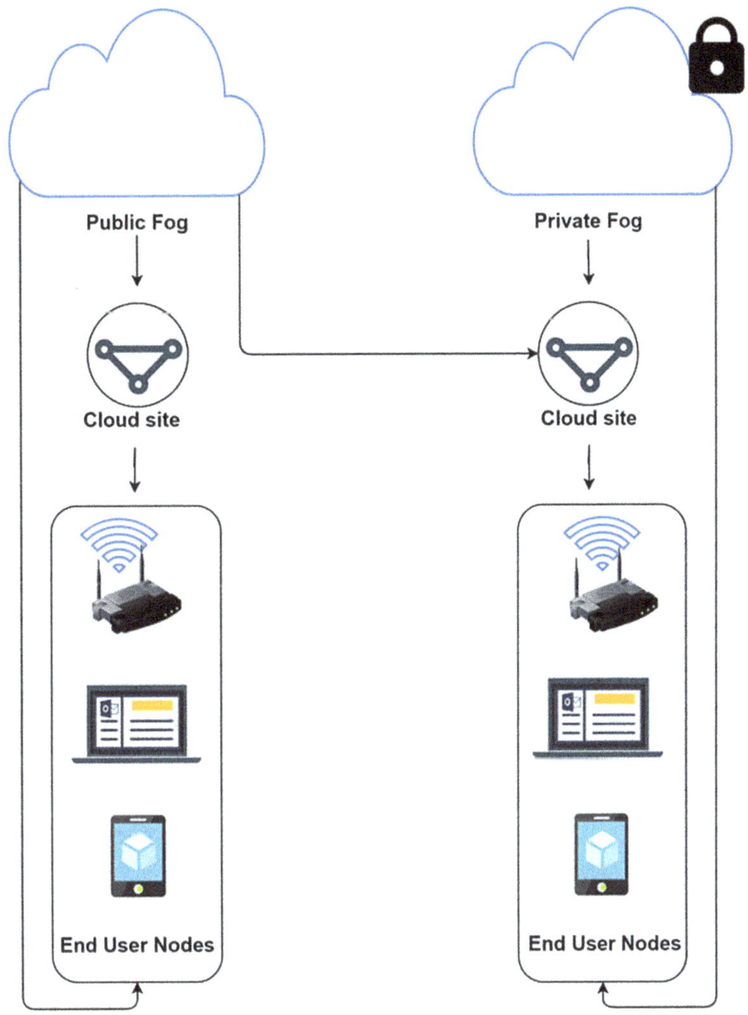

The private cloud model, in contrast to the public cloud model is aimed at providing the services to a selected few clients only, thus adding a layer of confidentiality to the critical data that might be of paramount importance to any organization or firm. Some of the key points of the private cloud model are listed down below

- As the name suggests, the private cloud model provides direct access of the services only to the client that requested for the same, thus concealing the services from the public intervention and adds a security layer
- The benefit of using a private cloud model is that we can add or remove any service anytime, without having the risk of data loss; which in case of public cloud might not be that convenient to do.

- Since the services are tailored to meet the needs of a specific client, the cost of operating and accessing the private cloud is generally higher than the public cloud infrastructure

Hybrid Cloud

Figure 3. Hybrid cloud

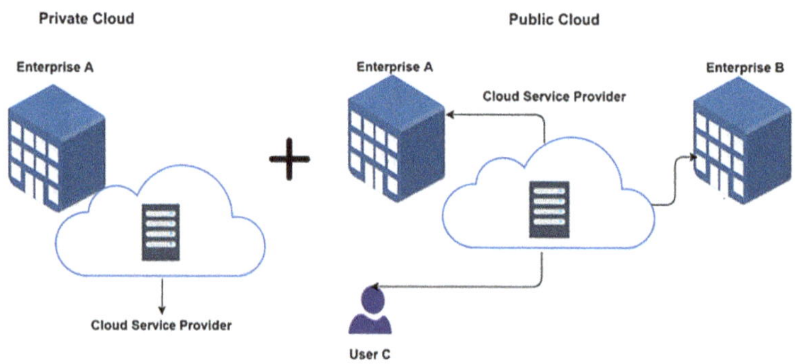

We can infer from the name itself, that this kind of deployment model can serve both public as well as private models as per the requirement of the users. Hybrid model is a combination of both public and private models and we have listed down the salient features of this model below

- One of the most obvious benefits offered by the hybrid cloud model is that the clients can make use of both the models simultaneously by exposing the public model to the users and use the private model for their internal usage.
- However, sometimes configuring the system and providing the abstraction between the two models can be a challenging task, which requires the expertise of the vendor or the clients themselves for managing.

Community Cloud

The community cloud model is generally used between the organizations and firms and is more or less an altered private cloud model, the only difference being that it is shared among some communities that share the same concern or have similar requirements. Some of the main points about the community cloud are

- Security is quite enhanced in case of community cloud as the services are being used by multiple organizations and the abstraction between their access level becomes imperative
- The management of this model is mostly done by any third party organization
- As mentioned, the main concern for the clients are the abstraction of their respective service, which although is managed well but sometimes can be daunting for the clients

So we just saw some of the most common deployment models available at the disposal of the clients and they can freely choose the model they think suits best for their needs. These services, as mentioned, have high availability and are highly scalable and they users can either opt in or out at any point in time which makes these services highly flexible to the user's needs Now we can quickly go through some of the most common service models in existence for the clients (Panigrahi et al., 2018).

Figure 4. Community cloud

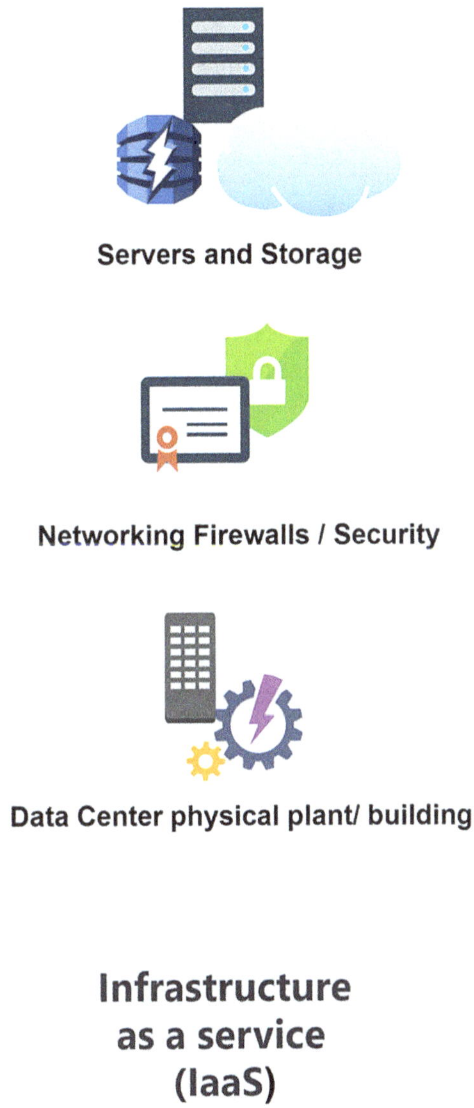

Types of Service Models

Service models are the models that define what kind of service the client needs, and once the users have figured out what kind of deployment model they wish to use, this question is of quite importance as in what service model to employ for the usage and it depends on what kind of application the clients are intending to use. We will go through some of the common service models briefly in the next paragraphs

Infrastructure as a Service

Figure 5. Infrastructure as a Service

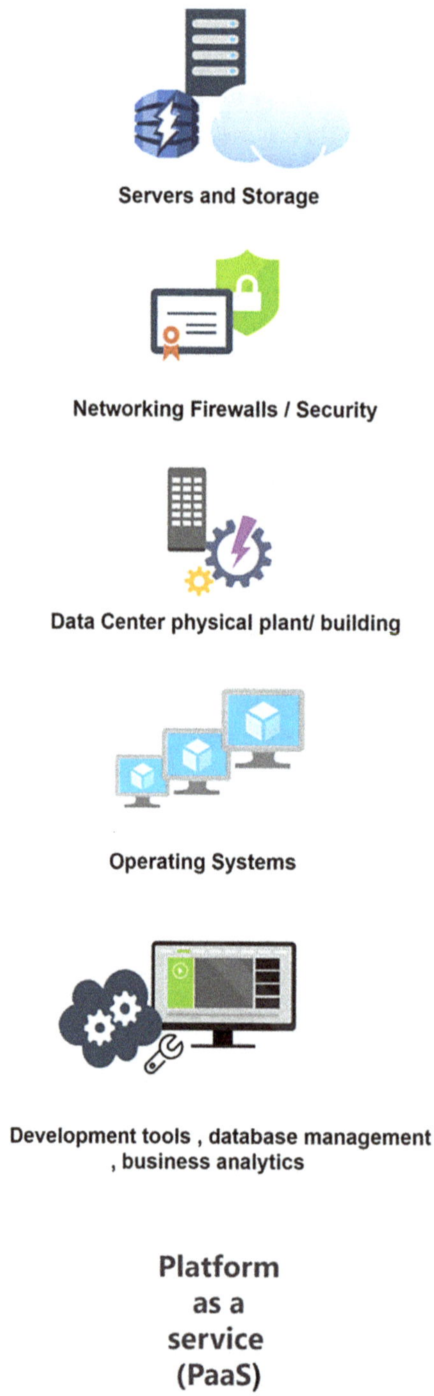

Infrastructure As a Service or commonly known as IaaS, aims at providing just the basic infrastructure upon which the clients can work upon to build their own cloud model which they can access the cloud services. In other words the users get the basic infrastructure which they can utilize for accessing the cloud services. Although generally the IaaS providers also give the users virtual storage and in some cases load balancers as well which essentially serve to divide the load amongst the multiple servers so that a particular server is not excessively loaded with requests which is essential when the server load is expected to be high. This is also a pay-per-use model and the clients can use the services as long as they wish to use. The main highlights of IaaS are listed down below:

- The headache of maintaining the data centers for deployment of the services is taken care of by the service providers which comes in handy for the clients and particularly for small businesses.
- Time saver for businesses as they can focus on other aspects rather than caring about load balancers .
- Economical as the users only need to pay for what they use
- The services are available all the time and thus provide excellent availability which is essential for any business

Platform as a Service

Figure 6. Platform as a service

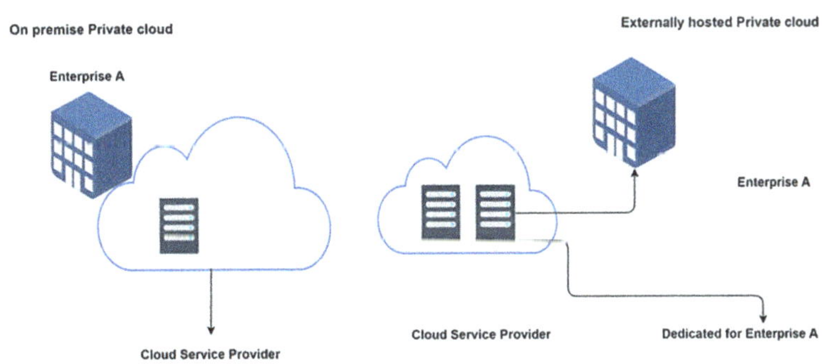

Platform as a service commonly termed as PaaS is a bit different from the IaaS because PaaS includes the infrastructure, something which comes under the purview of IaaS but on top of that provides the client with the choice of the deployment environment which again saves tonnes of time for the clients. They can choose from a variety of different environments which suits their requirements the best. Some of the salient features of PaaS are mentioned below

- PaaS provides the client a plethora of environment options to choose from whichever suits their requirement or whatever flavour they are most comfortable with
- Apart from the environment PaaS generally offers more than one deployment stacks which the clients can select based on their predilection and expertise
- The PaaS services like any other cloud service is readily available and is not dependent on geographical constraints and thus the team can work together irrespective of their locations

Software as a Service

Figure 7. Software as a service

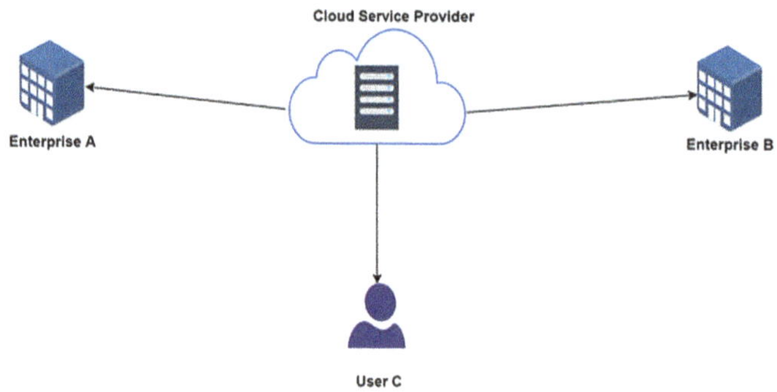

Software as a Service, or SaaS as called in the common language is another service model that is being used throughout the globe and in this service model the solution that is being offered to the end users is in the form of a Software which can be a web application or even a mobile application. The whole infrastructure, environment and security is managed by the service providers themselves. SaaS is used very commonly and we in our daily lives use them on literally a daily basis, for instance the mailing clients, online storage websites, and many more applications are being used by the masses on a daily basis and thus this makes SaaS as one of the most used cloud services. Although there can be public or private variants of the service, the most commonly used is the public SaaS. Some of the noteworthy features of SaaS are listed down below

- SaaS has been instrumental in providing the users the same experience without any dependency on platform, or in other words, using SaaS the developers deploy the application on the cloud and irrespective of the platform or the operating system, the users can access the services from anywhere in the globe by just opening their web browser
- The organizations can easily manage the applications and do the modifications which will work for all of the end users
- As with rest of the models as well, the clients have to pay only for what they use

There are also some other variants which have come into existence over the course of time, highlights amongst them being

- **Identity as a service** Identity as a Service or IaaS aims at providing identity, which is nothing but a token of validation or authentication, as a service. This is of immense use for many organizations which want to have a ready to use service for authentication. Some of the common identity services are as follows
    - Active Directory Services
    - Authentication Services
    - Single Sign On (SSO) Services

- **Network as a service** This service, aliased as NaaS, provides network as a service to the users, which generally includes providing virtual networks, network management or providing bandwidths on demand amongst others.

Hence these are some of the common service models that are being used actively by a large number of clients and the services benefit a large number of end users as well. These services are robust, dynamic and resilient which makes them perfect for usage in IoT applications, and by utilizing them wisely we can create a nice framework for their usage in the healthcare domain. The integration of cloud services would ensure seamless connectivity along with faster and robust data transfer which is essential for smooth running of healthcare services and also as some of the IoT devices are expected to run on a real time basis, a huge amount of data would be generated so channeling the data also becomes quite important so that we only send the most relevant data to the server for processing, something which comes under the purview of data pre-processing (Kleppmann, 2017). We will look into some of the latest developments and approaches in the next section for achieving this with IoT devices in mind.

DESIGNING HEALTHCARE IOT FRAMEWORK

So in the previous section we saw the concise overview of the cloud computing architecture which we can use with the IoT devices so that even the tiniest of the IoT devices is able to get the benefits of the ubiquitous cloud computing framework.(Erl, 2015) When it comes to healthcare the main parameters to focus on are the latency and faster and smarter processing of the data so that the final information that is being transferred from the devices connected with the patient reaches the organization in time and also maintains the data integrity (Vora, Devmurari, Tanwar et al, 2018). This is obviously not an easy task to do and inorder to achieve this level of capability in the whole system we need to have a robust and resilient framework in place which accommodates the major concerns and provides a seamless connectivity to the IoT devices which are connected to the patients (Panigrahi et al., 2018). There have been many proposals for designing the architecture for the IoT systems and the most promising one has been that of 'Fog' architecture, which we will explore in the next section.

Fog Computing for Healthcare IoT

Fog computing has been the recent candidate for designing the IoT framework and has shown significant potential. This technology which is also known as Edge computing is an enhanced and slightly modified version of the cloud computing architecture, where in the main focus is to keep the major computations as localized as possible, in other words the data processing and computation should take place to a point which is very near from the place data was generated and hence the name is Fog Computing (Kumari et al., 2018). The whole system has small decentralized nodes which can work independently and are located at some distance from each other. This has major implications for the healthcare industry and some of the high level areas that fog computing can address effectively are

Figure 8. General fog computing architecture

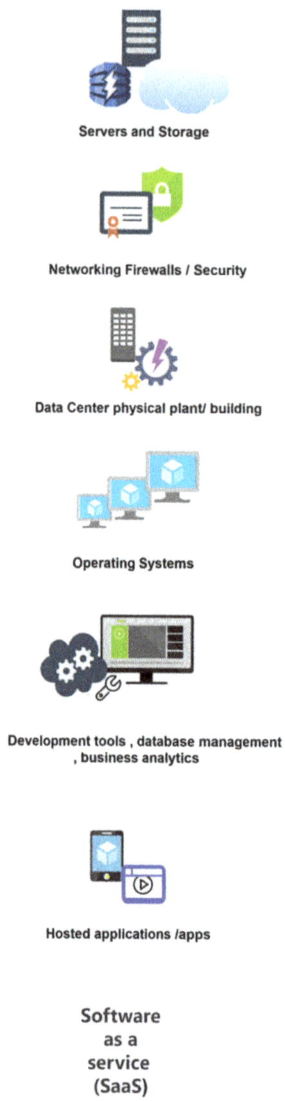

- **Latency** In areas like healthcare data loss due to latency can prove to be catastrophic hence it becomes extremely important to ensure strong connectivity and it becomes even more important to make sure that the servers are not excessively loaded with requests and data for processing because healthcare IoT devices would generate huge amount of raw data and the processing of the data might be resource intensive and thus the fog nodes can really help in taking the load off from the main server which will ultimately give the main cloud server a better resource pool and potentially lesser latency owing to computations (Kumari, Tanwar, Tyagi, Kumar, Obaidat et al, 2019).
- **Analysis** By localizing the data being transferred to the fog nodes, we get a better chance to analyze and extract the meaningful data from a smaller chunk of IoT devices as compared to a main cloud server being bombarded with exorbitant amount of data to process

- **Security** We can implement enhanced data security by using encryption algorithms before we send the data to the main cloud server, which essentially adds another layer of security to the whole architecture and ensures data safety.
- **Reliable** By combining all of the above attributes the whole system reliability increases and adds to the trust of the clients and the end users as well

Benefits of Fog Computing

Apart from the key points that we just discussed in the previous section, fog computing aims at enhancing and improving the cloud computing architecture by taking some of the load off the main cloud servers as they can hold and process the data momentarily before sending off the data to the server. Using these fog nodes we can also set up a framework where we can prioritize data from some categories of patients (Vora, Tanwar, Verma et al, 2018). For instance if an IoT device is sending the data of a patient marked as critical, then that data should get more priority over any patient whose general heart rate data is being transmitted. This would help in prioritizing the kind of data that we intend to send thus making the system more efficient. Fog computing shares a great deal of similarities with cloud computing. Fog nodes, like the cloud computing servers have the computational, logical and networking capabilities and they also function in the same way as a cloud server does. However sometimes setting up the whole architecture for fog computing can be resource intensive and their maintenance might also add up to the bill (Prasad et al., 2019). Also, setting up the structure all around the globe is another major challenge which although is time and resource consuming but can prove to be very beneficial in the long run. The current innovations and integrations of technology in the healthcare domain is now being coined as ''Healthcare 4.0' and is attributed to signify the movement of the healthcare domain with the mainstream technology (Tanwar & Parekh, 2019). Healthcare is mostly hit in many of the developing nations due to many reasons - sometimes it is the lack of expertise, sometimes people residing in remote areas of any country are not able to get access to healthcare due to unavailability of enough number of medical staff and in such situations remote attendance of the patients can prove to be highly beneficial as now most of the parts of the world are connected with the internet through mobile or broadband.(Tanwar et al., 2019) This way of telemedicine has been tried in some of the countries and the results have been encouraging. We will go through a case study elaborating the same.

IoT Devices and Remote Surgery

IoT powered surgical machines have also come into existence, and some of the surgical machines have been used to perform surgery on patients with the doctor remaining far away from the place of operation (David et al., 2017). This recent and advanced development in the medical science field is a herald of inclusion of modern technical solutions in the healthcare domain. In China, recently a brain surgery was performed on a patient with the surgeons being located thousands of miles away and the devices were connected all the time through the internet. Many such kinds of surgeries have taken place all over the globe and this is not just restricted to surgeries only. There has been a surge in telemedicine approach as well where the doctors could connect with the patients by means of any mobile or web application and this has major implications for people living in remote areas where access to quality healthcare is not present (Wilder, 2012).

However this also underscores the need of strong data connectivity along with a robust underlying architecture which can ensure reliable data connectivity all the time. There are many fields where data loss is intolerable and healthcare is one of those. For instance, if during a surgery there are some delays in the data streaming or latency issue along the way then it can really hamper the whole objective of the surgery.

IOT AS APPLIED IN HEALTHCARE

Healthcare has always been the top incorporator of latest technologies and latest developments in technology over a long period of time. Be it the application of X-Rays to the use of minute cameras for checking the internal injuries, Healthcare has put the potentially useful technological trends into use and this is something which holds true even now. The IoT ecosystem has opened a wide array of opportunities for the healthcare system to choose from.

Role of IoT in Advancing Healthcare

As mentioned earlier as well, IoT offers a huge range of benefits to the healthcare system which apart from sending real time updates to the healthcare providers also provides them with an efficient and effective data storage and management opportunities. It also helps the healthcare providers to understand the needs of the patients in a better way which is essential for patients with critical care. This also facilitates the dedicated team to make better and faster decisions based on the data acquired by these IoT devices. Using this IoT approach, the healthcare providers can create a whole roadmap for the treatment of patients which ranges from the initial monitoring of the patients to intelligent real time monitoring which can alert the healthcare service providers in advance without any manual intervention at all. Some of the major highlights of the IoT in healthcare are mentioned below:

- Keeping a real time overall record of the patient, which both the healthcare service provider and the patient can track
- Boon for chronically ill patients - equipped with mobile/wearable applications powered by IoT the patients can monitor their well being any time.
- Useful for research - the data collected by the patients can be fed to Machine Learning systems to identify or develop patterns which can potentially provide valuable information for the future patients.
- It also improves the all round efficacy and reliability of the healthcare providers.

Next, we see how and where IoT can be applied.

Implementation of IoT in Healthcare

With the promising prospects presented by IoT, an efficient implementation of these services becomes a necessity. However the road to achieve the same is still seemingly full of challenges. The IoT implementation relies heavily on technology and ofcourse Internet and as it turns out to be many of the healthcare providers are unable to perform this transition all of a sudden owing to limited resources and infrastructure needed to incorporate IoT in their existing systems. Apart from this the IoT use cases are different for different kinds of users, which needs to be implemented for each of the sections of users. The use-cases of the different kinds of users are listed below:

- **Patients**: Patients are the ones who need continuous tracking and monitoring at their disposal and this is what wearable devices and sensors do i.e capturing the data on a real time basis and let them track the progress at their fingertips.
- **Doctors** - Doctors can access the data of the patients and this greatly helps them make quick and informed decisions regarding the treatment.
- **Healthcare Providers** - The healthcare providers can 'upgrade' their existing system by incorporating IoT in their equipment such as oxygen pumps, wheelchairs etc for effective management of these resources.
- **Insurance Providers** - The IoT approach can come quite handy for the insurance providers, as they can easily alleviate the situations like false claims using the data from the smart monitoring devices worn by the patients.

So these were the main beneficiaries of the IoT ecosystem, however this by no means is an exhaustive list as many other disciplines can also get added to the list in future.

Examples of Real World Application of IoT Devices

There have been various IoT devices with their proof of concepts presented over last few years and some of the devices worth mentioning are listed down

- **Smart Monitoring Devices** - There are a lot of wearable devices in market which can detect the oxygen level in the blood and they can notify the users via mobile notifications in case there is a considerable drop in the blood oxygen levels
- **Disease Detectors:** A great deal of benefit is being drawn by the artificial intelligence and machine learning algorithms which run on IoT devices via the internet and they can predict the progression of a patient toward any particular illness.
- **Consumable Devices:** Recently small capsule shaped cameras have also come into existence which can be swallowed with water and these cameras are connected with the internet and they stream live video data to the servers and this approach can provide an alternative to the uncomfortable procedures like endoscopy
- **Robotic Surgeries:** In China and some other parts of the world robotic surgeries were performed by the means of these IoT devices which are connected to the operating end via the internet. As the surgeons move their hands, the robotic end also moves with the same precision providing an excellent solution to distance barriers in urgent and critical medical treatment (Gupta, 2019).
- **Smart Shoes:** In diseases associated with memory loss and impairment like Alzheimer's it is very common for the patients to get lost somewhere outside and this is where these smart shoes can prove to be effective as the relatives or the caretakers can track the patient's location on the associated mobile or web applications and can track the patients down safely.

We have also mentioned earlier that IoT implementation has some challenges and some of the major challenges are as below

- **Data Privacy Concerns:** Although the main intention of IoT in healthcare is to provide personalized and effective care to the patients by collecting and sending real time or historical data of the patient; it is also prone to data privacy concerns which can be raised by the patients. However, to avoid this the patients must be made aware about the type of data which would be collected and they must sign an agreement to provide their consent to share their data with the healthcare providers.
- **Data Security Concerns:** The security of data is another aspect that IoT service providers must be wary of. We have seen extensively the cloud computing approach in the previous sections which can be leveraged by the IoT devices to effectively communicate the data through the server and ensuring end to end security is of paramount importance for the IoT service providers.
- **Pricing Concerns:** Another challenging aspect is the cost-effectiveness of the whole system concerned with keeping the services within the realm of reasonable costs so that it can prove to be attractive to the potential healthcare providers.

Hence in this section we saw how IoT is an interesting addition to the healthcare system and what benefits it can offer to the healthcare providers and the patients as well although there are few challenges in the way which can be resolved prudently.

FUTURE RESEARCH DIRECTIONS

As mentioned previously, with the rise of the Internet of Things, plethora of fields are taking advantage of the geographical independence and real time data access aspects of the technology and this has broken many barriers that could have been considered as an impedance in the success of those fields and Healthcare is also not untouched by this. Healthcare domain is doing its much needed bit of leveraging on the benefits offered by technological advancements. The results are already encouraging to whatever extent the process has been tested as of now.(Tanwar et al., 2019a) Although this does not mean that the whole process of implementing such systems is free from challenges, surely the potential of such systems is immeasurable and can benefit mankind in general in the long run. Provided we have a strong underlying framework which can support the increasing load of incessant data which will get generated from the wearable devices from the patients, we will have a strong framework to track and manage patients all over the world at any particular instance. The most important research area would be to analyse how to expand the resources and utilize the ubiquitous cloud framework so that with minimal investment in additional resources we can elicit maximum benefit for connectivity of IoT devices.(Tanwar et al., 2019b)

SUMMARY

In this chapter we looked into how IoT devices are shaping the future of healthcare and how the healthcare domain has slowly and steadily moved towards embracing the technological advancements in the disparate field like computer science. Applications of machine learning and AI has enabled the medical professionals to predict and analyse the patterns in case of many diseases like cancer, where given the current stage of a patient one can predict the progress that would take place along with medication.(Mittal et al., 2019) We next looked into the type of IoT devices that we can potentially use for monitoring the well being of the patients. We also looked into the hardware and the software components of these IoT devices and how many different technological and protocol stacks can be integrated into these IoT devices for their effective communication.(Vora, Tanwar, Tyagi et al, 2019) Next we saw how IoT devices can make use of the existing cloud computing architecture for sending the data to any part of the globe, thanks to the availability of the cloud services. We also briefly waded through the basics of cloud computing and the different kinds of models that are being actively used. We looked into the popular deployment and the service models and how they can be used in the perspective of IoT devices. We also looked into some of the recent developments in the field of cloud computation, with the most recent proposal being that of the fog computing which aims to take the load off the main servers by channelling and dispersing the data among the fog nodes which can delegate some of the burden of the parent cloud servers.(Kumari, Tanwar, Tyagi, Kumar, Parizi et al, 2019) We also saw how IoT devices have started to play a monumental role in the healthcare of the future and has been proven to be the harbinger of a new revolution in the field of healthcare. In the times of pandemic like that of the COVID-19, availability of medical professionals via any app can prove to be extremely beneficial at the time when stepping out of the houses is not even feasible. Although some research has to be done in order to estimate how we can most efficiently elicit the benefits from the cloud computing framework and how much of resources have to be invested in order to fully develop this framework for the betterment of the masses.

REFERENCES

Ahmed, M. U. (2017). Internet of Things (IoT) Technologies for HealthCare. *4th International Conference, HealthyIoT 2017*, 50-78.

David, H., Gonzalo, S., & Patrick, G. (2017). *IoT Fundamentals: Networking Technologies, Protocols and Use Cases for the Internet of Things*. Pearson.

Erl, T. (2015). *Cloud Computing Design Patterns*. Prentice Hall.

Erl, T., Puttini, R., & Mahmood, Z. (2014). *Cloud Computing: Concepts, Technology & Architecture*. Pearson.

Gupta, R. (2019). Tactile Internet-based Telesurgery System for Healthcare 4.0: An Architecture, Research Challenges, and Future Directions. *IEEE Network*, 12–19.

Gupta, R., Tanwar, S., Tyagi, S., Kumar, N., Obaidat, M. S., & Sadoun, B. (2019). HaBiTs: Blockchain Based Telesurgery Framework for Healthcare 4.0. *International Conference on Computer, Information and Telecommunication Systems (IEEE CITS-2019)*, 6-10.

Kaneriya, S., Tanwar, S., Buddhadev, S., Verma, J. P., Tyagi, S., Kumar, N., & Misra, S. (2018). A Range-based approach for Long-Term Forecast of Weather Using Probabilistic Markov Model. *IEEE International Conference on Communication (IEEE ICC-2018)*, 1-6.

Kaneriya, S., Tanwar, S., Verma, J. P., Tyagi, S., Kumar, N., Obaidat, M. S., & Rodrigues, J. P. C. (2018). Data Consumption-Aware Load Forecasting Scheme for Smart Grid Systems. *IEEE Global Communications Conference (IEEE GLOBECOM-2018),* 1-6.

Kavis, M. J. (2014). *Architecting the Cloud.* Wiley. doi:10.1002/9781118691779

Kleppmann, M. (2017). *Designing Data-Intensive Applications: The Big Ideas Behind Reliable, Scalable, and Maintainable Systems.* O'Reilly.

Kumari, A., Tanwar, S., Tyagi, S., & Kumar, N. (2018). Fog Computing for Healthcare 4.0 Environment: Opportunities and Challenges. *Computers & Electrical Engineering*, *72*, 1–13. doi:10.1016/j.compeleceng.2018.08.015

Kumari, A., Tanwar, S., Tyagi, S., Kumar, N., Obaidat, M. S., & Rodrigues, J. J. P. C. (2019, June). Fog Computing for Smart Grid Systems in 5G Environment: Challenges and Solutions. *IEEE Wireless Communication Magazine*, *26*(3), 47–53. doi:10.1109/MWC.2019.1800356

Kumari, A., Tanwar, S., Tyagi, S., Kumar, N., Parizi, R. M., & Choo, K.-K. R. (2019). S. Tanwar., S. Tyagi, N. Kumar, R. Parizi, K. K. R. Choo, Fog Data Analytics: A Taxonomy and Process Model. *Journal of Network and Computer Applications*, *128*, 90–104. doi:10.1016/j.jnca.2018.12.013

Mistry, I., Tanwar, S., Tyagi, S., & Kumar, N. (2020). Blockchain for 5G-Enabled IoT for Industrial Automation: A Systematic Review, Solutions, and Challenges. *Mechanical Systems and Signal Processing*, *135*, 1–19. doi:10.1016/j.ymssp.2019.106382

Mittal, M., Tanwar, S., Agarwal, B., & Goyal, L. M. (Eds.). (2019). *Energy Conservation for IoT Devices: Concepts, Paradigms and Solutions, Studies in Systems, Decision and Control*. Springer Nature Singapore Pte Ltd. doi:10.1007/978-981-13-7399-2

Patel, D., Narmawala, Z., Tanwar, S., & Singh, P. K. (2018). A Systematic Review on Scheduling Public Transport Using IoT as Tool. In B. Panigrahi, M. Trivedi, K. Mishra, S. Tiwari, & P. Singh (Eds.), *Smart Innovations in Communication and Computational Sciences. Advances in Intelligent Systems and Computing* (Vol. 670, pp. 39–48). Springer. doi:10.1007/978-981-10-8971-8_4

Prasad, V. K., Bhavsar, M., & Tanwar, S. (2019). Influence of monitoring: Fog and Edge Computing", Scalable Computing. *Practice and Experience*, *20*(2), 365–376. doi:10.12694cpe.v20i2.1533

Rajput, D. S., & Gaur, R. (2017). *An IoT Framework for Healthcare Monitoring System*. LAP LAMBERT Academic Publishing.

Smart, E. (2019). Tourism and Hospitality Management. *International Conference on Computer, Information and Telecommunication Systems (IEEE CITS-2019),* 237-241.

Tanwar, S., & Parekh, K. (2019). Blockchain-based Electronic Healthcare Record System for Healthcare 4.0 Applications. *Journal of Information Security and Applications*, *50*, 1–14.

Tanwar, S., Thakkar, K., Thakor, R., & Singh, P. K. (2018). M-Tesla-Based Security Assessment in Wireless Sensor Network. In *International Conference on Computational Intelligence and Data Science (ICCIDS 2018).* NorthCap University.

Tanwar, S., Tyagi, S., & Kumar, N. (Eds.). (2019a). *Security and Privacy of Electronics Healthcare Records*. IET Book Series on e-Health Technologies.

Tanwar, S., Tyagi, S., & Kumar, N. (Eds.). (2019b). Multimedia Big Data Computing for IoT Applications: Concepts, Paradigms and Solutions. Intelligent Systems Reference Library. Springer Nature Singapore Pte Ltd.

Tanwar, S., Tyagi, S., & Kumar, S. (2017). The Role of Internet of Things and Smart Grid for the Development of a Smart City. *Intelligent Communication and Computational Technologies (Lecture Notes in Networks and Systems: Proceedings of Internet of Things for Technological Development, IoT4TD, 19*, 23-33.

Tanwar, S., Vora, J., Kanriya, S., Tyagi, S., Kumar, N., Sharma, V., & You, I. (2019). Human Arthritis Analysis in Fog Computing Environment using Bayesian Network Classifier and Thread Protocol. *IEEE Consumer Electronics Magazine*, *9*(1), 88–94. doi:10.1109/MCE.2019.2941456

Vohra, J., Kaneriya, S., Tanwar, S., & Tyagi, S. (2019). Standardising the use of Duplex Channels in 5G-WiFi Networking for Ambient Assisted Living. *IEEE Conference on Communications (IEEE ICC-2019)*, 1-6.

Vora, J., Devmurari, P., Tanwar, S., Tyagi, S., Kumar, N., & Obaidat, M. S. (2018). Blind Signatures Based Secured E-Healthcare System. *International Conference on Computer, Information and Telecommunication Systems (IEEE CITS-2018)*, 177-181.

Vora, J., Kanriya, S., Tanwar, S., Tyagi, S., Kumar, N., & Obaidat, M. S. (2019). TILAA: Tactile Internet Based Ambient Assistant Living In Fog Environment. *Future Generation Computer Systems*, *98*, 635–649. doi:10.1016/j.future.2019.01.035

Vora, J., Tanwar, S., Tyagi, S., Kumar, N., & Rodrigues, J. P. C. (2019). HRIDaY: Ballistocardiogram-based Heart Rate Monitoring Using Fog Computing. *IEEE Global Communications Conference (GLOBECOM-2019, 209*, 1-6.

Vora, J., Tanwar, S., Verma, J. P., Tyagi, S., Kumar, N., Obaidat, M. S., & Rodrigues, J. P. C. (2018). BHEEM: A Blockchain-based Framework for Securing Electronic Health Records. *IEEE Global Communications Conference (IEEE GLOBECOM-2018)*, 1-6.

Wilder, B. (2012). *Cloud Architecture Patterns: Develop Cloud-Native Applications*. O'Reilly.

KEY TERMS AND DEFINITIONS

Cloud Server: Cloud is a server located at a remote location used to provide different kinds of services to the clients.

Fog Computing: General term given to localized cloud servers which are located near to the data creation source and help in effective computation and transfer of data to the main cloud server.

IaaS: Cloud service model providing the core infrastructure as a service.

Internet of Things (IoT): IoT is the general term given to any device which has the capability to get connected to the internet.

PaaS: Cloud service model providing the platform as a service, which includes deployment environments.

Private Cloud: Cloud model intended to be used within a particular organization, for instance the file upload server of an organization.

Public Cloud: Cloud accessible to the general masses by the means of the internet, for instance online storage services.

SaaS: Cloud service model providing the complete software as a service, for instance the online mail clients.

Chapter 13
IoT on Healthcare Using Clinical Decision Support System

Manju Priya Sundaramurthy
Karpagam Academy of Higher Education, India

ABSTRACT

Most of the developing countries face major problems in providing quality healthcare. It is very essential to move the health stream to a higher level with more effective. Though medical care is improving, due to the enormous amount of data, making the decisions is more complex. The technology already links patients, providers, and customers in many ways that are converting the patient experience and delivery of care. This chapter reveals the importance of healthcare by using CDSS along with IoT. By combining connected devices with CDSS will help the clinicians to take decisions immediately for any disease. It provides an efficient, effective quality measurement and enhancement because of its ability to get the data of any patient at any time anywhere.

INTRODUCTION

At the moment, our electronic life is pinpointed approximately with smartphones and mobile technologies, but the research community is exigent to develop the scope of all potential applications. At present, the world has various kinds of health problems. Some problems are easily curable, whereas some problems are unknown to the doctors. In the emerging world, it is still an immense challenge to reach more people in all areas with not enough health care. Healthcare needs cannot be fulfilled in most countries due to the vast population. Information and communication technologies (IT) (Aggarwal V K et al., 1998) could revolutionize healthcare. Many healthcare organizations are exploring machine to machine communication and IoT.

Healthcare organizations provide the access to data and applications needed to everyone whenever and wherever, so it helps to improve the efficiency of curing the patients soon and to enhance patient care. The physician has the responsibility not only based on the knowledge but also in managing the huge amount of information.

DOI: 10.4018/978-1-7998-6527-8.ch013

IoT is going to revolve around the healthcare industry in the upcoming future with the integration of clinical DSS. Large healthcare organizations are international so that their connectivity services are also to be international. It is necessary to maintain consistent patient care across the work; healthcare providers need a reliable communications network.

This CDSS provides clinicians as well as patients with relevant medical information. Vital information is gathered from sensors are transmitted wirelessly through IoT devices is used as the input for the DSS. If the patient state is identified as critical, an alert can be generated to the physician. An electronic health record (EHR) of the patients can be documented with the help of the sensor data, patient feedback.

With the connected medicines, it will certainly help the physician to get the necessary information wherever and whenever and it helps the people to acquire eminence care through the development and progression in diagnostics, imaging, and treatment. This will let the patients attain high-quality medical care in real-time and at a reasonable price.

The technologies that enable the IoT promise to turn almost any objects into a source of information. The report from MarketReasearch.com states that by 2020, IoT in healthcare is to increase 117 billion dollars.

The main factors for boosting the healthcare industry are the growing adoption of wearable technology and the emergence of connected care. Research steered by a network provider company in Aruba, states that by the end of 2019, nearly 87% of the healthcare organizations around the world will implement IoT services (as shown in figure 1).

Nearly 3,100 IT enterprises were surveyed by the researchers including healthcare and business concerns across 20 countries. Their study remarks that most healthcare institutions have familiarized themselves with IoT for refining patient monitoring, nurturing innovations, and minimizing the cost (Market Analysis Report, 2019).

The clinical decision support systems market is largely going to be driven by the urgent need to reduce global healthcare costs and a rising number of deaths due to preventable medical errors (www.prnnewswire.com). In the upcoming years, the whole world will connect with the web or the internet, where the internet of things is an incorporated component of the next generation. This chapter aims to establish a framework for IoT with CDSS on healthcare to increase the lifetime of the patients. Before going in-depth on IoT on healthcare with CDSS, it is very essential to know the importance of IoT.

Introduction to IoT

In the olden days, people found it very difficult to communicate with people in faraway places. Later on, birds or persons practiced to travel and deliver the news from one place to the next place, but it also took more time to go from one person to another. Later, when the communications were developed with the help of vehicles, telephone, the information was sent faster (Subramaniam & Ganesh, 2014).

With the development of computers, using cable communications become much easier. The cables are connected along with a modem to form a network and hence internet has progressed to a remarkable evolution, making the world connect with everyone (David Niewolny, 2013).

Developing countries have more opportunities now because the current technology helps to provide more cost-effective solutions. IoT is changing the world. IT is a revolutionary change and this new technology connects, gathers data, and reacts according to the situations in the world. The main function of an IoT includes getting acquired facts from things to interchange the known data, process the data, and manage the report logically and to act at a very outsized level.

Figure 1. IoT Usage
(Market Analysis Report, 2019)

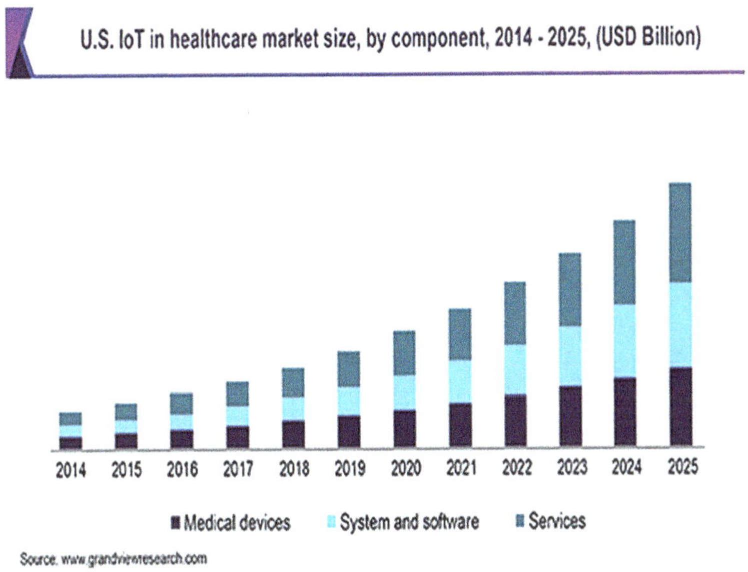

An important key to the success of IoT is the ability to provide users with the right information at the right time at anywhere (as shown in figure.2).

IoT has appeared as one of the modern advances of information and intelligent technologies and it has an immense impact when incorporated with health utility. IoT associates the internet with various objects in our day-to-day activity.

IoT is contemplated to encompass 4 layers of viable areas (Atzori et al., 2010):

First Layer: Recognition of each thing
Second Layer: Assistance for peoples need (healthcare)
Third Layer: Digital urbanization
Fourth Layer: Sensory world

IoT is moderately diverse from the common internet in communication. IoT is standardized into four main layers which are shown in the figure. 3:

1. **Sensing Layer:** This layer consists of entire sensors, RFIDs, and wireless sensor networks (WSN). Example: Google glass.
2. **Aggregated layer:** This layer consists of distinct types of aggregators based on the sensors of the Perceive layer. Example: Smartphones
3. **Processing Layer:** This layer processes the information received from the aggregated layer through servers.
4. **Cloud Platform:** It is a platform that allows on-demand network access to computing services (Bhömer et al., 2013). All the processed data are uploaded into the cloud, stored, and develop data for reasoning and findings. Then the data can be accessed by a large number of users.

Figure 2. Internet of things

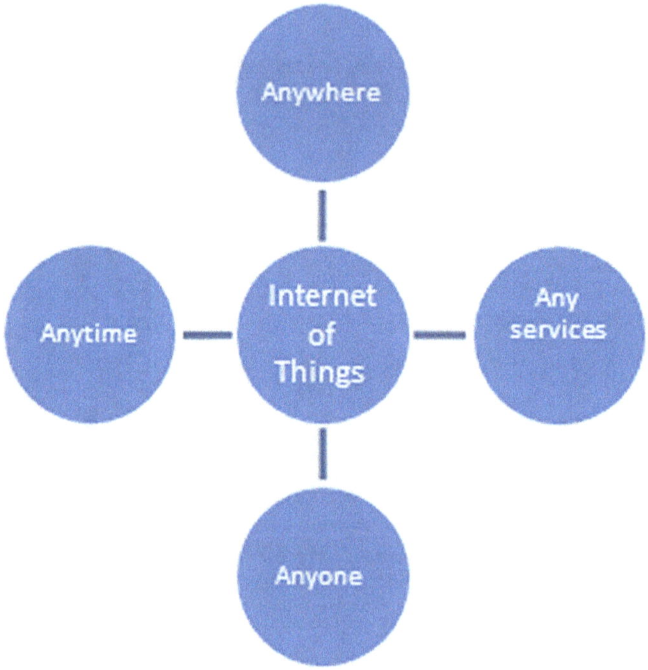

Figure 3. Layers in IoT

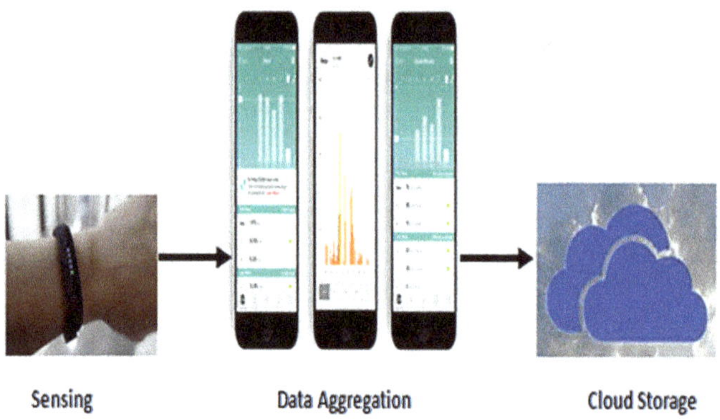

The concept of IoT has some specific characteristics that confirmed it in a multidimensional way.

- **Smart Sensing**: The devices are connected with sensors to detect the situations.
- **Intellect:** The IoT device is embedded with a few manipulative system and software which is used for making decisions, forecasting, and automatic management.
- **Interconnected:** The devices are linked to devices and sometimes from devices to other devices.
- **Data Sharing**: The data collected from one device is shared with all other connected devices. It provides enhanced communication between the user and the devices.

- **Assurance:** It ensures safety and assurance. For example, smart medical devices.
- Many things that were in our imaginations like smart cities, smart cars are now becoming real with modern technology. IoT proposes a lot of prospects transversely the healthcare industry where appropriate information is a deposit of fast and safe cure. As the scheme and elucidation for collecting, sending data, and investigate it are bettering all the time, by which a bigger number of internet of things had driven medical solutions for supervising patients (David Niewolny, 2013).

Why Healthcare Need IoT?

Qualified health is going to be the future of healthcare because health can be better improved. From the way of thinking of particular health providers, it is effortless to see as deserted episodes. Illness directly hurts the quality of life of the people. It is always extra pricey to get people well than to forbid them from getting hospitalized.

Quality health protections are main, essential for making rising to each person's condition of health, rapid approach into the healthcare system, forbidding the diseases and impairment, finding and taking care of health circumstances, and forbidding loss (https://www.healthypeople.gov/2020).

The benefit of contemporary technology in healthcare gives relives to victims and doctors because of its different utilizations such as real-time monitoring, patient information management systems, and healthiness (He & Zeadally, 2015).

With the help of IoT's by updating personal health data of patients, by considering every tiny detail, it makes a more advantageous decision for patients as well as physicians. Since healthcare expenses are going higher, it is very essential for the prevention of many diseases. The widespread access to real-time, high-qualified data of each health, will reform healthcare by helping people to live a longer life and prevent disease. Furthermore, it could provide patient satisfaction too in all ways.

IoT with clinical DSS can ensure less time for taking decisions for the physicians. It can reduce the need for direct patient-physician interaction devices that are interconnected through the internet which could deliver valuable data.

IoT Healthcare System Architecture

The data is transformed in a very fast and accurate manner in IoT healthcare. The architecture of an IoT healthcare system is as shown in figure.4:

- **Sensors:** IoT in healthcare has different sensors like pulse-oximeter, thermometer, blood pressure sensors that read the current patient data. The sensors might also function as a standalone sensing device or it can act as a component of larger equipment for sensing and control.
- **Product Infrastructure:** This includes the hardware/software components that read the sensor signals and display them to the device.
- **Connectivity:** A better connectivity is needed to connect the devices or sensors from the micro-controller to the server to read the data.
- **Analytics:** IoT healthcare system analyzes the collected raw data from the sensors and it is converted into an actionable format, which helps to make the decisions by the clinicians. Various data science and analytics methods along with machine-learning innovations can be utilized to generate a sense of information and implement a desirable reaction.

- **Application Platform:** IoT system accesses the data to healthcare providers on their device with all the necessary details of the patients.

Figure 4. IoT Healthcare system architecture

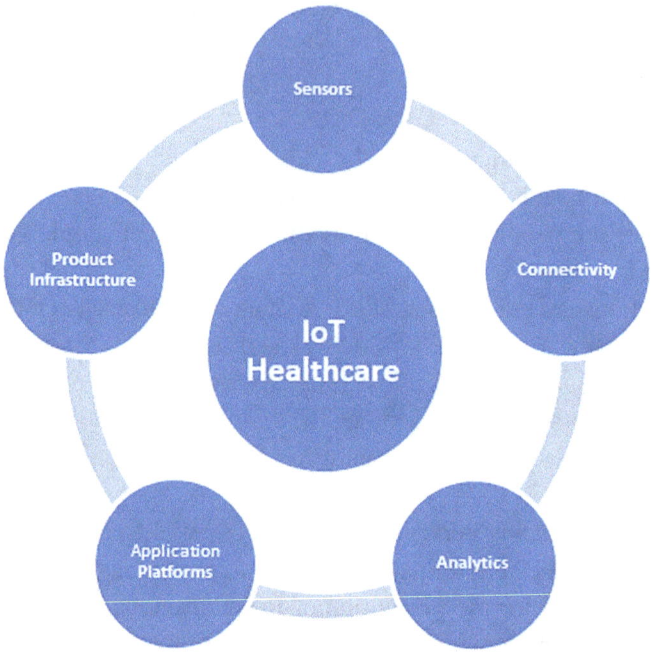

Benefits of Health IoT

The primary goal of IoT healthcare is to collect all essential data. It can deliver a wide range of benefits, including system-level benefits, better delivery of data, improved patient safety. IoT can especially improve patient monitoring. IoT will completely revolutionize our daily lives and as such, you should stay informed and aware of all of the changes it will bring.

By using IoT, allied devices can compile medical and more health data and can transfer the information to a physician. IoT enables the physicians to collect and connect billions of devices and can collect the data and diagnose the disease and provide the treatment.

If a heart attack person enters an emergency place, it is significant for the clinic to do their task great. It is crucial to view the previous records of the patients. The use of present state-of-art technology and modernization should be used to progress the access to provide quality healthcare services to the patients.

Connecting with all the devices and things within the world will bring a huge impact on human life in different environments.

Presently about 87% of healthcare organizations have adopted the Internet of Things to improve patient monitoring, faster innovations, and to reduce costs.

The Motivation for Clinical Healthcare IoT

Managing health and the quality of life for a long time remains a vital task for several people. IoT endows in many ways by affording access to healthcare services, enhancing the quality of living, and decreases the cost. By applying smart things, it benefits the patients and the doctors to work ingeniously in diagnosis and further treatment process. Normally a physician has to analyze the collected data to give the treatment to the patient.

Present technologies permit us to handle the vast amount of data than historic methods. IoT makes the potential to vaguely conduct examinations with outstanding experts, which hike the comprehensive excellence of health care.

Already the present IoT healthcare monitors the patients' health, reminds patients to take medicine, monitors blood pressure, sugar, heartbeats, and sends the data to the physician. It is very essential to prepare the document about the critical cases which the physician has never treated.

IoT has the potential to transform managed healthcare by providing the way for delivering new models that help to improve the health of the patient and efficiency. The information collected through the sensors is stored in the databases in a distributed manner. By using this, the physicians can check the symptoms of the patients and the doctor can conclude the disease and how it occurred and what treatment has to be followed. After analyzing the things, the doctor can start his treatment by specifying the medicines to be given and the dosage limits.

IoT healthcare with CDSS is gaining increased usage in various domains of healthcare. It can provide intelligent access to relevant medical knowledge, provides an important, applicable checkpoint asked upon the previous record's assistance. (Regin Joy Conejar and Haeng-konkim, 2014)

Smart wearables, wearable biometric sensors, glucose monitors are some of the ways of the IoT technologies which are already running, and shortly, it can influence more and improved managed care.

The below statistics report (shown in figure.5) shows the estimated healthcare IoT devices which are to be used globally from 2015 to 2020. Nearly 161 million IoT devices are likely to be used universally in the year 2020.

Introduction to Clinical DSS

CDSS is an important application for the healthcare industry. It helps to analyze the data and helps the doctors in making decisions related to patients. It provides hospital staff, patients, clinicians, and other people to improve healthcare. It also improves the safety, efficiency, and quality of healthcare. It helps in providing timely information about the patient. It takes the whole data recorded in HER and notices the changes required for a particular patient.

A particular patient can be given reminders, advice, or interpretation on time by a computer program that is defined as Clinical DSS (Wyatt. JC, 2000).

It can also be stated as a system that gives an accurate amount of significant knowledge at a suitable time and context and the end contributing to enhancing the quality of clinical care and results (Osheroff et al., 2007).

CDSS is a part of the clinical workflow. It is triggered by computerized data analysis. CDSS is also defined by the office of the National Co-Ordinator for Health Information Technology (ONC) as it gives doctors, nurses, patients, and other persons with information and person precise data intelligently filtered or given at the correct time, to improve health and healthcare (https://www.healthit.gov).

Figure 5. Expected installations of IoT healthcare devices globally from 2015 to 2020 (https://www.statista.com)

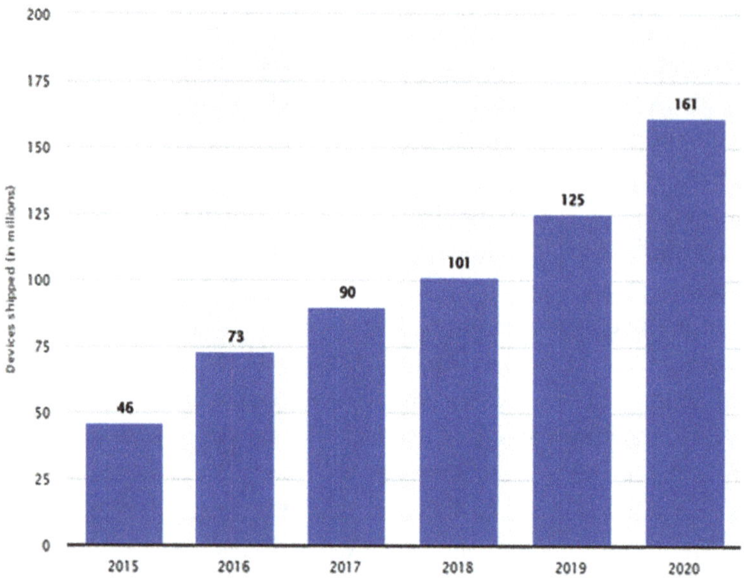

As medical care is becoming complex, it is more important to have full information from a reliable resource that can be accessed from multiple devices.

An overlooked tool is CDSS which has been defined as systems that give clinicians or patients through computer-generated clinical facts and patient-related information, intelligently filtered or accessible at suitable times to improve patient care (Osheroff et al., 2012).

CDSS provides biomedical information, person-specific data that links data and knowledge to give useful information to clinician patients. The collected information must be processed and systematized in a proper way that helps to take correct decisions soon and take action on those decisions.

CDSS has not impelled to effects clinician decision but to render data to assist the physicians in handling any complex and growing size of biomedical and person-centric data required to make appropriate, knowledgeable, and advanced value decisions based on present clinical knowledge. CDSS strengthen their decision-making procedure by adding a lack of data or intellectual biases. It can provide the most up to date information to facilitate decisions regarding patient well-being and healthcare delivery.

It is impossible to make good decisions without information. Studies have proved that well-executed CDSS can reduce harmful events from drug-drug interactions. It is determined that clinical DSS improves the quality of health care. New technologies can extend and replace existing clinical processes in health.

In specific, based on the health information technology (HIT), CDSSs play an important task in smoothing the progress of the application of evidence-based medicine to patient care by permitting persons to access information and clinical evidence more resourcefully and successfully.

Asper HIT, CDSS can be classified into three categories namely (Musen, 2014)

- Information management
- Situational awareness
- Patient-specific

The information management type of CDSS lets the users access medical data or clinical evidence data. The situational awareness enhances the decision-makers based on the situations by making an alarming. This type of CDSS can also help to endorse the care provider's clinical imminent by efficiently visualizing the multifaceted and elevated amount of data. This helps the patients to know their health information very easily. The last type of CDSS offers patient-specific proposals or involvement from finding to action. The clinicians' confidence in their predictions also increased when using CDSS (http://medinform.jmir.org). CDSS have to be efficient, able to integrate with the workflow, avoiding overload. They should keep advice only for relevant information, reducing alert fatigue, should avoid the need for manual data collection, and should ease the needed tasks when different computer systems and medical devices that hinder the extraction work together (Antonio et al., 2020).

Benefits of CDSS

Healthcare organizations that use CDSS can get more responses from the users in an easier way. Few benefits of CDSS and how it is helping healthcare professionals are as follows:

Error Reduction

When a patient is in critical condition, it is very challenging to find accurate information and the doses to be given. It is reported, some of the errors in the hospitals are caused by improper dosage. This CDSS could help the physicians the idea of dosage to be given when they know the detailed information of the patient. When accurate medicine is given, it reduces the error.

Progresses the Efficiency

Determining a treatment plan and monitoring a patient is a complex task. It requires a lot of effort and experience in collecting accurate data. With the help of CDSS, the physicians can deliver a good outcome without committing any mistakes.

Data at Fingertips

By following CDSS, the organizations can assure reliable information about the specific patient. This helps them to treat the patient accordingly without wasting time. It also reduces costs by avoiding unnecessary tests. It helps to provide anyone with the right information at the right time.

Existing Techniques in Healthcare

Prabha Sundaravadivel et.al., (2015) have discussed the connected health which refers to any digital healthcare solution which can operate remotely, with other components like continuous health monitoring, emergency detection, and give the alarm to the user. In paper (Mostafa Haghi, 2017), the author had introduced several types of wearable devices for IoT and illustrated their applications in health care segments.

Ahmed Abdelgawad et.al., (2016) have discussed the remote healthcare for senior citizen. They designed a manageable and customizable IoT system that can be used to gather the information which is required to assist the self-determining living of senior and challenged citizens to enhance their excellence of life.

In paper (Syeda Faiza Unnisa Begum, Imtiyazunnisa Begum, 2017), the author proposed a design of how to build a healthcare system on the internet of things using a lot of network-layer systems and computer software. On the whole, they designed an IoT healthcare network (IoThNet) which is one of the essentials of IoT healthcare.

In paper (Riazul Islam et al., 2015), the authors have designed a wearable healthcare context to determine how people get amenities by economic and societies in terms of sustainability.

P.Anooj (2011) has proposed how to predict the risk level of heart diseases, using a clinical decision support system.

Nowadays smart wearables are designed as electronic devices that are located near, or in the body to collect the data. Smart clothes are also fashioned by inserting smart wearables into garments. Smart clothes can monitor, document, augment and motivate on our survives by providing extraordinary opportunities for attempting global social tasks in health (Haghi et al., 2017), aging (Bhömer et al., 2013), work safety (Bonfiglio et al., 2011), or personal productivity (Feito et al., 2018).

For example, in (Joshi et al., 2016), the authors contemporary IoT-embedded system to avoid obesity, which accumulates sensor data through smartphones.

In (Trindade et al., 2016), the authors present a wearable T-shirt that helps to monitor the ECG signals through a BLE connection. It reads the information through a smartphone and later the data can be uploaded to the server.

For assessing the daily activities during rehabilitation, smart garments can be used (Spulber et al., 2015). Besides, some researchers have projected a Bluetooth-enabled smart garment based on Adafruit Flora for rehabilitating shoulders in physical therapy treatments (Wang et al., 2017), some people have engrossed on knee osteoarthritis rehabilitation (Chen et al., 2015). Furthermore, for the rehabilitation of patients with sensory impairments, the haptic wearables can be used (Shull et al., 2015).

Smart garments are also designed for babies and elders to follow their activities, falls, or health. The authors (Perego et al., 2014) have designed a smart garment through which the newborn babies can be monitored. It collects health data and transfers to Bluetooth gateways and alters it is uploaded to the server.

Another existing work is also presented in (Morales, et al., 2017), where a harness for avoiding accidents in babies that crawl is given. The dangerous occasion is detected by the system, which uploads the information to an IoT server and an alert is sent to the caretakers. The authors in (Ferreira et al., 2016) have aimed to monitor the child's temperature, heart, and breath rate to prevent infant death syndrome.

The authors in (Frydrysiak & Tesiorowski, 2016) have designed a smart shirt for monitoring the elderly persons, which can collect the heart rate, respiration rate, and underwear temperature. A related approach is proposed in (Burns, 2012) but collecting ECG and accelerometer data related to walking is gathered and transferred to the smartphone through Bluetooth, where it processes and permits for emergency alerts.

For instance, presently hospitals use IoT for security purposes (shown in figure.6). Newborn babies are given wrist bands using sensors. If the child is taken away the door will automatically give an alarm. The pill-sized sensors are the ingestible sensors that observe the medication of the body and alarm us if any abnormality occurs in the body.

Figure 6. Hospitals with IoT

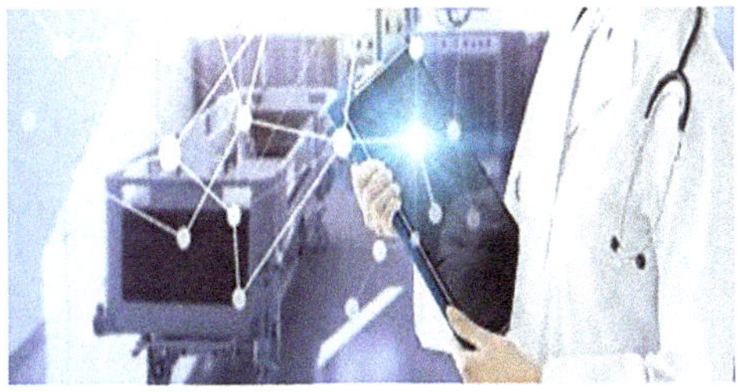

How Do Wearables Differ From Smartphone Apps?

There is a lot of difference in using these IoT based wearables when compared to a normal smart app. The first things are the size. The most noticeable contrast in wearables is the size of the display screen, assuming there is one, and the device itself. Next its functionality and the user interaction with the wearables. A wearable device can be designed to communicate with any apps on a mobile device. It may not have any display at all, only connecting the data it receives and sends it with other places.

Architectural Framework Model of IoT With CDSS

The proposed frame is developed to help the physician in monitoring the patient. (as shown in figure.7)

Figure 7. Framework representation of IoT with CDSS

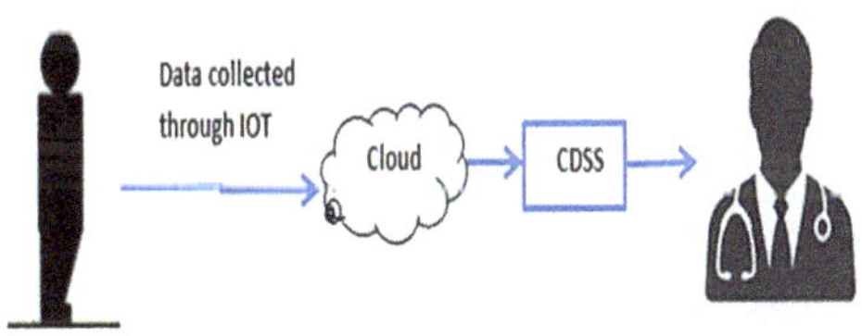

With the help of IoT, diagnosis of the disease can be done. It is important for almost every disease because it indicates how the symptoms should be treated. The collected data would be unstructured data, which should be organized into structured data. Unstructured data is a free form of text; it is more extensive to predictive.

Normally structured data is extremely ordered and formatted data, which can be searched easily in the database. There is no pre-defined format in unstructured data, so it makes it more difficult to collect, process, and analyze.

Before forming the CDSS, the data must be loaded from the database into a computing workspace. Using the workspace, it allows the users to manipulate the data and build models for CDSS.

With the IoT based CDSS, it helps to assess and evaluate the data from the database to achieve a good result. Since different kinds of data are processed, it is very important to analyze and then produce the results (as shown in figure.8)

Figure 8. Processes from data to decisions

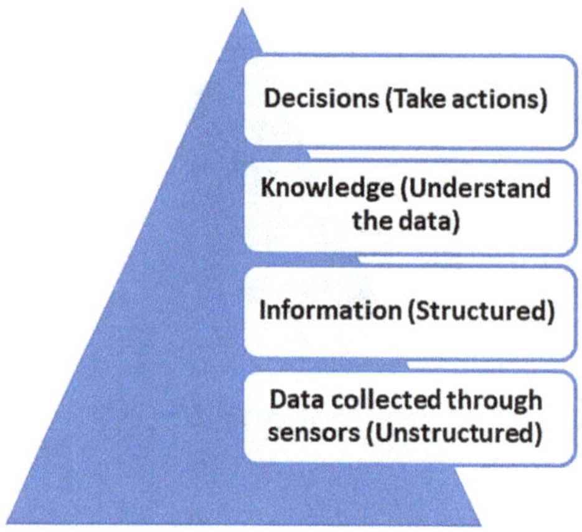

Generally, there are five steps procedures to collect the data from the patients:

Step 1: In the first step, the data is collected through wearable sensor devices that are attached to the patient's body.
Step 2: Usually the data will be in the analog form which has to be aggregated and changed to digital form.
Step 3: Then the digitized data is stimulated to the cloud or data center.
Step 4: By using Decision Support Systems or algorithms, the data can be analyzed.
Step 5: The resultant data can be sent to the physicians to take the action immediately to the patients.

The above procedure can be utilized for any kind of health issue. Some of the common health issues are as follows:

Cancer

Nowadays cancer is the foremost cause of death among the disease. Existing and upcoming cancer cares are not enough to tackle the increasing burden of cancer care. The most common categories of cancers are lung cancer, breast cancer, prostate cancer, liver cancer, colorectal cancer, and stomach cancer and the more top cause for death in women is breast cancer (Mcguire, 2015).

Overall, 1 in 28 women is affected by breast cancer. Breast cancer trouble is not only restricted to disease burden and humanity but also shows the way to an economic loss of the nation.

According to the Indian Council of Medical Research in India, about 413,519 men and 371,302 women died of cancer in 2018. Current methods outside of the mastectomy are not always able to grasp cancer early. Yet, wearable's can be used as an alternative to the radical operation.

Wearables are intended to turn out to be a vital indicative tool for cardiovascular and cancer detection. This will ignite into every feature of the detection of diseases. One such has been developed by Rob Royea (https://www.arrow.com).

The product is iTBra, which helps in detecting breast cancer at the early stage. This device is a bra, which is embedded with sensors to detect even small temperature changes in breast tissues for a certain period. Inspired with the possibilities, a film based on the technology called Detected has been sponsored by Cisco.(as shown in figure 9).

Figure 9. Seven sensors positioned within the bra
(https://www.arrow.com)

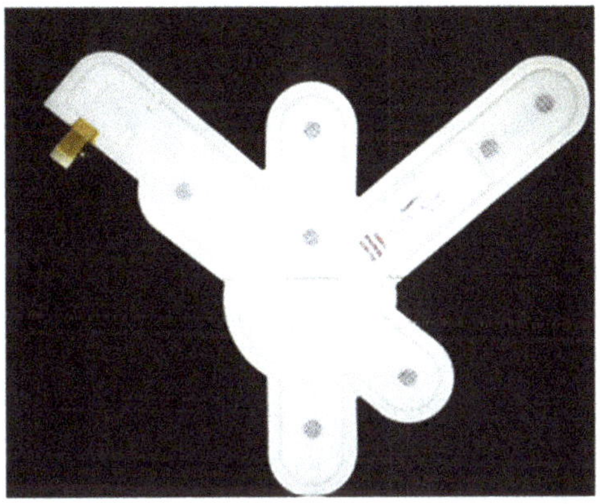

Elderly Persons

There are many tracking devices to track the child, elderly persons, and inform about their safety. Home monitoring of elderly people through IoT helps them to live at home safely (shown in fig. 10).

It is also a fact that the ratio of elderly persons is increasing. For an elderly person, it is very essential to monitor the parameters like systolic and diastolic blood pressure, pulse rate, heart rate, body temperature, sugar level, human brain activity.

Imagine an elderly patient suddenly has chest pain. The chest pain varies in intensity with the heartbeat and might have high blood pressure.

Figure 10. Elderly monitoring using IoT

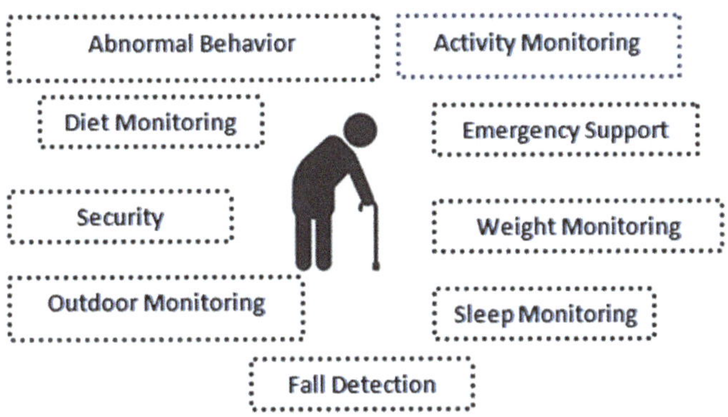

A smart wearable device such as a smartwatch, fitness tracker, and smart hat helps to get the user status. The collected data is transmitted to the cloud for further processing.

It is very crucial to extend the care services to elderly people by giving health monitoring services. It helps to share the elderly information with the medical experts to help them improve the quality of life.

Diabetes

Diabetes mellitus is normally referred to as diabetes, which has become a universal epidemic. It occurs due to the inability of the body to produce insulin for its own needs, either due to weakening in insulin secretion, impaired insulin action, or together. About 300 million persons globally are affected by diabetes and it is still increasing.

Diabetes is a long-standing metabolic disorder in which blood glucose (BG) level differs and it is occurred due to lack of insulin (Type 1 diabetes, T1D) or due to the lack of ability of the body to make use of the produced insulin (Type 2 diabetes, T2D) (Acciaroli et al., 2018).

Mainly in the developing countries, the diagnosis of T1D and T2D has extended, but the increase has been more for T2D, which nears about 90-95% of every case of diabetes. (Rubino, 2008).

It is predicted, nearly 366 million people would have diabetes from the total population in the year 2030(Wild et al., 2004).

In paper (Regin Joy Conejar & Haeng-konkim, 2014), it states that from the total population it is expected to have 171 million in 2000 to 366 million people with diabetes in 2030.

To diagnose the diabetes patients the glucose sensor, pulse, temperature, and blood pressure sensors are used. By using these sensors the data can be collected from the patients. The Arduino board can be used to convert the analog to digital conversion. The collected data can be transmitted to the cloud storage (shown in fig.11).

Figure 11. Diagnose diabetes patients

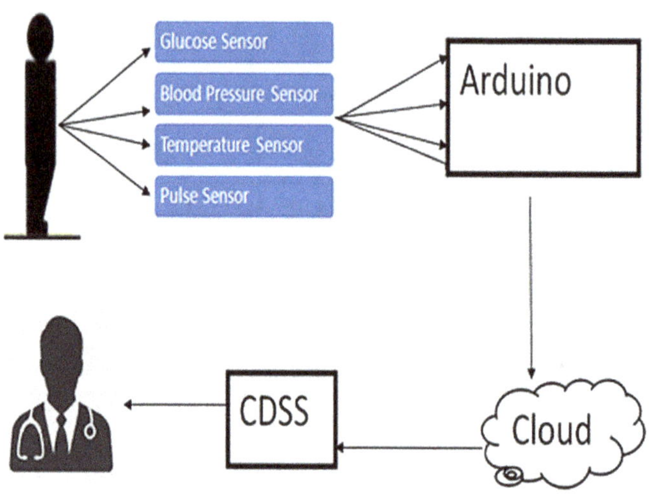

The glucose sensor is a division of a continuous glucose monitoring (CGM) system that is inserted under the skin and measures the glucose levels. The sensor monitors the level of glucose in the interstitial fluid every 10 seconds and converts it into an electrical signal. The signal signifies the amount of sugar in the blood.

To measure systemic arterial blood pressure in humans, blood pressure sensors can be used. The arterial blood pressure can also be measured and by using the oscillometric method and can calculate both the systolic and diastolic blood pressure (shown in fig.12).

Figure 12. Blood pressure sensor

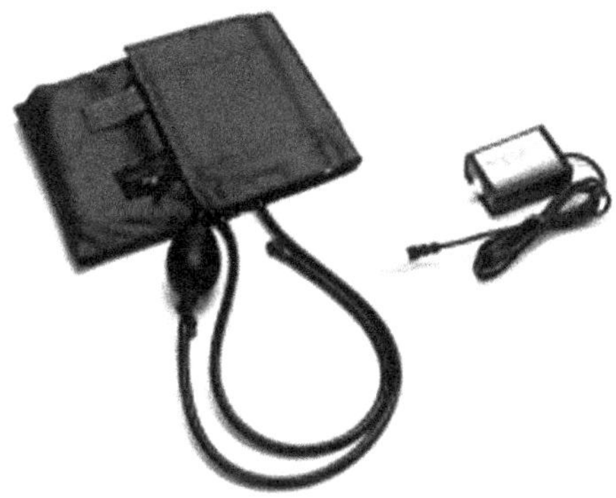

The temperature sensor can be applied to the skin surface and it specifies the body temperature. To measure the heart rate of the human the pulse sensor can be used. It works on the principle of photoplethysmography (shown in fig.13). The movement of blood volume is determined by the rate of heart pulses and since light is absorbed by the blood, the signal pulses are equal to the heartbeat pulses. The pulse reading of the patient is read by infrared lighting by sensing the fingertip.

Figure 13. Temperature sensor

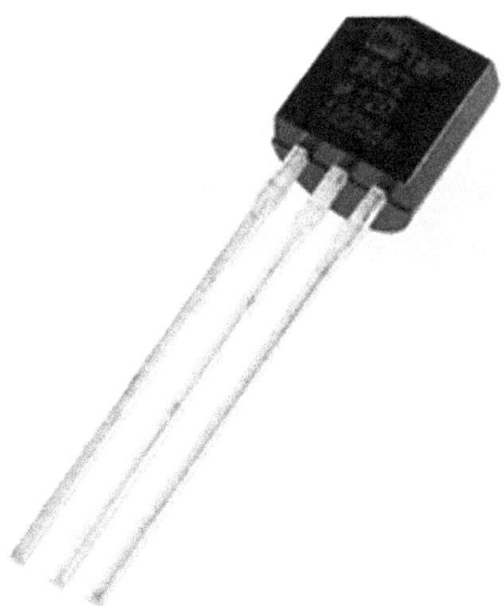

Through wrist band or smart watches the data can be collected and delivered to the cloud. The patient readings are collected by the sensors like a wrist band or smartwatches and are transmitted through the internet to the cloud database. The collected data is analyzed to make decisions. There can be many attributes for all the diseases and by using these above-mentioned sensors, we could predict for diabetes.

Any diastolic blood pressure under 60 is considered hypotension, which needs to be treated immediately as it specifies not enough blood is reaching the person's organ. When a person is sleeping, the diastolic blood pressure can be low too. Normally the plasma glucose levels range from 3.9 to 7.2 for non-diabetic patients even after fasting.

Mostly diabetes inclines to lesser the "good" cholesterol levels and increases triglyceride and "bad" cholesterol levels, which lead to the threat of heart disease and stroke. Even earlier to the diagnoses also, these conditions can occur.

The below table shows the data values for a diabetes patient, taken Pima-Indians-diabetes-dataset-part-1 from which the clinicians can take the decisions.

Table 1. Datasets for a diabetes patient

S. No.	Age	Blood Pressure (mm/Hg)	Glucose (mg/DL)	BMI
1	50	72	148	33.6
2	31	66	85	26.6
3	32	64	183	23.3
4	21	66	89	28.1
5	33	40	137	43.1

In case, if these were received through IoT, the clinicians can decide the effect of diabetes on the patients and provide the necessary treatment immediately.

People with diabetes should maintain both their blood sugar and cholesterol at a low level to avoid the risk of having a heart attack. It is also compulsory to maintain healthy weight and low blood pressure.

Adults should have the entire cholesterol levels less than 200 milligrams per deciliter (mg/dL). When the range is from 200 to 239 mg/dL it is treated as borderline high and a value of about 240 mg/dL and more is treated as high. When the value is 240 mg/dL and above it is treated as high blood cholesterol. At this level, the person is considered to have more risk for heart disease.

The persons having diabetes and no known coronary heart disease, the LDL levels in the blood are supposed to be less than 100 milligrams per deciliter (mg/dL), and HDL levels are supposed to be more than 50mg/dL and triglycerides less than 150 mg/dL. In the HA1C test, the level of blood sugar or glucose level should be below 7% is recommended.

For people having diabetes and known heart disease, the LDL is supposed to be below 70mg/dL. Triglyceride levels are supposed to be less than 150 mg/dL and HDL above 40 mg/dL. The HDL levels should be more than 50mg/dL for women with diabetes and coronary heart disease.

Challenges Faced in Healthcare

Though there are many advantages in using IoT with CDSS, there exist some challenges faced by the healthcare service providers. The main thing is security, most of the healthcare industry lacks it. Next are the integration and implementation of the existing systems. Another big challenge is the awareness of this technology among the patients.

ADVANTAGES OF USING IOT CDSS IN HEALTHCARE

Improved Treatment

It helps the physicians make the decision at a faster time and give the treatment soon. The connected healthcare solutions with CDSS enable the care providers to provide real-time information that makes them take good decisions and provide confirmation- based treatments. This provides improved treatment results.

Diagnosing the Disease

As the data is in the cloud, it can be viewed by any of the physicians. So anyone can give suggestions and in the meantime can monitor the patients continuously. It also assists in diagnosing the disease at an early-bird stage even by knowing the symptoms earlier; it helps to prevent the disease further.

Reduction of Cost

By this feature, it helps the patients to reduce the cost by visiting the doctors directly and could also save time.

Error Reduction

Data that is generated through IoT devices ensures to give smooth healthcare with less error and waste

Saves Time

The capability to easily monitor and manage the patient's health, saves precious minutes, without visiting each patient manually.

Customization

With dedicated IoT solutions, the health of each patient is analyzed well and the treatment is given to their needs. This enriches a patient's experience at a healthcare facility and leaves them feeling satisfied and cared for.

Enhanced Patient Experience

Healthcare is all about for a patient, so their comfort is the first. The IoT CDSS helps to improve that experience by giving wise intercession and diagnosis, proactive treatments, and good outcomes.

LIMITATIONS OF IOT CDSS IN HEALTHCARE

Though the IoT in healthcare has reached to a great extent, still it has some pitfalls.

Technical Requirements

From the technical point of view, IoT is often fragmented and it lacks interoperability. The platforms must be able to work across devices regardless of the manufacture and make.

Regulatory Concerns

A large volume of data is collected that could be harmful or sensitive if exposed, as the data might contain personal information. On the regulatory side, for security purpose, who can access IoT data and how it can be used, must be addressed. The government needs to set proper instructions and protocols for the healthcare industries to confirm that the data is not misused.

Security

Due to poor design, IoT devices are often susceptible to security. It needs strong authentication methods and a platform to track irregularities. Many healthcare organizations are not aware of the barrier they will encounter when trying to detain and harness the huge volume of data.

Data Avalanche

The most noteworthy merit is connecting devices in healthcare. But, due to the lack of experience and knowledge is holding back the use of connecting devices with healthcare organizations. Healthcare providers should find a proper way to handle large volumes of data and store it for further processing and analytics.

Improvement Cost

The efficient deployment of IoT based healthcare saves lots of life and money. But before that, its developments and implementations require lots of investments and a clear understanding of its purpose.

End Users

Most of the patients are unfair against the use of IoT applications in healthcare. It is more important to give awareness about the benefits of using IoT in healthcare to the people.

CONCLUSION

Technology is changing how the healthcare industry diagnoses, monitors, and gives treatments to patients. IoT healthcare with CDSS would indeed a boon in the health sector. Despite security concerns and privacy issues, the IoT healthcare has brought tremendous improvement to society. The IoT healthcare with CDSS has the potential to reach every individual at one time or another in their lifetime. With its vast applications, IoT has been smoothing the progress of healthcare providers including doctors, hospitals, and clinics to take care of the patients with precise treatment. This technology IoT healthcare with CDSS is very essential to counterpart with the growing needs of the digital world.

REFERENCES

Abdelgawad, A., Yelamarthi, K., & Khattab, A. (2016), IoT-Based Health Monitoring System for Active and Assisted Living. GOODTECHS 2016, 11-20.

Acciaroli, G., Vettoretti, M., Facchinetti, A., & Sparacino, G. (2018). Calibration of Minimally Invasive Continuous Glucose Monitoring Sensors: State-of-the-art and current perspectives. *Biosensors (Basel)*, *8*(1), 13–24. doi:10.3390/bios8010024 PMID:29534053

Aggarwal, V. K. (Ed.). (1998). *Institutional Designs for a complex world: Bargaining, Linkages and Nesting*. Cornell University. doi:10.7591/9781501733123

American Diabetes Association. (2006). Standards of medical care in diabetes–2006. *Diabetes Care*, *29*(Suppl. 1), s4–s42. PMID:16373931

Anooj, A. (2011). Clinical Decision Support System: Risk Level Prediction of Heart Disease using Weighted Fuzzy Rules and Decision Tree Rules. *Open Computer Science*, *1*(4). Advance online publication. doi:10.247813537-011-0032-y

Atzori, L., Iera, A., & Morabito, G. (2010). The Internet of Things: A Survey. *Computer Networks*, *54*(15), 2787–2805. doi:10.1016/j.comnet.2010.05.010

Bhömer, M., Tomico, O., & Hummels, C. (2013), Smart textile services to support rehabilitation. *Proceedings of the Nordic Design Research Conference (NORDES 2013)*, *9*, 12.

Bonfiglio, A., Curone, D., Secco, E. L., Magenes, G., & Tognetti, A. (2011). Emergency and work. In *Wearable Monitoring Systems* (pp. 205–219). Springer. doi:10.1007/978-1-4419-7384-9_10

Burns, W. P. (2012). Evaluation of a technology enabled garment for older walkers. *Proceedings of the Annual International Conference of the IEEE Engineering in Medicine and Biology Society*, 2100–2103. 10.1109/EMBC.2012.6346374

Chen, K. H., Chen, P. C., Liu, K. C., & Chan, C. T. (2015). Wearable Sensor-Based Rehabilitation Exercise Assessment for Knee Osteoarthritis. *Sensors (Basel)*, *15*(2), 4193–4211. doi:10.3390150204193 PMID:25686308

Conejar. (2014). Medical Decisions Support System (DSS) for Ubiquitous Healthcare Diagnosis System. *International Journal of Software Engineering and Its Applications*, *8*(10), 237–244.

Feito, Y., Moriarty, T. A., Mangine, G., & Monahan, J. (2018). The Use Of A Smart-Textile Garment During High-Intensity Functional Training. A Pilot Study. *The Journal of Sports Medicine and Physical Fitness*. PMID:30024125

Ferreira, A. G., Fernandes, D., Branco, S., Monteiro, J. L., Cabral, J., Catarino, A. P., & Rocha, A. M. (2016), A Smart Wearable System For Sudden Infant Death Syndrome Monitoring. *Proceedings of the 2016 IEEE International Conference on Industrial Technology (ICIT)*, 1920–1925. 10.1109/ICIT.2016.7475060

Frydrysiak, M., & Tesiorowski, L. (2016), Health monitoring system for protecting elderly people. *Proceedings of the International Multidisciplinary Conference on Computer and Energy Science*, 1–6. 10.1109/SpliTech.2016.7555935

Geng, H. (2017). *Internet of Things and Data Analytics Handbook*. John Wiley & Sons. doi:10.1002/9781119173601

Haghi, M., Thurow, K., & Stoll, R. (2017). Wearable Devices in Medical Internet of Things: Scientific Research and Commercially Available Devices, Review Article. *Healthcare Informatics Research*, *23*(1), 4–15. doi:10.4258/hir.2017.23.1.4 PMID:28261526

Haghi, M., Thurow, K., & Stoll, R. (2017). Wearable Devices In Medical Internet-Of-Things: Scientific Research And Commercially Available Devices. *Healthcare Informatics Research*, *23*(1), 4–15. doi:10.4258/hir.2017.23.1.4 PMID:28261526

He, D., & Zeadally, S. (2015). An Analysis of RFID Authentication Scheme for Internet of Things in Healthcare Environment using Elliptic curve cryptography. *IEEE Internet of Things Journal*, *2*(1), 72–83. doi:10.1109/JIOT.2014.2360121

Joshi, J., Kurian, D., Bhasin, S., Mukherjee, S., Awasthi, P., Sharma, S., & Mittal, S. (2016), Health Monitoring Using Wearable Sensor and Cloud Computing. *Proceedings of the International Conference on Cybernetics, Robotics and Control*, 104–108. 10.1109/CRC.2016.031

Market Analysis Report. (2019). *Internet of Things (IoT) in Healthcare Market Size, Share & Trends Analysis Report By Component (Service, System & Software), By Connectivity Technology (Satellite, Cellular), By End Use (CRO, Hospital & Clinic), By Application, And Segment Forecasts, 2019 – 2025*. Author.

Mcguire, S. (2015). *World Cancer report 2014*. World Health Organization, International Agency for Research on Cancer, Who Press.

Morales, I. J. C., Pupiales, S. K. N., Criollo, A. C. U., & Montalvo, P. D. R. (2017). Wearable Textile for Accident Prevention for Babies in Crawl Phase. *Proceedings of the International Conference on Information Systems and Computer Science (INCISCOS)*, 66–72. 10.1109/INCISCOS.2017.55

Musen, M. A., Middleton, B., & Greenes, R. A. (2014). Clinical Decision-Support Systems. In E. H. Shortlife & J. J. Cimino (Eds.), *Biomedical Informatics Springer* (pp. 643–674). doi:10.1007/978-1-4471-4474-8_22

Naharro-Abellán & Lobo-Valbuena. (2020). Clinical Decision Support Systems: Future or Present in ICU? *ICU Management & Practice, 19*(4).

Niewolny, D. (2013). *How the Internet of Things Is Revolutionizing Healthcare*. Freescale Semiconductors.

Osheroff, J. A., & Teich, J. (2012). Improving Outcomes with Clinical Decision Support: An Implementer's Guide (2nd ed.). Chicago: Healthcare Information and Management Systems Society (HIMSS).

Osheroff, J. A., Teich, J. M., Middleton, B., Steen, E. B., Wright, A., & Detmer, D. E. (2007). A Roadmap for National Action on Clinical Decision Support. *Journal of the American Medical Informatics Association, 14*(2), 141–145. doi:10.1197/jamia.M2334 PMID:17213487

Perego, P., Andreoni, G., Zanini, R., & Bellù, R. (2014) Wearable Biosignal Monitoring System For Newborns. *Proceedings Of The 4th International Conference On Wireless Mobile Communication and Healthcare—Transforming Healthcare Through Innovations in Mobile and Wireless Technologies (MOBIHEALTH),* 271–274. 10.4108/icst.mobihealth.2014.257403

Riazul Islam, S., Daehan Kwak, Humaun Kabir, M., Hossain, M., & Kyung-Sup Kwak. (2015). The Internet of Things for Health Care: A Comprehensive Survey. *IEEE Access: Practical Innovations, Open Solutions, 3*, 678–708. doi:10.1109/ACCESS.2015.2437951

Rubino, F. (2008). Is type 2 diabetes an operable intestinal disease? A Provocative Yet Reasonable Hypothesis. *Diabetes Care, 31*(Suppl. 2), S290–S296. doi:10.2337/dc08-s271 PMID:18227499

Shull, P. B., & Damian, D. D. (2015). Haptic Wearables As Sensory Replacement, Sensory Augmentation And Trainer—A Review. *Journal of Neuroengineering and Rehabilitation, 12*(1), 595. doi:10.118612984-015-0055-z PMID:26188929

Spulber, I., Chen, Y. M., Papi, E., Anastasova Ivanova, S., Bergmann, J., McGregor, A. H., & Georgiou, P. (2015). Live Demonstration: Wearable Electronics For A Smart Garment Aiding Rehabilitation. *Proceedings of the IEEE International Symposium on Circuits and Systems (ISCAS).* 10.1109/ISCAS.2015.7169045

Subramaniam,, M., & Ganesh,, B. (2014). Origin and Applications of Internet of Things. *CSI Communications, 38*(1).

Sundaravadivel, P., Kougianos, E., Mohanty, S. P., & Ganapathiraju, M. K. (2018). Everything You Wanted to Know about Smart Health Care: Evaluating the different technologies and components of the Internet of Things for better healthcare. *IEEE Consumer Electronics Magazine, 7*(1), 18–28. doi:10.1109/MCE.2017.2755378

Syeda, F. U. B., & Begum, I. (2017). Smart Health Care Solutions Using IOT, International Journal and Magazine of Engineering, Technology. *Management and Research, 4*(3), 10–15.

Trindade, I. G., Machado da Silva, J., Rui, M., Pereira, M., Lucas, J., Oliveira, L., Valentim, B., Barreto, J., & Santos Silva, M. (2016). Design and Evaluation of Novel Textile Wearable Systems for the Surveillance of Vital Signals. *Sensors (Basel), 16*(10), 1573. doi:10.339016101573 PMID:27669263

Wang, Q., De Baets, L., Timmermans, A., Chen, W., Giacolini, L., Matheve, T., & Markopoulos, P. (2017). Motor Control Training for the Shoulder with Smart Garments. *Sensors (Basel)*, *17*(7), 1687. doi:10.339017071687 PMID:28737670

Wild, S., Roglic, G., Green, A., Sicree, R., & King, H. (2004). Global Prevalence of Diabetes: Estimates for the Year 2000 and projections for 2030. *Diabetes Care*, *2004*(27), 1047–1053. doi:10.2337/diacare.27.5.1047 PMID:15111519

World Health Organization. (1999). *Definition, Diagnosis, and Classification of Diabetes Mellitus and Its Complications. Part 1: Diagnosis and Classification of Diabetes Mellitus*. World Health Organization.

Wyatt, J. C. (2000). Decision Support Systems. *Journal of the Royal Society of Medicine*, *93*(12), 629–633. doi:10.1177/014107680009301206 PMID:11193060

Compilation of References

AAMC Reporter. (2012, Oct.). Available online: https://www.aamc.org/newsroom/reporter/october2012/308516/health-care-apps.html

Abadi, M., Barham, P., Chen, J., Chen, Z., Davis, A., Dean, J., & Kudlur, M. (2016). Tensorflow: A system for large-scale machine learning. In *12th {USENIX} Symposium on Operating Systems Design and Implementation ({OSDI} 16)* (pp. 265-283). USENIX.

Abbas, Q., Garcia, I. F., Emre Celebi, M., Ahmad, W., & Mushtaq, Q. (2013). A perceptually oriented method for contrast enhancement and segmentation of dermoscopy images. *Skin Research and Technology*, *19*(1), e490–e497. doi:10.1111/j.1600-0846.2012.00670.x PMID:22882675

Abdelgawad, A., Yelamarthi, K., & Khattab, A. (2016), IoT-Based Health Monitoring System for Active and Assisted Living. GOODTECHS 2016, 11-20.

AbdelKader, W., & Elnakeeb, M. (2017). The relationship between the use of media and emotional intelligence among youth nursing students. *Journal of Nursing and Health Science*, *6*(5), 63–77.

Acciaroli, G., Vettoretti, M., Facchinetti, A., & Sparacino, G. (2018). Calibration of Minimally Invasive Continuous Glucose Monitoring Sensors: State-of-the-art and current perspectives. *Biosensors (Basel)*, *8*(1), 13–24. doi:10.3390/bios8010024 PMID:29534053

Acharya, U. R., Oh, S. L., Hagiwara, Y., Tan, J. H., & Adeli, H. (2018). Deep convolutional neural network for the automated detection and diagnosis of seizure using EEG signals. *Computers in Biology and Medicine*, *100*, 270–278. doi:10.1016/j.compbiomed.2017.09.017 PMID:28974302

Adabor, E. S., & Acquaah-Mensah, G. K. (2019). Machine learning approaches to decipher hormone and HER2 receptor status phenotypes in breast cancer. *Briefings in Bioinformatics*, *20*(2), 504–514. doi:10.1093/bib/bbx138 PMID:29045694

Adam, A., Hellig, J. C., Perera, M., Bolton, D., & Lawrentschuk, N. (2018). Prostate Cancer Risk Calculator' mobile applications (Apps): A systematic review and scoring using the validated user version of the Mobile Application Rating Scale (uMARS). *World Journal of Urology*, *36*(4), 565–573. doi:10.100700345-017-2150-1

Adams, S. K., Piekiel, N. W., Ervin, M. H., & Morris, C. J. (2018). Silicon quantum dots for energetic material applications. *Applied Physics Letters*, *112*(23), 233108. doi:10.1063/1.5022587

Aggarwal, N., & Aggarwal, K. (2012). Comparative Analysis of kmeans and Enhanced Kmeans clustering algorithm for data mining. *International Journal of Scientific & Engineering Research.*

Aggarwal, V. K. (Ed.). (1998). *Institutional Designs for a complex world: Bargaining, Linkages and Nesting*. Cornell University. doi:10.7591/9781501733123

Ahmed, M. U. (2017). Internet of Things (IoT) Technologies for HealthCare. *4th International Conference, HealthyIoT 2017*, 50-78.

Ahmed, F. E. (2005). Artificial neural networks for diagnosis and survival prediction in colon cancer. *Molecular Cancer*, *4*(1), 29. doi:10.1186/1476-4598-4-29 PMID:16083507

Ahr, A., Holtrich, U., Solbach, C., Scharl, A., Strebhardt, K., Karn, T., & Kaufmann, M. (2001). Molecular classification of breast cancer patients by gene expression profiling. *The Journal of Pathology: A Journal of the Pathological Society of Great Britain and Ireland, 195*(3), 312-320.

Akay, M. F. (2009). Support vector machines combined with feature selection for breast cancer diagnosis. *Expert Systems with Applications*, *36*(2), 3240–3247. doi:10.1016/j.eswa.2008.01.009

Akyel, C., & Arici, N. (2020). *Cilt Kanserinde Kıl Temizliği ve Lezyon Bölütlemesinde Yeni Bir Yaklaşım. Politeknik Dergisi*. Early Access.

Akyol, K. (2020). Stacking ensemble based deep neural networks modeling for effective epileptic seizure detection. *Expert Systems with Applications*, *148*, 113239. doi:10.1016/j.eswa.2020.113239

Alabi, O. F. (2013). A survey of Facebook addiction level among selected Nigerian university undergraduates. *New Media and Mass Communication, 10*, 70–80.

Albahar, M. A. (2019). Skin lesion classification using convolutional neural network with novel regularizer. *IEEE Access: Practical Innovations, Open Solutions*, *7*, 38306–38313. doi:10.1109/ACCESS.2019.2906241

Al-Hadeethi, H., Abdulla, S., Diykh, M., Deo, R. C., & Green, J. H. (2020). Adaptive boost LSSVM classification approach for time-series signal classification in epileptic seizure diagnosis applications. *Expert Systems with Applications*, *161*, 113676. doi:10.1016/j.eswa.2020.113676

Aličković, E., & Subasi, A. (2017). Breast cancer diagnosis using GA feature selection and Rotation Forest. *Neural Computing & Applications*, *28*(4), 753–763. doi:10.100700521-015-2103-9

Alizadeh, A. A., Eisen, M. B., Davis, R. E., Ma, C., Lossos, I. S., Rosenwald, A., ... Powell, J. I. (2000). Distinct types of diffuse large B-cell lymphoma identified by gene expression profiling. *Nature*, *403*(6769), 503–511. doi:10.1038/35000501 PMID:10676951

Allen, N. L., Karlson, E. W., Malspeis, S., Lu, B., Seidman, C. E., & Lehmann, L. S. (2014). Biobank participants' preferences for disclosure of genetic research results: Perspectives from the OurGenes, OurHealth, OurCommunity project. *Mayo Clinic Proceedings*, *89*(6), 738–746. doi:10.1016/j.mayocp.2014.03.015 PMID:24943692

Allen, V. D., Weissman, A., Hellwig, S., MacCann, C., & Roberts, R. D. (2014). Development of the situational test of emotional understanding–brief (STEU-B) using item response theory. *Personality and Individual Differences*, *65*, 3–7. doi:10.1016/j.paid.2014.01.051

Alon, U., Barkai, N., Notterman, D. A., Gish, K., Ybarra, S., Mack, D., & Levine, A. J. (1999). Broad patterns of gene expression revealed by clustering analysis of tumor and normal colon tissues probed by oligonucleotide arrays. *Proceedings of the National Academy of Sciences of the United States of America*, *96*(12), 6745–6750. doi:10.1073/pnas.96.12.6745 PMID:10359783

Alpaydın, E. (2020). *Introduction to machine learning*. MIT Press.

Al-Rawi, M., & Karajeh, H. (2007). Genetic algorithm matched filter optimization for automated detection of blood vessels from digital retinal images. Comput. Methods Programs Biomed., 87, 248–253.

Alsaba, M. T., Al Dushaishi, M. F., & Abbas, A. K. (2020). A comprehensive review of nanoparticles application in the oil and gas industry. *Journal of Petroleum Exploration and Production Technology*, *10*(4), 1389–1300. doi:10.100713202-019-00825-z

Altaf, Shahbaz, & Guergachi. (2017). Applications of association rule mining in health informatics, *AI Journal Under Springer, 47*, 313-340.

Alzu'bi, A. A., Zhou, L., & Watzlaf, V. J. M. (2019, April 1). Genetic Variations and Precision Medicine. *Perspectives in Health Information Management*, 16. PMID:31019429

American Diabetes Association. (2006). Standards of medical care in diabetes–2006. *Diabetes Care*, *29*(Suppl. 1), s4–s42. PMID:16373931

Amin, H. U., Yusoff, M. Z., & Ahmad, R. F. (2020). A novel approach based on wavelet analysis and arithmetic coding for automated detection and diagnosis of epileptic seizure in EEG signals using machine learning techniques. *Biomedical Signal Processing and Control*, *56*, 101707. doi:10.1016/j.bspc.2019.101707

Amor-García, M. Á., Collado-Borrell, R., Escudero-Vilaplana, V., Melgarejo-Ortuño, A., Herranz-Alonso, A., Arranz Arija, J. Á., & Sanjurjo-Sáez, M. (2020). Assessing apps for patients with genitourinary tumors using the Mobile Application Rating Scale (MARS): Systematic search in app stores and content analysis. *JMIR mHealth and uHealth*, *8*(7), e17609. doi:10.2196/17609

Anand, V., & Koundal, D. (2020). Computer-Assisted Diagnosis of Thyroid Cancer Using Medical Images: A Survey. In *Proceedings of ICRIC 2019* (pp. 543-559). Springer. 10.1007/978-3-030-29407-6_39

Andersson, G., & Cuijpers, P. (2008). Pros and cons of online cognitive-behavioural therapy. *The British Journal of Psychiatry*, *193*(4), 270–271. doi:10.1192/bjp.bp.108.054080

Andino, J. J., Guduguntla, V., Weizer, A., Roberts, W. W., Wittmann, D., Miller, D., Morgan, T. M., & Ellimoottil, C. (2007). Examining the value of video visits to patients in an outpatient urology clinic. *Urology*, *110*, 31–35. doi:10.1016/j.urology.2017.07.050

Andriole, G. L., Crawford, E. D., Grubb, R. L. III, Buys, S. S., Chia, D., Church, T. R., Fouad, M. N., Gelmann, E. P., Kvale, P. A., Reding, D. J., Weissfeld, J. L., Yokochi, L. A., O'Brien, B., Clapp, J. D., Rathmell, J. M., Riley, T. L., Hayes, R. B., Kramer, B. S., Izmirlian, G., ... Berg, C. D. (2009). Mortality results from a randomized prostate-cancer screening trial. *The New England Journal of Medicine*, *360*(13), 1310–1319. doi:10.1056/NEJMoa0810696

Andrzejak, R. G., Lehnertz, K., Mormann, F., Rieke, C., David, P., & Elger, C. E. (2001). Indications of nonlinear deterministic and finite-dimensional structures in time series of brain electrical activity: Dependence on recording region and brain state. *Physical Review. E*, *64*(6), 061907. doi:10.1103/PhysRevE.64.061907 PMID:11736210

Anonymous. (2016). *The key differences between Telehealth and mHealth*. https://liveclinic.com/blog/key-differences-telehealth-mhealth/

Anonymous. (2017). *Why mHealth is Essential for Patient Engagement*. https://liquid-state.com/why-mhealth-is-essential-for-patient-engagement/

Anooj, A. (2011). Clinical Decision Support System: Risk Level Prediction of Heart Disease using Weighted Fuzzy Rules and Decision Tree Rules. *Open Computer Science*, *1*(4). Advance online publication. doi:10.247813537-011-0032-y

Ansari, S. M., Bhor, R. D., Pai, K. R., Sen, D., Mazumder, D., Ghosh, K., Kolekar, Y. D., & Ramana, C. V. (2017). Cobalt nanoparticles for biomedical applications: Facile synthesis, physiochemical characterization, cytotoxicity behavior and biocompatibility. *Applied Surface Science*, *414*, 171–187. doi:10.1016/j.apsusc.2017.03.002

Argenziano, G., Fabbrocini, G., Carli, P., De Giorgi, V., Sammarco, E., & Delfino, M. (1998). Epiluminescence microscopy for the diagnosis of doubtful melanocytic skin lesions: Comparison of the ABCD rule of dermatoscopy and a new 7-point checklist based on pattern analysis. *Archives of Dermatology*, *134*(12), 1563–1570. doi:10.1001/archderm.134.12.1563 PMID:9875194

Arita, I., Nakane, M., Kojima, K., Yoshihara, N., Nakano, T., & El-Gohary, A. (2004). Role of a sentinel surveillance system in the context of global surveillance of infectious disease. *The Lancet. Infectious Diseases*, *4*(3), 171–177. doi:10.1016/S1473-3099(04)00942-9 PMID:14998504

Arjun. (2017). *Retinopathy Dataset.* Retrieved from https://github.com/javathunderman/retinopathy-dataset

Armstrong, B. K., & Kricker, A. (1995). Skin cancer. *Dermatologic Clinics*, *13*(3), 583–594. doi:10.1016/S0733-8635(18)30064-0 PMID:7554506

Armstrong, B., & Doll, R. (1975). Environmental factors and cancer incidence and mortality in different countries, with special reference to dietary practices. *International Journal of Cancer*, *15*(4), 617–631. doi:10.1002/ijc.2910150411

Aronson, S. J., & Rehm, H. L. (2015, October 15). Building the foundation for genomics in precision medicine. *Nature*, *526*(7573), 336–342. doi:10.1038/nature15816 PMID:26469044

Astefanei, A., Nunez, O., & Galceran, M. (2015). Characterization and Determination of Fullerenes: A Critical Review. *ChemInform*, *46*(33), 19–21. doi:10.1002/chin.201533304

Atzori, L., Iera, A., & Morabito, G. (2010). The Internet of Things: A Survey. *Computer Networks*, *54*(15), 2787–2805. doi:10.1016/j.comnet.2010.05.010

Aungst, T. D. (2013). Medical applications for pharmacists using mobile devices. *The Annals of Pharmacotherapy*, *47*(7–8), 1088–1095. doi:10.1345/aph.1S035 PMID:23821609

Ayan, E., & Ünver, H. M. (2018). *Data augmentation importance for classification of skin lesions via deep learning. In Electric Electronics, Computer Science, Biomedical Engineerings' Meeting (EBBT).* IEEE.

Azar, A. T., & El-Said, S. A. (2014). Performance analysis of support vector machines classifiers in breast cancer mammography recognition. *Neural Computing & Applications*, *24*(5), 1163–1177. doi:10.100700521-012-1324-4

Baba, Y., & Nakamura, T. (2002). Time dependent principal component analysis. In *Measurement and Multivariate Analysis* (pp. 155–162). Springer. doi:10.1007/978-4-431-65955-6_16

Bahrami, A., Hasanzadeh, M., Shahidsales, S., Farazestanian, M., Hassanian, S. M., Moetamani Ahmadi, M., Maftouh, M., Gharib, M., Yousefi, Z., Kadkhodayan, S., Ferns, G. A., & Avan, A. (2018). Genetic susceptibility in cervical cancer: From bench to bedside. *Journal of Cellular Physiology*, *233*(3), 1929–1939. doi:10.1002/jcp.26019 PMID:28542881

Bailie, K. (2005). *An exploration of the utility of a self-report emotional intelligence measure* (Doctoral dissertation). Stellenbosch: University of Stellenbosch.

Banaie, M., Soltanian-Zadeh, H., Saligheh-Rad, H. R., & Gity, M. (2018). Spatiotemporal features of DCE-MRI for breast cancer diagnosis. *Computer Methods and Programs in Biomedicine*, *155*, 153–164. doi:10.1016/j.cmpb.2017.12.015 PMID:29512495

Bao, F. S., Lie, D. Y. C., & Zhang, Y. (2008, November). A new approach to automated epileptic diagnosis using EEG and probabilistic neural network. In *2008 20th IEEE International Conference on Tools with Artificial Intelligence* (Vol. 2, pp. 482-486). IEEE. 10.1109/ICTAI.2008.99

Barata, C., & Marques, J. S. (2019). Deep Learning For Skin Cancer Diagnosis With Hierarchical Architectures. In *IEEE 16th International Symposium on Biomedical Imaging (ISBI 2019)* (pp. 841-845). IEEE.

Bar-On, R. (2006). The Bar-On model of emotional-social intelligence (ESI). *Psicothema*, *18*, 13–25. PMID:17295953

Bar-On, R., & Parker, J. D. A. (2000). *BarOn emotional quotient inventory: Youth version*. Multi-Health System, Incorporated.

Barreto, M. L. (2006). Comentário: Tecnologias Em saúde E o sempre tenue equilíbrio entre riscos E benefícios. *Revista de Saude Publica*, *40*(3), 397–399. doi:10.1590/S0034-89102006000300005 PMID:16810361

Basch, E., Deal, A. M., Dueck, A. C., Scher, H. I., Kris, M. G., Hudis, C., & Schrag, D. (2017). Overall survival results of a trial assessing patient-reported outcomes for symptom monitoring during routine cancer treatment. *Journal of the American Medical Association*, *318*(2), 197–198. doi:10.1001/jama.2017.7156

Bekish, Y. N., Poznyak, S. K., Tsybulskaya, L. S., & Gaevskaya, T. V. (2010). Electrodeposited Ni–B alloy coatings: Structure, corrosion resistance and mechanical properties. *Electrochimica Acta*, *55*(7), 2223–2231. doi:10.1016/j.electacta.2009.11.069

Belarmino, A., Walsh, R., Alshak, M., Patel, N., Wu, R., & Hu, J. C. (2019). Feasibility of a mobile health application to monitor recovery and patient-reported outcomes after robot-assisted radical prostatectomy. *Eur. Urol. Oncol.*, *2*(4), 425–428. doi:10.1016/j.euo.2018.08.016

Bender, J. L., Feldman-Stewart, D., Tong, C., Lee, K., Brundage, M., Pai, H., Robinson, J., & Panzarella, T. (2019). Health-related internet use among men with prostate cancer in Canada: Cancer registry survey study. *Journal of Medical Internet Research*, *21*(11), e14241. doi:10.2196/14241

Ben-Dor, A., Bruhn, L., Friedman, N., Nachman, I., Schummer, M., & Yakhini, Z. (2000, April). Tissue classification with gene expression profiles. In *Proceedings of the fourth annual international conference on Computational molecular biology* (pp. 54-64). Academic Press.

Beyzay, F., Hosseini, A. Z., & Soudi, S. (2017). Alpha alumina nanoparticle conjugation to cysteine peptidase A and B: An efficient method for autophagy induction. *Avicenna Journal of Medical Biotechnology*, *9*(2), 71–81.

Bhardwaj, A., Tiwari, A., Krishna, R., & Varma, V. (2016). A novel genetic programming approach for epileptic seizure detection. *Computer Methods and Programs in Biomedicine*, *124*, 2–18. doi:10.1016/j.cmpb.2015.10.001 PMID:26645791

Bhatkar, A. P., & Kharat, G.U. (2015). Detection of Diabetic Retinopathy in Retinal Images using MLP Classifier. *2015 IEEE International Symposium on Nanoelectronic and Information Systems*, 331-335. 10.1109/iNIS.2015.30

Bhömer, M., Tomico, O., & Hummels, C. (2013), Smart textile services to support rehabilitation. *Proceedings of the Nordic Design Research Conference (NORDES 2013)*, *9*, 12.

Birkhead, G. S., & Maylahn, C. M. (2000). State and Local Public Health Surveillance. In Principles and Practices of Public Health Surveillance. Oxford University Press.

Birkhead, G. S., & Maylahn, C. M. (2010). State and local public health surveillance in the United States. *Principles & Practice of Public Health Surveillance*, 381-398. . doi:10.1093/acprof:oso/9780195372922.003.0018

Blackadar, C. B. (2016). Historical review of the causes of cancer. *World Journal of Clinical Oncology*, *7*(1), 54–86. doi:10.5306/wjco.v7.i1.54 PMID:26862491

Blomberg, K., Wengström, Y., Sundberg, K., Browall, M., Isaksson, A. K., Nyman, M. H., & Langius-Eklöf, A. (2016). Symptoms and self-care strategies during and six months after radiotherapy for prostate cancer - scoping the perspectives of patients, professionals and literature. *European Journal of Oncology Nursing*, *21*, 139–145. doi:10.1016/j.ejon.2015.09.004

Bogart, L.K., Morozov, I.G., Parkin, I.V., & Kuznetcov, M.V. (2018). Fe Mössbauer study of NiFe2O4 nanoparticles produced by the levitation-jet aerosol technique. *Journal of Materials Science: Materials in Electronics, 29*(10). 1007/s10854-018-9569

Bokhorst, L. P., Valdagni, R., Rannikko, A., Kakehi, Y., Pickles, T., Bangma, C. H., & Roobol, M. J. (2016). A decade of active surveillance in the PRIAS Study: An update and evaluation of the criteria used to recommend a switch to active treatment. *European Urology*, *70*(6), 954–960. doi:10.1016/j.eururo.2016.06.007

Bonfiglio, A., Curone, D., Secco, E. L., Magenes, G., & Tognetti, A. (2011). Emergency and work. In *Wearable Monitoring Systems* (pp. 205–219). Springer. doi:10.1007/978-1-4419-7384-9_10

Borbane, S. A., Pande, V. V., Vibhute, S. K., Kendre, P. N., & Dange, V. U. (2015). Design and Fabrication of ordered meso-porous alumina scaffold for drug delivery of poorly water-soluble drug. *Austin Therapeutics*, *2*(1), 1015.

Borda, F.L.G., Oliveria, S.J.R., Lazaro, L.M.S.M., & Leiroz, A.J.K. (2018). *Experimental investigation of the tribological behavior of lubricants with additive containing copper nanoparticles*. Academic Press.

Borosund, E., Cvancarova, M., Ekstedt, M., Moore, S. M., & Ruland, C. M. (2013). How user characteristics affect use patterns in web-based illness management support for patients with breast and prostate cancer. *Journal of Medical Internet Research*, *15*(3), e34. doi:10.2196/jmir.2285

Boser, B. E., Guyon, I. M., & Vapnik, V. N. (1992). A training algorithm for optimal margin classifiers. In *Proceedings of the Fifth Annual Workshop on Computational Learning Theory*. ACM.

Bourke, L., Boorjian, S. A., Briganti, A., Klotz, L., Mucci, L., Resnick, M. J., Rosario, D. J., Skolarus, T. A., & Penson, D. F. (2015). Survivorship and improving quality of life in men with prostate cancer. *European Urology*, *68*(3), 374–383. doi:10.1016/j.eururo.2015.04.023

Brachman, P. S. (2009). Public health surveillance. *Bacterial Infections of Humans*, 51-67. doi:10.1007/978-0-387-09843-2_2

Bradski, G., & Kaehler, A. (2008). *Learning OpenCV: Computer vision with the OpenCV library*. O'Reilly Media, Inc.

Brambilla, D., Chiari, M., Gori, A., & Cretich, M. (2019). Towards precision medicine: the role and potential of protein and peptide microarrays. *The Analyst, 144.*

Bray, F., Ferlay, J., Soerjomataram, I., Siegel, R. L., Torre, L. A., & Jemal, A. (2018). Global cancer statistics 2018: GLOBOCAN estimates of incidence and mortality worldwide for 36 cancers in 185 countries. *CA: a Cancer Journal for Clinicians*, *68*(6), 394–424. doi:10.3322/caac.21492

Breiman, L. (1996). Arcing classifiers. *Annals of Statistics*, *26*, 123–140.

Brownson, R. C., Fielding, J. E., & Maylahn, C. M. (2009). Evidence-based public health: A fundamental concept for public health practice. *Annual Review of Public Health*, *30*(1), 175–201. doi:10.1146/annurev.publhealth.031308.100134 PMID:19296775

Brownson, R. C., & Petitti, D. B. (2006). *Applied epidemiology: Theory to practice*. Oxford University Press. doi:10.1093/acprof:oso/9780195187410.001.0001

Buckeridge, D. L. (2007). Outbreak detection through automated surveillance: A review of the determinants of detection. *Journal of Biomedical Informatics*, *40*(4), 370–379. doi:10.1016/j.jbi.2006.09.003 PMID:17095301

Buehler, J. W., Hopkins, R. S., Overhage, J. M., Sosin, D. M., & Tong, V. (2004). Framework for Evaluating Public Health Surveillance Systems for Early Detection of Outbreaks: Recommendations from CDC Working Group. *MMWR. Recommendations and Reports*, *53*(RR-5), 1–11. PMID:15129191

Burkle, F. M. (1999). Fortnightly review: Lessons learnt and future expectations of complex emergencies. *BMJ (Clinical Research Ed.)*, *319*(7207), 422–426. doi:10.1136/bmj.319.7207.422 PMID:10445925

Burns, W. P. (2012). Evaluation of a technology enabled garment for older walkers. *Proceedings of the Annual International Conference of the IEEE Engineering in Medicine and Biology Society*, 2100–2103. 10.1109/EMBC.2012.6346374

Byambasuren, O., Sanders, S., Beller, E., & Glasziou, P. (2018). Prescribable mHealth apps identified from an overview of systematic reviews. *NPJ Digital Medicine*, *1*(1), 12. doi:10.103841746-018-0021-9

Cao, Y., Chen, Y., & Khosla, D. (2015). Spiking deep convolutional neural networks for energy-efficient object recognition. *International Journal of Computer Vision*, *113*(1), 54–66. doi:10.100711263-014-0788-3

Carter, C. L., Allen, C., & Henson, D. E. (1989). Relation of tumor size, lymph node status, and survival in 24,740 breast cancer cases. *Cancer*, *63*(1), 181–187. doi:10.1002/1097-0142(19890101)63:1<181::AID-CNCR2820630129>3.0.CO;2-H PMID:2910416

Catan, G., & Espanha, R., Veloso, Mendes, R., Toren, O. & Chinitz, D. (2015). The impact of eHealth and mHealth on doctor behavior and patient involvement: An Israeli and Portuguese comparative approach. *Studies in Health Technology and Informatics*, *210*, 813–817.

Centers for Disease Control and Prevention (CDC). (n.d.). *Encyclopedia of Public Health.* doi:10.1007/978-1-4020-5614-7_343

Cha, B. G., & Kim, J. (2019). Functional mesoporous silica nanoparticles for bio-imaging applications. *Wiley Interdisciplinary Reviews. Nanomedicine and Nanobiotechnology*, *11*(1), 1–22. doi:10.1002/wnan.1515

Chambers, S. K., Hyde, M. K., Smith, D. P., Hughes, S., Yuill, S., Egger, S., O'Connell, D. L., Stein, K., Frydenberg, M., Wittert, G., & Dunn, J. (2017). New challenges in psycho-oncology research III: A systematic review of psychological interventions for prostate cancer survivors and their partners: clinical and research implications. *Psycho-Oncology*, *26*(7), 873–913. doi:10.1002/pon.4431

Chambers, S. K., Schover, L., Halford, K., Ferguson, M., Gardiner, R. A., Occhipinti, S., & Dunn, J. (2013). ProsCan for Couples: A feasibility study for evaluating peer su pport within a controlled research design. *Psycho-Oncology*, *22*(2), 475–479. doi:10.1002/pon.2110

Chandaka, S., Chatterjee, A., & Munshi, S. (2009). Cross-correlation aided support vector machine classifier for classification of EEG signals. *Expert Systems with Applications*, *36*(2), 1329–1336. doi:10.1016/j.eswa.2007.11.017

Chattopadhyay, D. P., & Patel, B. H. (2010). Effect of Nanosized Colloidal Copper on Cotton Fabric. *Journal of Engineered Fibers and Fabrics*, *5*(3), 1–6. doi:10.1177/155892501000500301

Chaudhuri, S., Chatterjee, S., Katz, N., Nelson, M., & Goldbaum, M. (1989). Detection of blood vessels in retinal images using two-dimensional matched filters. IEEE Trans. Med. Imag., 8(3), 263–269.

Chen, H., Engkvist, O., Wang, Y., Olivecrona, M., & Blaschke, T. (2018). The rise of deep learning in drug discovery. *Drug Discovery Today*, *23*(6), 1241–1250. doi:10.1016/j.drudis.2018.01.039 PMID:29366762

Chen, J., Ou, L., & Hollis, S. J. (2013). A systematic review of the impact of routine collection of patient reported outcome measures on patients, providers and health organizations in an oncologic setting. *BMC Health Services Research*, *13*(1), 21. doi:10.1186/1472-6963-13-211

Chen, K. H., Chen, P. C., Liu, K. C., & Chan, C. T. (2015). Wearable Sensor-Based Rehabilitation Exercise Assessment for Knee Osteoarthritis. *Sensors (Basel)*, *15*(2), 4193–4211. doi:10.3390150204193 PMID:25686308

Chetoui, M., Akhloufi, M. A., & Kardouchi, M. (2018). Diabetic Retinopathy Detection Using Machine Learning and Texture Features. *2018 IEEE Canadian Conference on Electrical & Computer Engineering (CCECE)*. 10.1109/CCECE.2018.8447809

Choi, B. C. (2012). The past, present, and future of public health surveillance. *Scientifica*, *2012*, 1–26. doi:10.6064/2012/875253 PMID:24278752

Chou, Cao, Weng, & Tsai. (2020). Mixed integer optimization approach to learning association rules for unplanned ICU transfer. *AI in Medicines Journal, 103*.

Chow, P. I., Drago, F., Kennedy, E. M., & Cohn, W. F. (2020). A novel mobile phone app intervention with phone coaching to reduce symptoms of depression in survivors of women's cancer: Pre-post pilot study. *JMIR Cancer*, *6*(1), e15750. doi:10.2196/15750

Christian Nordqvist. (2017). *What to know about diabetic retinopathy*. Retrieved from https://www.medicalnewstoday.com/articles/183417.php

Chudin, E., Walker, R., Kosaka, A., Wu, S. X., Rabert, D., Chang, T. K., & Kreder, D. E. (2001). Assessment of the relationship between signal intensities and transcript concentration for Affymetrix GeneChip® arrays. *Genome Biology, 3*(1).

Chui, P. L. (2019). Cancer- and chemotherapy-related symptoms and the use of complementary and alternative medicine. *Asia-Pacific Journal of Oncology Nursing*, *6*(1), 4–6. doi:10.4103/apjon.apjon_51_18

Chu, L. W., Ritchey, J., Devesa, S. S., Quraishi, S. M., Zhang, H., & Hsing, A. W. (2011). Prostate cancer incidence rates in Africa. *Prostate Cancer*.

Chu, S., Boxer, R., Madison, P., Kleinman, L., Skolarus, T., Altman, L., Bennett, C., & Shelton, J. (2015). Veterans affairs telemedicine: Bringing urologic care to remote clinics. *Urology*, *86*(2), 255–260. doi:10.1016/j.urology.2015.04.038

Cianfrocca, M., & Goldstein, L. J. (2004). Prognostic and predictive factors in early-stage breast cancer. *The Oncologist*, *9*(6), 606–616. doi:10.1634/theoncologist.9-6-606 PMID:15561805

Cinsdikici, M. G., & Aydin, D. (2009). Detection of blood vessels in ophthalmoscope images using MF/ant (matched filter/ant colony) algorithm. Comput. Methods Programs Biomed., 96, 85–95.

Collins, C., Xu, J., & Tang, S. (2012). Schistosomiasis control and the health system in P.R. China. *Infectious Diseases of Poverty*, *1*(1), 8. doi:10.1186/2049-9957-1-8 PMID:23849320

Collins, S. F., & Varmus, H. (2015). A New Initiative on Precision Medicine. *The New England Journal of Medicine*, *372*(9), 793–795. doi:10.1056/NEJMp1500523 PMID:25635347

Colman, A. M. (2015). *A dictionary of psychology*. Oxford Quick Reference.

Combi & Pozzi. (2019). Clinical information systems and artificial intelligence: Recent research trends. *Yearbook of Medical Infirmatics Thieme Journal, 28*(1), 83-94.

Conejar. (2014). Medical Decisions Support System (DSS) for Ubiquitous Healthcare Diagnosis System. *International Journal of Software Engineering and Its Applications*, *8*(10), 237–244.

Cooper, C. S. (2001). Applications of microarray technology in breast cancer research. *Breast Cancer Research*, *3*(3), 158. doi:10.1186/bcr291 PMID:11305951

Crane, R. A., Pullin, H., Macfarlane, J., Silion, M., Popescu, I. C., Andersen, M., Calen, V., & Scott, T. B. (2015). Field Application of Iron and Iron-Nickel Nanoparticles for the Ex Situ Remediation of a Uranium-Bearing Mine Water Effluent. *Journal of Environmental Engineering*, *141*(8), 8. doi:10.1061/(ASCE)EE.1943-7870.0000936

Dahlke, D. V., Fair, K., & Hong, Y. A. (2015). Apps seeking theories: Results of a study on the use of health behavior change theories in cancer survivorship mobile apps. *JMIR mHealth and uHealth*, *3*(1), e31. doi:10.2196/mhealth.3861

Daliri. (2017). Data Mining for Health Care Industry: A Practical Machine Learning Tool. *Int. Res. J. Multidiscip. Stud.*, *3*(4).

Dalton, L. W., Page, D. L., & Dupont, W. D. (1994). Histologic grading of breast carcinoma. A reproducibility study. *Cancer*, *73*(11), 2765–2770. doi:10.1002/1097-0142(19940601)73:11<2765::AID-CNCR2820731119>3.0.CO;2-K PMID:8194018

Das, A. B., Bhuiyan, M. I. H., & Alam, S. S. (2014, May). A statistical method for automatic detection of seizure and epilepsy in the dual tree complex wavelet transform domain. In *2014 International Conference on Informatics, Electronics & Vision (ICIEV)* (pp. 1-6). IEEE. 10.1109/ICIEV.2014.6850758

Das, A. B., Bhuiyan, M. I. H., & Alam, S. S. (2016). Classification of EEG signals using normal inverse Gaussian parameters in the dual-tree complex wavelet transform domain for seizure detection. *Signal, Image and Video Processing*, *10*(2), 259–266. doi:10.100711760-014-0736-2

Datar, M., Padfield, D., & Cline, H. (2008). Color and texture based segmentation of molecular pathology images using HSOMs. In *5th IEEE International Symposium on Biomedical Imaging: From Nano to Macro* (pp. 292-295). IEEE. 10.1109/ISBI.2008.4540990

Datta, S., Barua, R., & Das, J. (2019). Application of Artificial Intelligence in Modern Healthcare System. *Alginates - Recent Uses of This Natural Polymer.* https://www.intechopen.com/books/alginates-recent-uses-of-this-natural-polymer/application-of-artificial-intelligence-in-modern-healthcare-system

David, H., Gonzalo, S., & Patrick, G. (2017). *IoT Fundamentals: Networking Technologies, Protocols and Use Cases for the Internet of Things*. Pearson.

Davis, T. L., DiClemente, R., & Prietula, M. (2016). Taking mHealth forward: Examining the core characteristics. *JMIR mHealth and uHealth*, *4*(3), e97. doi:10.2196/mhealth.5659

de Koning, H. J., Gulati, R., Moss, S. M., Hugosson, J., Pinsky, P. F., Berg, C. D., Auvinen, A., Andriole, G. L., Roobol, M. J., Crawford, E. D., Nelen, V., Kwiatkowski, M., Zappa, M., Luján, M., Villers, A., de Carvalho, T. M., Feuer, E. J., Tsodikov, A., Mariotto, A. B., ... Etzioni, R. (2018). The efficacy of prostate-specific antigen screening: Impact of key components in the ERSPC and PLCO trials. *Cancer*, *124*(2), 1197–1206. doi:10.1002/cncr.31178

Dehuri, S., Jagadev, A. K., & Cho, S. B. (2013). Epileptic seizure identification from electroencephalography signal using DE-RBFNs ensemble. *Procedia Computer Science*, *23*, 84–95. doi:10.1016/j.procs.2013.10.012

DeLeonardis, K., Hogan, L., Cannistra, S. A., Rangachari, D., & Tung, N. (2019, September). When Should Tumor Genomic Profiling Prompt Consideration of Germline Testing? *Journal of Oncology Practice / American Society of Clinical Oncology*, *15*(9), 465–473. doi:10.1200/JOP.19.00201 PMID:31509718

Deroo, B. J., & Korach, K. S. (2006). Estrogen receptors and human disease. *The Journal of Clinical Investigation*, *116*(3), 561–570. doi:10.1172/JCI27987 PMID:16511588

Devijver, P. A., & Kittler, J. (1982). *Pattern recognition: A statistical approach.* Prentice hall.

Domadia, N., & Rao, U. P. (2019). Privacy preserving distributed association rule minning approach on vertically partitioned health care data. Procedia Computer Science, 148, 303-312.

Donegan, W. L. (1997). Tumor-related prognostic factors for breast cancer. *CA: a Cancer Journal for Clinicians*, *47*(1), 28–51. doi:10.3322/canjclin.47.1.28 PMID:8996077

Dorn, V., Chopa, A., & Radivoy, G. (2016). Mild bottom-up synthesis of indium (0) nanoparticles: Characterization and application in the allylation of carbonyl compounds. *RSC Advances*, *6*(28), 23798–23803. doi:10.1039/C5RA27928C

Do, T. T., Hoang, T., Pomponiu, V., Zhou, Y., Chen, Z., Cheung, N. M., Koh, D., Tan, A., & Tan, S. H. (2018). Accessible melanoma detection using smartphones and mobile image analysis. *IEEE Transactions on Multimedia*, *20*(10), 2849–2864. doi:10.1109/TMM.2018.2814346

Draisma, G., Boer, R., Otto, S. J., van der Cruijsen, I. W., Damhuis, R. A. M., Schroder, F. H., & de Koning, H. J. (2003). Lead times and over-detection due to prostate-specific antigen screening: Estimates from the European Randomized Study of Screening for Prostate Cancer. *Journal of the National Cancer Institute*, *95*(12), 868–878. doi:10.1093/jnci/95.12.868

Dreiseitl, S., & Ohno-Machado, L. (2002). Logistic regression and artificial neural network classification models: A methodology review. *Journal of Biomedical Informatics*, *35*(5-6), 352–359. doi:10.1016/S1532-0464(03)00034-0 PMID:12968784

Drost, F.-J. H., Rannikko, A., Valdagni, R., Pickles, T., Kakehi, Y., Remmers, S., van der Poel, H. G., Monique, C. H., & Roobol, J. (2018). PRIAS study group. Can active surveillance really reduce the harms of over-diagnosing prostate cancer? A reflection of real life clinical practice in the PRIAS Study. *Translational Andrology and Urology*, *7*(1), 98–105. doi:10.21037/tau.2017.12.28

Dutz, S., Buske, N., Landers, J., Grafe, C., Wende, H., & Clement, J. H. (2020). Biocompatible Magnetic Fluids of Co-Doped Iron Oxide Nanoparticles with Tunable Magnetic Properties. *Nanomaterials (Basel, Switzerland)*, *10*(6), 1019. doi:10.3390/nano10061019

El Zowalaty, M. E., Hussein-Al-Ali, S. H., Husseiny, M. I., Geilich, B. M., Webster, T. J., & Hussein, M. Z. (2015). The ability of streptomycin-loaded chitosan-coated magnetic nanocomposites to possess antimicrobial and antituberculosis activities. *International Journal of Nanomedicine*, *10*, 3269–3274. doi:10.2147/IJN.S74469

Ellimoottil, C., Polcari, A., Kadlec, A., & Gupta, G. (2012). Readability of websites containing information about prostate cancer treatment options. *The Journal of Urology*, *188*(6), 2171–2175. doi:10.1016/j.juro.2012.07.105

Ellimoottil, C., Skolarus, T., Gettman, M., Boxer, R., Kutikov, A., Lee, B. R., Shelton, J., & Morgan, T. (2016). Telemedicine in urology: State of the art. *Urology*, *94*, 10–16. doi:10.1016/j.urology.2016.02.061

Erl, T. (2015). *Cloud Computing Design Patterns.* Prentice Hall.

Erl, T., Puttini, R., & Mahmood, Z. (2014). *Cloud Computing: Concepts, Technology & Architecture.* Pearson.

Estape, Ortiz, Mays, & Laras. (2020). Data mining to transform clinical & translational research findings into precision health, AI in precision health under academic press. *Science Direct Journal*, 149-173.

Esteban, Tablado, Peper, Mahumud, & Ricci, Kopitowski, & Terrasa. (2017). Development and validation of various phenotyping algorithms for diabetes mellitus using data from EHR's. *Computer Method and Program in Bio-Medicine of Elsevier Journal*, *152*, 53–70.

Estelrich, J., Escribano, E., Queralt, J., & Busquets, M. A. (2015). Iron oxide nanoparticles for magnetically guided and magnetically responsive drug delivery. *International Journal of Molecular Sciences*, *16*(4), 8070–8101. doi:10.3390/ijms16048070

Eton, D. T., & Lepore, S. J. (2002). Prostate cancer and health-related quality of life: A review of the literature. *Psycho-Oncology*, *11*(4), 307–326. doi:10.1002/pon.572

European Commission. (2012). *eHealth Action Plan 2012-2020: Innovative healthcare for the 21st century*. Available online: https://ec.europa.eu/digital-single-market/en/news/ehealth-action-plan-2012-2020-innovative-healthcare-21st-century

Eye Care. (2019). *OCT Göz Cihazı*. Retrieved from http://www.clairhursteyecare.com/retinal-digital-imaging

Fakhri, A., & Nejad, A. P. (2016). Antimicrobial, antioxidant and cytotoxic effect of Molybdenum trioxide nanoparticles and application of this for degradation of ketamine under different light illumination. *Journal of Photochemistry and Photobiology*, *159*, 211–217. doi:10.1016/j.jphotobiol.2016.04.002

Fan, X., Peters, B. A., Jacobs, E. J., Gapstur, S. M., Purdue, M. P., Freedman, N. D., Alekseyenko, A. V., Wu, J., Yang, L., Pei, Z., Hayes, R. B., & Ahn, J. (2018). Drinking alcohol is associated with variation in the human oral microbiome in a large study of American adults. *Microbiome*, *6*(1), 59. doi:10.118640168-018-0448-x PMID:29685174

Fan, Y., Guo, L., Zheng, H., Ji, C., Wang, W., & Sun, H. (2020, January). BMP-9 is a novel marker for colorectal tumorigenesis undergoing the normal mucosa-adenoma-adenocarcinoma sequence and is associated with colorectal cancer prognosis. *Oncology Letters*, *19*(1), 271–282. PMID:31897139

Fauci, A. S. (2001). *Infectious diseases: considerations for the 21st century*. Clin Infect.

Fazio, E., Speciale, A., Spadaro, S., Bonsignore, M., Cimino, F., Cristani, M., Trombetta, D., Saija, A., & Neri, F. (2018). Evaluation of biological response induced by molybdenum oxide nanocolloids on in vitro cultured NIH/3T3 fibroblast cells by micro-Raman spectroscopy. *Colloids and Surfaces. B, Biointerfaces*, *1*(170), 233–241. doi:10.1016/j.colsurfb.2018.06.028

FDA. (n.d.). *Novel drug approvals for 2019*. https://www.fda.gov/drugs/new-drugs-fda-cders-new-molecular-entities-and-new-therapeutic-biological-products/novel-drug-approvals-2019

Feigin, V. L., Nichols, E., Alam, T., Bannick, M. S., Beghi, E., Blake, N., ... Fisher, J. L. (2019). Global, regional, and national burden of neurological disorders, 1990–2016: A systematic analysis for the Global Burden of Disease Study 2016. *Lancet Neurology*, *18*(5), 459–480. doi:10.1016/S1474-4422(18)30499-X PMID:30879893

Feito, Y., Moriarty, T. A., Mangine, G., & Monahan, J. (2018). The Use Of A Smart-Textile Garment During High-Intensity Functional Training. A Pilot Study. *The Journal of Sports Medicine and Physical Fitness*. PMID:30024125

Ferlay, J. E. M., Lam, F., Colombet, M., Mery, L., Pineros, M., Znaor, A., Soerjomataram, I., & ... . (2011). *Global cancer observatory: cancer today*. International Agency for Research on Cancer. Available from https://gco.iarc.fr/today

Fernández-Abascal, E. G., & Martín-Díaz, M. D. (2015). Dimensions of emotional intelligence related to physical and mental health and to health behaviors. *Frontiers in Psychology*, *6*, 317. doi:10.3389/fpsyg.2015.00317 PMID:25859229

Ferreira, A. G., Fernandes, D., Branco, S., Monteiro, J. L., Cabral, J., Catarino, A. P., & Rocha, A. M. (2016), A Smart Wearable System For Sudden Infant Death Syndrome Monitoring. *Proceedings of the 2016 IEEE International Conference on Industrial Technology (ICIT)*, 1920–1925. 10.1109/ICIT.2016.7475060

Field, J., Holmes, M. M., & Newell, D. (2019). PROMs data: Can it be used to make decisions for individual patients? A narrative review. *Patient Related Outcome Measures*, *10*, 233–241. doi:10.2147/PROM.S156291

Filella, X., Fernández-Galan, E., Fernández Bonifacio, R., & Foj, L. (2018). Emerging biomarkers in the diagnosis of prostate cancer. *Pharmacogenomics and Personalized Medicine*, *11*, 83–94. doi:10.2147/PGPM.S136026

Firebase. (2020). *Firebase is Google's mobile platform that helps you quickly develop high-quality apps and grow your business.* Retrieved from https://firebase.google.com/

Fisher, R. S., Boas, W. V. E., Blume, W., Elger, C., Genton, P., Lee, P., & Engel, J. Jr. (2005). Epileptic seizures and epilepsy: Definitions proposed by the International League Against Epilepsy (ILAE) and the International Bureau for Epilepsy (IBE). *Epilepsia*, *46*(4), 470–472. doi:10.1111/j.0013-9580.2005.66104.x PMID:15816939

Flutter. (2019). *Flutter*. Retrieved from https://flutter.dev/

Folaranmi, T. (2014). mHealth in Africa: Challenges and opportunities. *Perspectives in Public Health*, *134*(1), 14–15. doi:10.1177/1757913913514703

Forbes, C. C., Finlay, A., McIntosh, M., Siddiquee, S., & Short, C. E. (2019). A systematic review of the feasibility, acceptability, and efficacy of online supportive care interventions targeting men with a history of prostate cancer. *Journal of Cancer Survivorship: Research and Practice*, *13*(1), 75–96. doi:10.100711764-018-0729-1

Forman, A., & Sotelo, J. (2019, September 30). Tumor-Based Genetic Testing and Familial Cancer Risk. *Cold Spring Harbor Perspectives in Medicine*. Advance online publication. doi:10.1101/cshperspect.a036590 PMID:31570381

Fratoddi, I., Matassa, R., Fontana, L., Venditti, I., Familiari, G., Battocchio, C., Magnono, E., Nappini, S., Leahu, G., Belardini, A., & … . (2017). Electronic Properties of a Functionalized Noble Metal Nanoparticles Covalent Network. *The Journal of Physical Chemistry C*, *121*(33), 18110–18119. doi:10.1021/acs.jpcc.7b07176

Freudenthaler, H. H., Neubauer, A. C., Gabler, P., Scherl, W. G., & Rindermann, H. (2008). Testing and validating the trait emotional intelligence questionnaire (TEIQue) in a German-speaking sample. *Personality and Individual Differences*, *45*(7), 673–678. doi:10.1016/j.paid.2008.07.014

Frydrysiak, M., & Tesiorowski, L. (2016), Health monitoring system for protecting elderly people. *Proceedings of the International Multidisciplinary Conference on Computer and Energy Science*, 1–6. 10.1109/SpliTech.2016.7555935

Fujiki, H., Suganuma, M., Okabe, S., Sueoka, N., Komori, A., Sueoka, E., Kozu, T., Tada, Y., Suga, K., Imai, K., & Nakachi, K. (1998). Cancer inhibition by green tea. *Mutation Research*, *402*(1-2), 307–310. doi:10.1016/S0027-5107(97)00310-2

Furasova, A. D., Zakhiodov, A. A., Di Carlo, A., & Makarov, S. V. (2018). Resonant Silicon Nanoparticles for Enhanced Light Harvesting in Halide Pervskite Solar Cells. *Journal of Physics: Conference Series*, *1092*(012038).

Gadkar-Sable, S., Shah, C., Rosario, G., Sachdeva, G., & Puri, C. (2005). Progesterone receptors: Various forms and functions in reproductive tissues. *Frontiers in Bioscience*, *10*(2118), 30. doi:10.2741/1685 PMID:15970482

Gallagher, R. P., & Fleshner, N. (1998). Prostate cancer: 3. Individual risk factors. *Canadian Medical Association Journal*, *159*(7), 807–813.

Galley, C. (1995). Terence ranger and Paul slack, EDS., epidemics and ideas. Essays on the historical perception of Pestilence. (Cambridge: Cambridge university press, 1992.) pages ix + 346. £35.00. *Continuity and Change*, *10*(2), 301–303. doi:10.1017/S0268416000002708

Gang, L., Chutatape, O., & Krishnan, S. M. (2002). Detection and measurement of retinal vessels in fundus images using amplitude modified second-order Gaussian filter. IEEE Trans. Biomed. Eng., 49, 168–172.

Gao, X., Yan, X., Gao, P., Gao, X., & Zhang, S. (2020). Automatic detection of epileptic seizure based on approximate entropy, recurrence quantiðcation analysis and convolutional neural networks. *Artificial Intelligence in Medicine*, *102*, 101711. doi:10.1016/j.artmed.2019.101711 PMID:31980085

Garcia, M., Millat-Carus, R., Bertucci, F., Finetti, P., Birnbaum, D., & Bidaut, G. (2012). Interactome–transcriptome integration for predicting distant metastasis in breast cancer. *Bioinformatics (Oxford, England)*, *28*(5), 672–678. doi:10.1093/bioinformatics/bts025 PMID:22238264

García-Sancho, E., Salguero, J. M., & Fernández-Berrocal, P. (2014). Relationship between emotional intelligence and aggression: A systematic review. *Aggression and Violent Behavior*, *19*(5), 584–591. doi:10.1016/j.avb.2014.07.007

Gardner, G. G., Keating, D., Williamson, T. H., & Elliott, A. T. (1996). Automatic detection of diabetic retinopathy using an artificial neural network: A screening tool. Br. J. Ophthalmol., 80, 940–944.

Garg, N., & Sharma, K. (2020). Sentiment Analysis of Events on Social Web. *International Journal of Innovative Technology and Exploring Engineering*, *9*(6).

Gay, H. A., & Michalski, J. M. (2018). Radiation therapy for prostate cancer. *Missouri Medicine*, *115*(2), 146–150.

Geng, H. (2017). *Internet of Things and Data Analytics Handbook*. John Wiley & Sons. doi:10.1002/9781119173601

Ghanchi, J. (2019). 7 Reasons Why A Smartwatch Can Be Beneficial For Your Health With AI. *becominghuman*. https://becominghuman.ai/7-reasons-why-a-smartwatch-can-be-beneficial-for-your-health-with-ai-27e994620b10

Ghoto, S. A., Khuhawar, M. Y., Jahangir, T. M., & Mangi, J. D. (2019). Applications of copper nanoparticles for colorimetric detection of dithiocarbamate pesticides. *Journal of Nanostructure in Chemistry*, *1*(2), 1–17. doi:10.100740097-019-0299-4

Giannoula, E., Iakovou, I., Katsikavelas, I., Antoniou, P., Raftopoulos, V., Chatzipavlidou, V., Papadopoulos, N., & Bamidis, P. (2020). A mobile app for thyroid cancer patients aiming to enhance their quality of life: Protocol for a quasi-experimental interventional pilot study. *JMIR Research Protocols*, *9*(3), e13409. doi:10.2196/13409

Gignac, G. E. (2010). Genos Emotional Intelligence Inventory. Technical Manual (2nd ed.). Sydney: Academic Press.

Ginsburg, G. S., & Phillips, K. A. (2018). Precision Medicine: From Science to Value. *Health Affairs (Project Hope)*, *37*(5), 694–701. doi:10.1377/hlthaff.2017.1624 PMID:29733705

Giunti, G., Giunta, D., Guisado-Fernandez, E., Bender, J., & Fernandez-Luque, L. (2018). A biopsy of breast cancer mobile applications: State of the practice review. *International Journal of Medical Informatics*, *110*, 1–9. doi:10.1016/j.ijmedinf.2017.10.022

Global Web Index Data. (2020). Retrieved from https://www.cybermagonline.com/turkiye-internette-vakit-gecirmede-dunya-dorduncusu

Goel, S., Chen, F., & Cai, W. (2013). Synthesis and biomedical applications of copper sulfide nanoparticles: From sensors to theranostics. *Small*, *10*(4), 631–645. doi:10.1002mll.201301174

Goleman. (1995). *Emotional Intelligence: Why It Can Matter More Than IQ*. Bantam Books. https://en.wikipedia.org/wiki/David_Wechsler

Golsteijn, R. H. J., Bolman, C., Volders, E., Peels, D. A., de Vries, H., & Lechner, L. (2017). Development of a computer-tailored physical activity intervention for prostate and colorectal cancer patients and survivors: OncoActive. *BMC Cancer*, *17*(1), 446. doi:10.118612885-017-3397-z

Golub, T. R., Slonim, D. K., Tamayo, P., Huard, C., Gaasenbeek, M., Mesirov, J. P., ... & Bloomfield, C. D. (1999). Molecular classification of cancer: class discovery and class prediction by gene expression monitoring. *Science, 286*(5439), 531-537.

Golub, T., Mukherjee, S., Ramaswamy, S., Rifkin, R., & Tamayo, P. (2003). *U.S. Patent Application No. 10/294,453*. US Patent Office.

Gonzales, R. C., & Woods, R. E. (2002). *Digital image processing*. Pearson.

Google. (2019). *Googletrends*. Retrieved from https://www.googletrends.com

GradesFixer. (2019). *A literature review of Emotional Intelligence*. Author.

Grinnell, F. (2020). Biomedical ethics 2.0: Redefining the meaning of disease, patient and treatment. *Nature Reviews. Molecular Cell Biology*, *10*(8), 1038. doi:10.103841580-020-0247-7 PMID:32303724

Groseclose, S. L., & Buckeridge, D. L. (2017). Public health surveillance systems: Recent advances in their use and evaluation. *Annual Review of Public Health*, *38*(1), 57–79. doi:10.1146/annurev-publhealth-031816-044348 PMID:27992726

Grundmann, O. (2014). The current state of bioterrorist attack surveillance and preparedness in the US. *Risk Management and Healthcare Policy*, *177*, 177. Advance online publication. doi:10.2147/RMHP.S56047 PMID:25328421

Gruvberger, S., Ringnér, M., Chen, Y., Panavally, S., Saal, L. H., Borg, Å., ... Meltzer, P. S. (2001). Estrogen receptor status in breast cancer is associated with remarkably distinct gene expression patterns. *Cancer Research*, *61*(16), 5979–5984. PMID:11507038

Gugliandolo, M. C., Costa, S., Cuzzocrea, F., Larcan, R., & Petrides, K. V. (2015). Trait emotional intelligence and behavioral problems among adolescents: A cross-informant design. *Personality and Individual Differences*, *74*, 16–21. doi:10.1016/j.paid.2014.09.032

Gulati, R., Inoue, L. Y., Gore, J. L., Katcher, J., & Etzioni, R. (2014). Individualized estimates of over-diagnosis in screen-detected prostate cancer. *Journal of the National Cancer Institute*, *106*(2), 1–5. doi:10.1093/jnci/djt367

Guo, L., Rivero, D., Dorado, J., Rabunal, J. R., & Pazos, A. (2010). Automatic epileptic seizure detection in EEGs based on line length feature and artificial neural networks. *Journal of Neuroscience Methods*, *191*(1), 101–109. doi:10.1016/j.jneumeth.2010.05.020 PMID:20595035

Gupta, R., Tanwar, S., Tyagi, S., Kumar, N., Obaidat, M. S., & Sadoun, B. (2019). HaBiTs: Blockchain Based Telesurgery Framework for Healthcare 4.0. *International Conference on Computer, Information and Telecommunication Systems (IEEE CITS-2019),* 6-10.

Gupta, R. (2019). Tactile Internet-based Telesurgery System for Healthcare 4.0: An Architecture, Research Challenges, and Future Directions. *IEEE Network*, 12–19.

Guyon, I., Weston, J., Barnhill, S., & Vapnik, V. (2002). Gene selection for cancer classification using support vector machines. *Machine Learning*, *46*(1-3), 389–422. doi:10.1023/A:1012487302797

Haghi, M., Thurow, K., & Stoll, R. (2017). Wearable Devices in Medical Internet of Things: Scientific Research and Commercially Available Devices, Review Article. *Healthcare Informatics Research*, *23*(1), 4–15. doi:10.4258/hir.2017.23.1.4 PMID:28261526

Haibe-Kains, B. (2009). *Identification and assessment of gene signatures in human breast cancer*. Academic Press.

Halevas, E. G., & Pantazaki, A. A. (2018). Copper Nanoparticles as Therapeutic Anticancer Agents. *Nanomedicine and Nanotechnology Journal*, *2*(1), 119.

Hameed, N., Ruskin, A., Hassan, K. A., & Hossain, M. A. (2016). A comprehensive survey on image-based computer aided diagnosis systems for skin cancer. In *10th International Conference on Software, Knowledge, Information Management & Applications (SKIMA)* (pp. 205-214). IEEE. 10.1109/SKIMA.2016.7916221

Hamilton, E., Van Veldhuizen, E., Brown, A., Brennan, S., & Sabesan, S. (2018). Telehealth in radiation oncology at the Townsville Cancer Centre: Service evaluation and patient satisfaction. *Clin. Transl. Radiat. Oncol.*, *15*, 20–25. doi:10.1016/j.ctro.2018.11.005

Han, J., Pei, J., & Kamber, M. (2011). *Data mining: concepts and techniques*. Elsevier.

Hanley, C., Layne, J., Punnoose, A., Reddy, K. M., Coombs, I., Coombs, A., Feris, K., & Wingett, D. (2008). Preferential killing of cancer cells and activated human T cells using ZnO nanoparticles. *Nanotechnology*, *19*(29), 295103. doi:10.1088/0957-4484/19/29/295103

Harahap, M., Husein, A. M., & Lubis, F. R. (2017). Mining association rule based on the disease population for recommendations of medical need. Journal of Physics, 1007.

Hasan, A. (2012). Evaluation of Decision Tree Classifiers and Boosting Algorithm for Classifying High Dimensional Cancer Datasets. *International Journal of Modeling and Optimization*, *2*(2), 92–96. doi:10.7763/IJMO.2012.V2.92

Hassan, A. R., Siuly, S., & Zhang, Y. (2016). Epileptic seizure detection in EEG signals using tunable-Q factor wavelet transform and bootstrap aggregating. *Computer Methods and Programs in Biomedicine*, *137*, 247–259. doi:10.1016/j.cmpb.2016.09.008 PMID:28110729

Hassan, A. R., Subasi, A., & Zhang, Y. (2020). Epilepsy seizure detection using complete ensemble empirical mode decomposition with adaptive noise. *Knowledge-Based Systems*, *191*, 105333. doi:10.1016/j.knosys.2019.105333

Hassanpour, P., Panahi, Y., Ebrahimi-Kalan, A., Akbarzadeh, A., Davaran, S., Nasibova, A. N., Khalilov, R., & Kavetskyy, T. (2018). Biomedical applications of aluminium oxide nanoparticles. *Micro & Nano Letters*, *13*(9), 1227–1231. doi:10.1049/mnl.2018.5070

Hastie, T., Tibshirani, R., & Friedman, J. (2009). *The elements of statistical learning: data mining, inference, and prediction*. Springer Science & Business Media. doi:10.1007/978-0-387-84858-7

Haveman-Nies, A., Jansen, M., Oers, J. A., & Veer, P. V. (2017). *Epidemiology in public health practice*. Academic Press.

Hawi, N. S., & Samaha, M. (2017). The relations among social media addiction, self-esteem, and life satisfaction in university students. *Social Science Computer Review*, *35*(5), 576–586. doi:10.1177/0894439316660340

Health Protection Agency. (n.d.). *Health protection in the 21st century*. Available from: http://www.hpa.org.uk/ publications/2005/burden disease/default.htm

He, D., & Zeadally, S. (2015). An Analysis of RFID Authentication Scheme for Internet of Things in Healthcare Environment using Elliptic curve cryptography. *IEEE Internet of Things Journal*, *2*(1), 72–83. doi:10.1109/JIOT.2014.2360121

Herikstad, H., Motarjemi, Y., & Tauxe, R. V. (2002). Salmonella Surveillance: A Global Survey of Public Health Serotyping. *Epidemiology and Infection*, *129*(1), 1–8. doi:10.1017/S0950268802006842 PMID:12211575

Herland, Khoshgoftaar, & Wald. (2014). A review of data mining using big data in health informatics. *Journal of Big Data*.

Heymann, D. (2006). *Control, elimination, eradication and the re-emergence of infectious diseases: getting the message right.* Retrieved from Bulletin of the World Health Organization. https://www.who.int/bulletin/volumes/84/2/editorial-10206html/en/

Heymann, D. L. (2004). *Control of Communicable Diseases Manual*. American Public Health Association.

Hinton, G. E., Osindero, S., & Teh, Y. W. (2006). A fast learning algorithm for deep belief nets. *Neural Computation, 18*(7), 1527–1554. doi:10.1162/neco.2006.18.7.1527 PMID:16764513

Hipwell, J. H., Strachan, F., Olson, J. A., McHardy, K. C., Sharp, P. F., & Forrester, J. V. (2000). Automated Detection of Microaneurysms in Digital Red-free Photographs: A Diabetic Retinopathy Screening Tool. *Diabetic Medicine, 17*(8), 588–594. doi:10.1046/j.1464-5491.2000.00338.x PMID:11073180

Hockings, J. K., Pasternak, A. L., Erwin, A. L., Mason, N. T., Eng, C., & Hicks, J. K. (2020). Pharmacogenomics: An evolving clinical tool for precision medicine. *Cleveland Clinic Journal of Medicine, 87*(2), 91–99. doi:10.3949/ccjm.87a.19073 PMID:32015062

Holmboe, E. S., & Concato, J. (2000). Treatment decisions for localized prostate cancer: Asking men what's important. *Journal of General Internal Medicine, 15*(10), 694–701. doi:10.1046/j.1525-1497.2000.90842.x

Hong, J. H., & Cho, S. B. (2006). The classification of cancer based on DNA microarray data that uses diverse ensemble genetic programming. *Artificial Intelligence in Medicine, 36*(1), 43–58. doi:10.1016/j.artmed.2005.06.002 PMID:16102956

Howard Gardner. (n.d.). https://en.wikipedia.org/wiki/Howard_Gardner

Howell, D., Molloy, S., Wilkinson, K., Green, E., Orchard, K., Wang, K., & Liberty, J. (2015). Patient-reported outcomes in routine cancer clinical practice: A scoping review of use, impact on health outcomes, and implementation factors. *Annals of Oncology: Official Journal of the European Society for Medical Oncology, 26*(9), 1846–1858. doi:10.1093/annonc/mdv181

Huang, D. M., Hsiao, J. K., Chen, Y. C., Chien, L. Y., Yao, M., Chen, Y. K., Ko, B. S., Hsu, S. C., Tai, L. A., Cheng, H. Y., Wang, S. W., Yang, C. S., & Chen, Y. C. (2009). The promotion of human mesenchymal stem cell proliferation by superparamagnetic iron oxide nanoparticles. *Biomaterials, 30*(22), 3645–3651. doi:10.1016/j.biomaterials.2009.03.032

Hubel, D. H., & Wiesel, T. N. (1968). Receptive Fields and Functional Architecture of Monkey Striate Cortex. *The Journal of Physiology, 195*(1), 215–243. doi:10.1113/jphysiol.1968.sp008455 PMID:4966457

Hu, Z., Tang, J., Wang, Z., Zhang, K., Zhang, L., & Sun, Q. (2018). Deep learning for image-based cancer detection and diagnosis– a survey. *Pattern Recognition, 83*, 134–149. doi:10.1016/j.patcog.2018.05.014

Hyde, M. K., Newton, R. U., Galvão, D. A., Gardiner, R. A., Occhipinti, S., Lowe, A., Wittert, G. A., & Chambers, S. K. (2017). Men's help-seeking in the first year after diagnosis of localized prostate cancer. *European Journal of Cancer Care, 26*(2), e12497. doi:10.1111/ecc.12497

IEEE DataPort. (2019). *Indian diabetic retinopathy image dataset (IDRID)*. Retrieved from https://ieee-dataport.org/open-access/indian-diabetic-retinopathy-image-dataset-idrid

Ilkin, S., Tayfur, T., & Şahin, S. (2018). Ortalama Kayma Algoritması Kullanılarak Dermatolojik Görüntüler Üzerindeki Melanomlu Alanların Tespiti. *IMASCON Uluslararası Marmara Fen ve Sosyal Bilimler Kongresi*, 780-787.

Ilkin, S., Aytar, O., Gençtürk, T. H., & Şahin, S. (2020). Dermoskopik Görüntülerde Lezyon Bölütleme İşlemlerinde K-ortalama Kümeleme Algoritmasının Kullanımı. *Gazi Üniversitesi Fen Bilimleri Dergisi Part C: Tasarım ve Teknoloji, 8*(1), 182–191. doi:10.29109/gujsc.625378

Inbavalli. (2015). Efficient Analysis of Frequent item set Association Rule Mining Methods. *International Journal of Scientific & Engineering Research, 6*(4), 1-23. http://www.ijser.org/researchpaper%5cefficient-Analysis-of-Frequent-itemset-Association-Rule-Mining-Methods.pdf

International Health Regulations. (2008). (2nd ed.). Geneva: World Health Organization. https://www.who.int/ihr/publications/9789241596664/en

Ito, T., Matsuda, Y., Jinba, T., Asai, N., Shimizu, T., & Shingubara, S. (2017). Fabrication and Characterization of nonoporous lattice biosensor using anodic aluminum oxide substrate. *Japan Society of Applied Physics, 56*, 6S1.

Ito, N., Kawahira, H., Nakashima, H., Uesato, M., Miyauchi, H., & Matsubara, H. (2019). Endoscopic diagnostic support system for ct1b colorectal cancer using deep learning. *Oncology, 96*(1), 44–50. doi:10.1159/000491636 PMID:30130758

Ivshina, A. V., George, J., Senko, O., Mow, B., Putti, T. C., Smeds, J., ... Wong, J. E. (2006). Genetic reclassification of histologic grade delineates new clinical subtypes of breast cancer. *Cancer Research, 66*(21), 10292–10301. doi:10.1158/0008-5472.CAN-05-4414 PMID:17079448

Jain, D., Kumar, V., Khanduja, D., Sharma, K., & Bateja, R. (2019). A detailed study of big data in health care: case study of Brenda and IBM Watson. *International Journal of Recent Technology and Engineering, 7*(5).

Jain, A., Tayal, D. K., Yadav, D., & Arora, A. (2020). Research Trends for Named Entity Recognition in Hindi Language. In *Data Visualization and Knowledge Engineering* (pp. 223–248). Springer. doi:10.1007/978-3-030-25797-2_10

Jain, S., Loblaw, A., Vesprini, D., Zhang, L., Kattan, M. W., Mamedov, A., Jethava, V., Sethukavalan, P., Yu, C., & Klotz, L. (2015). Gleason upgrading with time in a large prostate cancer active surveillance cohort. *The Journal of Urology, 194*(1), 79–84. doi:10.1016/j.juro.2015.01.102

Jaiswal, A. K., & Banka, H. (2017). Local pattern transformation based feature extraction techniques for classification of epileptic EEG signals. *Biomedical Signal Processing and Control, 34*, 81–92. doi:10.1016/j.bspc.2017.01.005

Jaiswal, A. K., & Banka, H. (2018). Local transformed features for epileptic seizure detection in EEG signal. *Journal of Medical and Biological Engineering, 38*(2), 222–235. doi:10.100740846-017-0286-5

Jarrell, D. K., Drake, S., & Brown, M. A. (2020). Advancing Therapies for Cancer—From Mustard Gas to CAR T. *Sci, 2*(2), 42. doi:10.3390ci2020042

Jensen, R. E., Snyder, C. F., Abernethy, A. P., Basch, E., Potosky, A. L., Roberts, A. C., Loeffler, D. R., & Reeve, B. B. (2014). Review of electronic patient-reported outcomes systems used in cancer clinical care. *Journal of Oncology Practice / American Society of Clinical Oncology, 10*(4), e215–e222. doi:10.1200/JOP.2013.001067

Jiang, F., Jiang, Y., Zhi, H., Dong, Y., Li, H., Ma, S., Wang, Y., Dong, Q., Shen, H., & Wong, Y. (2017). Artificial intelligence in healthcare: past, present and future. *Stroke and Vascular Neurology.* https://svn.bmj.com/content/2/4/230

Jiang, X., & Mojon, D. (2003), Adaptive local thresholding by verificationbased multithreshold probing with application to vessel detection in retinal images. IEEE Trans. Pattern Anal. Mach. Intell., 25(1), 131–137.

Jiang, M. Y., Feng, R. M., & Wang, L. (2018). Performance of Combined Liquid Based Cytology and HPV Nucleic Acid Test for Detecting Cervical Precancer Among Women Attending Screening. *Zhonghua Zhong Liu Za Zhi, 40*(10), 750–756. PMID:30392339

Jindal & Sharma. (2018). A Review on Sentiment Classification: Natural Language Understanding. *Bentham Science Journal, Recent Patents on Engineering.*

Joseph, M. A., Moysich, K. B., Freudenheim, J. L., Shields, P. G., Bowman, E. D., Zhang, Y., Marshall, J. R., & Ambrosone, C. B. (2004). Cruciferous vegetables, genetic polymorphisms in glutathione S-transferases M1 and T1, and prostate cancer risk. *Nutrition and Cancer, 50*(2), 206–213. doi:10.120715327914nc5002_11

Joshi, J., Kurian, D., Bhasin, S., Mukherjee, S., Awasthi, P., Sharma, S., & Mittal, S. (2016), Health Monitoring Using Wearable Sensor and Cloud Computing. *Proceedings of the International Conference on Cybernetics, Robotics and Control*, 104–108. 10.1109/CRC.2016.031

Juengst, E., & McGowan, M. (2018). Why Does the Shift from 'Personalized Medicine' to 'Precision Health' and 'Wellness Genomics' Matter? *AMA Journal of Ethics*, *20*(9), e881–e890. doi:10.1001/amajethics.2018.881 PMID:30242820

Kamen, C., Mustian, K. M., Heckler, C., Janelsins, M. C., Peppone, L. J., Mohile, S., McMahon, J. M., Lord, R., Flynn, P. J., Weiss, M., Spiegel, D., & Morrow, G. R. (2015). The association between partner support and psychological distress among prostate cancer survivors in a nationwide study. *Journal of Cancer Survivorship: Research and Practice*, *9*(3), 492–499. doi:10.100711764-015-0425-3

Kaneriya, S., Tanwar, S., Buddhadev, S., Verma, J. P., Tyagi, S., Kumar, N., & Misra, S. (2018). A Range-based approach for Long-Term Forecast of Weather Using Probabilistic Markov Model. *IEEE International Conference on Communication (IEEE ICC-2018),* 1-6.

Kaneriya, S., Tanwar, S., Verma, J. P., Tyagi, S., Kumar, N., Obaidat, M. S., & Rodrigues, J. P. C. (2018). Data Consumption-Aware Load Forecasting Scheme for Smart Grid Systems. *IEEE Global Communications Conference (IEEE GLOBECOM-2018),* 1-6.

Kangethe & Wagacha. (2014). Extracting diagnosis patterns in electronic medical records using association rule mining. *International Journal of Computer Applications, 108.*

Kang, I., Cui, H., & Son, J. (2019). Conformity consumption behavior and FoMO. *Sustainability*, *11*(17), 4734. doi:10.3390u11174734

Kang, J. H., Chung, Y. G., & Kim, S. P. (2015). An efficient detection of epileptic seizure by differentiation and spectral analysis of electroencephalograms. *Computers in Biology and Medicine*, *66*, 352–356. doi:10.1016/j.compbiomed.2015.04.034 PMID:25982199

Karaboğa, D. (2011). *Yapay Zeka Optimizasyon Algoritmaları*. Nobel Yayın Dağıtım.

Karim, M. N., Anderson, S. R., Singh, S., Ramanathan, R., & Bansal, V. (2018). Nanostructured silver fabric as a free-standing NanoZyme for colorimetric detection of glucose in urine. *Biosensors & Bioelectronics*, *110*, 8–15. doi:10.1016/j.bios.2018.03.025

Kasap, S., Pektaş, M. L., Dere, Y., & Altıparmak, M. (2015). Retrospective Evaluation of Skin Cancer Patients in Muğla. *Muğla Sıtkı Koçman Üniversitesi Tıp Dergisi*, *2*(3), 34-7. Retrieved from https://dergipark.org.tr/tr/download/article-file/409758

Kasmi, R., & Mokrani, K. (2016). Classification of malignant melanoma and benign skin lesions: Implementation of automatic ABCD rule. *IET Image Processing*, *10*(6), 448–455. doi:10.1049/iet-ipr.2015.0385

Katrien, Groenhof, Koers, Blasse, de Groot, Grobbee, Bots, Asselbergs, Lely, & Haitjema. (2020). Data mining information from EHR producing high yield and accuracy for current smoking status. *Journal of Clinical Epidemiology, 118*, 100-106.

Kavakiotis, I. (2017). *Machine learning and data mining methods in diabetes research. Computational and Structural Biotechnology, 15.*

Kavis, M. J. (2014). *Architecting the Cloud.* Wiley. doi:10.1002/9781118691779

Kaya, Y., Uyar, M., Tekin, R., & Yıldırım, S. (2014). 1D-local binary pattern based feature extraction for classification of epileptic EEG signals. *Applied Mathematics and Computation*, *243*, 209–219. doi:10.1016/j.amc.2014.05.128

Kermani, F., Orooji, A., & Sheikhtaheri, A. (2020). Teleoncology for children with cancer: A scoping review on applications and outcomes. *International Journal of Medical Informatics*, *139*, 104–118. doi:10.1016/j.ijmedinf.2020.104118

Kessel, K. A., Vogel, M. M., Schmidt-Graf, F., & Combs, S. E. (2016). Mobile apps in oncology: A survey on health care professionals' attitude toward telemedicine, mHealth, and oncological apps. *Journal of Medical Internet Research*, *18*(11), e312. doi:10.2196/jmir.6399

Khan, A., Sohail, A., Zahoora, U., & Qureshi, A. S. (2019). *A survey of the recent architectures of deep convolutional neural networks*. arXiv preprint arXiv:1901.06032.

Khani, Y., Pourgholam-Amiji, N., Afshar, M., Otroshi, O., Sharifi-Esfahani, M., Sadeghi-Gandomani, H., Vejdani, M., & Salehiniya, H. (2018). Tobacco Smoking and Cancer Types: A Review. *Biomedical Research and Therapy*, *5*(4), 2142–2159. doi:10.15419/bmrat.v5i4.428

Khan, J., Wei, J. S., Ringner, M., Saal, L. H., Ladanyi, M., Westermann, F., Berthold, F., Schwab, M., Antonescu, C. R., Peterson, C., & Meltzer, P. S. (2001). Classification and diagnostic prediction of cancers using gene expression profiling and artificial neural networks. *Nature Medicine*, *7*(6), 673–679. doi:10.1038/89044 PMID:11385503

King, C. E., & Sarrafzadeh, M. (2017). A survey of smartwatches in remote health monitoring. *Journal of Healthcare Informatics Research*, *2*(1-2), 1–24. doi:10.100741666-017-0012-7 PMID:30035250

Kleppmann, M. (2017). *Designing Data-Intensive Applications: The Big Ideas Behind Reliable, Scalable, and Maintainable Systems*. O'Reilly.

Knobler, S., Mahmoud, A., Lemon, S., Mack, A., Sivitz, L., & Oberholtzer, K. (2004). Workshop summary. In *Learning from SARS: Preparing for the Next Disease Outbreak* (p. 11). National Academies Press.

Kohavi, R., & John, G. H. (1997). Wrappers for feature subset selection. *Artificial Intelligence*, *97*(1-2), 273–324. doi:10.1016/S0004-3702(97)00043-X

Kondylakis, H., Koumakis, L., Hänold, S., Nwankwo, I., Forgó, N., Marias, K., Tsiknakis, M., & Graf, N. (2017). Donor's support tool: Enabling informed secondary use of patient's biomaterial and personal data. *International Journal of Medical Informatics*, *97*, 282–292. doi:10.1016/j.ijmedinf.2016.10.019

Kondylakis, H., Koumakis, L., & Tsiknakis, M. (2013). Smart recommendation services in support of patient empowerment and personalized medicine *BT*. In G. A. Tsihrintzis, M. Virvou, & L. C. Jain (Eds.), *Multimedia services in intelligent environments: Recommendation services* (pp. 39–61). Springer International Publishing. doi:10.1007/978-3-319-00375-7_4

Koprowski, R., & Skufca, J. D. (2014). Machine learning, medical diagnosis, and biomedical engineering research-commentary. *Biomedical Engineering Online*, *13*(1), 94. doi:10.1186/1475-925X-13-94 PMID:24998888

Kourou, K., Exarchos, T. P., Exarchos, K. P., Karamouzis, M. V., & Fotiadis, D. I. (2015). Machine learning applications in cancer prognosis and prediction. *Computational and Structural Biotechnology Journal*, *13*, 8–17. doi:10.1016/j.csbj.2014.11.005 PMID:25750696

Kranse, R., Roobol, M., & Schröder, F. H. (2008). A graphical device to represent the outcomes of a logistic regression analysis. *The Prostate*, *68*(15), 1674–1680. doi:10.1002/pros.20840

Krebs, K., & Milani, L. (2019). Translating pharmacogenomics into clinical decisions: Do not let the perfect be the enemy of the good. *Human Genomics*, *13*(1), 39. doi:10.118640246-019-0229-z PMID:31455423

Krizhevsky, A., Sutskever, I., & Hinton, G. E. (2012). Imagenet classification with deep convolutional neural networks. *Advances in Neural Information Processing Systems*, 1097–1105.

Kruger, S., Ilmer, M., Kobold, S., Cadilha, B. L., Endres, S., Ormanns, S., Schuebbe, G., Renz, B. W., D'Haese, J. G., Schloesser, H., Heinemann, V., Subklewe, M., Boeck, S., Werner, J., & von Bergwelt-Baildon, M. (2019). Advances in cancer immunotherapy. *Journal of Experimental & Clinical Cancer Research*, *38*(1), 268. doi:10.118613046-019-1266-0 PMID:31217020

Krzyszczyk, P., Acevedo, A., Davidoff, E. J., Timmins, L. M., Marrero-Berrios, I., Patel, M., White, C., Lowe, C., Sherba, J. J., Hartmanshenn, C., O'Neill, K. M., Balter, M. L., Fritz, Z. R., Androulakis, I. P., Schloss, R. S., & Yarmush, M. L. (2018). The growing role of precision and personalized medicine for cancer treatment. Technology. *Singap World Sci*, *6*(3-4), 79–100. PMID:30713991

Kulkarni & Mundhe. (2017). Data mining technique: an implementation of association rule mining in healthcare. *IARJSET Journal, 4*(7).

Kumari, A., Tanwar, S., Tyagi, S., & Kumar, N. (2018). Fog Computing for Healthcare 4.0 Environment: Opportunities and Challenges. *Computers & Electrical Engineering*, *72*, 1–13. doi:10.1016/j.compeleceng.2018.08.015

Kumari, A., Tanwar, S., Tyagi, S., Kumar, N., Obaidat, M. S., & Rodrigues, J. J. P. C. (2019, June). Fog Computing for Smart Grid Systems in 5G Environment: Challenges and Solutions. *IEEE Wireless Communication Magazine*, *26*(3), 47–53. doi:10.1109/MWC.2019.1800356

Kumari, A., Tanwar, S., Tyagi, S., Kumar, N., Parizi, R. M., & Choo, K.-K. R. (2019). S. Tanwar., S. Tyagi, N. Kumar, R. Parizi, K. K. R. Choo, Fog Data Analytics: A Taxonomy and Process Model. *Journal of Network and Computer Applications*, *128*, 90–104. doi:10.1016/j.jnca.2018.12.013

Kumar, Y., Dewal, M. L., & Anand, R. S. (2014). Epileptic seizures detection in EEG using DWT-based ApEn and artificial neural network. *Signal, Image and Video Processing*, *8*(7), 1323–1334. doi:10.100711760-012-0362-9

Kuss, D. J., & Griffiths, M. D. (2017). Social networking sites and addiction: Ten lessons learned. *International Journal of Environmental Research and Public Health*, *14*(3), 311. doi:10.3390/ijerph14030311 PMID:28304359

Kuznetcov, M. V., Morozov, Y. G., & Belousova, O. V. (2012). Levitation jet synthesis of nickel ferrite nanoparticles. *Inorganic Materials*, *48*(10), 1044–1051. doi:10.1134/S0020168512100020

Lahmiri, S., & Shmuel, A. (2019). Accurate classification of seizure and seizure-free intervals of intracranial EEG signals from epileptic patients. *IEEE Transactions on Instrumentation and Measurement*, *68*(3), 791–796. doi:10.1109/TIM.2018.2855518

Lakshmi, K. S., & Vadivu, G. (2017). Extracting association rule from medical health records using multi criteria decision analysis. Procedia Computer Science, 115, 290–295.

Lamba, M., Munjal, G., & Gigras, Y. (2018). Feature Selection of Micro-array expression data (FSM)-A Review. *Procedia Computer Science*, *132*, 1619–1625. doi:10.1016/j.procs.2018.05.127

Lancaster Cancer Center. (2020). *Review Types of Cancer.* Retrieved from http://www.lancastercancercenter.com/disease-drug-information/review-types-of-cancer/

Lange, L., Fink, J., Bleich, C., Graefen, M., & Schulz, H. (2017). Effectiveness, acceptance and satisfaction of guided chat groups in psychosocial aftercare for outpatients with prostate cancer after prostatectomy. *Internet Interventions: the Application of Information Technology in Mental and Behavioural Health*, *9*, 57–64. doi:10.1016/j.invent.2017.06.001

Langius-Eklöf, A., Christiansen, M., Lindström, V., Blomberg, K., Hälleberg Nyman, M., Wengström, Y., & Sundberg, K. (2017). Adherence to report and patient perception of an interactive app for managing symptoms during radiotherapy for prostate cancer: Descriptive study of logged and interview data. *JMIR Cancer*, *3*(2), e18. doi:10.2196/cancer.7599

Langius-Eklöf, A., Crafoord, M. T., Christiansen, M., Fjell, M., & Sundberg, K. (2017). Effects of an interactive mHealth innovation for early detection of patient-reported symptom distress with focus on participatory care: Protocol for a study based on prospective, randomized, controlled trials in patients with prostate and breast cancer. *BMC Cancer*, *17*(1), 466. doi:10.118612885-017-3450-y

Langmuir, A. D. (1963). The surveillance of communicable diseases of national importance. *The New England Journal of Medicine*, *268*(4), 182–192. doi:10.1056/NEJM196301242680405 PMID:13928666

Le, D., Holt, C. L., Saunders, D. R., Wang, M. Q., Coriolan, A., Savoy, A. D., Slade, J. L., Muwwakkil, B., & Atkinson, N. L. (2018). Feasibility and acceptability of SMS text messaging in a prostate cancer educational intervention for African American men. *Health Informatics Journal*, *22*(4), 932–947. doi:10.1177/1460458215598636

Lee, T., Ng, V., Gallagher, R., Coldman, A., & McLean, D. (1997). Dullrazor®: A software approach to hair removal from images. *Computers in Biology and Medicine*, *27*(6), 533–543. doi:10.1016/S0010-4825(97)00020-6 PMID:9437554

Lerman, C., Schnoll, R. A., Hawk, L. W. Jr, Cinciripini, P., George, T. P., Wileyto, E. P., Swan, G. E., Benowitz, N., Heitjan, D. F., & Tyndale, R. F. (2015). Use of the Nicotine Metabolite Ratio as a Genetically Informed Biomarker of Response to Nicotine Patch or Varenicline for Smoking Cessation: A Randomised, Double-Blind Placebo-controlled Trial. *The Lancet. Respiratory Medicine*, *3*(2), 131–138. doi:10.1016/S2213-2600(14)70294-2 PMID:25588294

Leslie, S. W., Soon-Sutton, T. L., Sajjad, H., & Siref, L. E. (2020). Prostate cancer. In *StatPearls*. StatPearls Publishing.

Lewandowska, A. M., Rudzki, M., Rudzki, S., Lewandowski, T., & Laskowska, B. (2019). Environmental risk factors for cancer – review paper. *Annals of Agricultural and Environmental Medicine*, *26*(1), 1–7. doi:10.26444/aaem/94299 PMID:30922021

Lewis, J., Ray, P., & Liaw, S.-T. (2016). Recent worldwide developments in eHealth and mHealth to more effectively manage cancer and other chronic diseases - a systematic review. *Yearbook of Medical Informatics*, *1*, 93–108.

Li, Y. (2014). *Sparse machine learning models in bioinformatics*. Academic Press.

Liao, T. W. (2011). Diagnosis of bladder cancers with small sample size via feature selection. *Expert Systems with Applications*, *38*(4), 4649–4654. doi:10.1016/j.eswa.2010.09.135

Liberman, D., Mehus, B., & Elliott, S. P. (2014). Urinary adverse effects of pelvic radiotherapy. *Translational Andrology and Urology*, *3*(2), 186–195.

Lidington, E., McGrath, S. E., Noble, J., Stanway, S., Lucas, A., Mohammed, K., van der Graaf, W., & Husson, O. (2020). Evaluating a digital tool for supporting breast cancer patients: A randomized controlled trial protocol (ADAPT). *Trials*, *21*(1), 86. doi:10.118613063-019-3971-6

Li, M., Chen, W., & Zhang, T. (2017). Classification of epilepsy EEG signals using DWT-based envelope analysis and neural network ensemble. *Biomedical Signal Processing and Control*, *31*, 357–365. doi:10.1016/j.bspc.2016.09.008

Limonero, J. T., Tomás-Sábado, J., & Fernández-Castro, J. (2006). Perceived emotional intelligence and its relation to tobacco and cannabis use among university students. *Psicothema*, *18*, 95–100. PMID:17295964

Lin, D. W., Porter, M., & Montgomery, B. (2009). Treatment and survival outcomes in young men diagnosed with prostate cancer: A Population-based Cohort Study. *Cancer*, *115*(13), 2863–2871. doi:10.1002/cncr.24324

Lin, F. P., Pokorny, A., Teng, C., Dear, R., & Epstein, R. J. (2016). Computational prediction of multidisciplinary team decision-making for adjuvant breast cancer drug therapies: A machine learning approach. *BMC Cancer*, *16*(1), 929. doi:10.118612885-016-2972-z PMID:27905893

Lin, P. H., Chen, M., Tsai, L. W., Lo, C., Yen, T.-C., Huang, T. Y., Chen, C.-K., Fan, S.-C., Kuo, S.-H., & Huang, C.-S. (2020). Using next-generation sequencing to redefine BRCAness in triple-negative breast cancer. *Cancer Science, 111*(4), 1375–1384. doi:10.1111/cas.14313 PMID:31958182

Lin, R., Li, Y., MacDonald, T., Wu, H., Provenzale, J., Peng, X., Huang, J., Wang, L., Wang, A. Y., Yang, J., & Mao, H. (2017). Improving sensitivity and specificity of capturing and detecting targeted cancer cells with anti-biofouling polymer coated magnetic iron oxide nanoparticles. *Colloids and Surfaces. B, Biointerfaces, 150*, 261–270. doi:10.1016/j.colsurfb.2016.10.026

Litjens, G., Kooi, T., Bejnordi, B. E., Setio, A. A. A., Ciompi, F., Ghafoorian, M., & Sánchez, C. I. (2017). A survey on deep learning in medical image analysis. *Medical Image Analysis, 42*, 60–88. doi:10.1016/j.media.2017.07.005 PMID:28778026

Liu I. & Sun Y. (1993). Recursive tracking of vascular networks in angiograms based on the detection-deletion scheme. *IEEE Trans. Med. Imag., 12*(2), 334–341.

Li, X., & O'Malley, B. W. (2003). Unfolding the action of progesterone receptors. *The Journal of Biological Chemistry, 278*(41), 39261–39264. doi:10.1074/jbc.R300024200 PMID:12893816

Louie, K. S., Seigneurin, A., Cathcart, P., & Sasieni, P. (2015). Do prostate cancer risk models improve the predictive accuracy of PSA screening? A meta-analysis. *Annals of Oncology: Official Journal of the European Society for Medical Oncology, 26*(5), 848–864. doi:10.1093/annonc/mdu525

Lu, S., & Lim, J. H. (2010). Automatic Optic Disc Detection Through Background Estimation. *17th IEEE International Conference on Image Processing*, 833-836. 10.1109/ICIP.2010.5653473

Lu, A. H., Salabas, E. L., & Schüth, F. (2007). Magnetic nanoparticles: Synthesis, protection, functionalization, and application. *Angewandte Chemie International Edition in English, 46*(8), 1222–1244. doi:10.1002/anie.200602866

Lui, H-J., & Xu, P. (2019). Smart Mesoporous Silicon Nanoparticles for Protein Delivery. *Nanomaterials, 9*(511), 1-23.

Lupascu, C. A., Tegolo, D., & Rosa, L. D. (2008). Automated Detection of Optic Disc Location in Retinal Images. *21st IEEE International Symposium on Computer Based Medical Systems*, 17-22. 10.1109/CBMS.2008.15

Lu, Y., & Han, J. (2003). Cancer classification using gene expression data. *Information Systems, 28*(4), 243–268. doi:10.1016/S0306-4379(02)00072-8

Mabena, L. F., Sinha, R. S., Mhlanga, S. D., & Coville, N. J. (2011). Nitrogen-doped carbon nanotubes as a metal catalyst support. *Applied Nanoscience, 1*(2), 67–77. doi:10.100713204-011-0013-4

Mackay, A., Weigelt, B., Grigoriadis, A., Kreike, B., Natrajan, R., A'Hern, R., Tan, D. S. P., Dowsett, M., Ashworth, A., & Reis-Filho, J. S. (2011). Microarray-based class discovery for molecular classification of breast cancer: Analysis of interobserver agreement. *Journal of the National Cancer Institute, 103*(8), 662–673. doi:10.1093/jnci/djr071 PMID:21421860

Maguire, Morris, Parikh-Patel, Cress, Keegan, Li, Lin, & Kizer. (2019). A text mining approach to obtain detailed treatment information from free text fields in population based cancer registries: a study of non-small cell lung cancer in California. *Plos One Journal, 14*(2).

Maguire, R., Ream, E., Richardson, A., Connaghan, J., Johnston, B., Kotronoulas, G., Pedersen, V., McPhelim, J., Pattison, N., Smith, A., Webster, L., Taylor, A., & Kearney, N. (2015). Development of a novel remote patient monitoring system: The advanced symptom management system for radiotherapy to improve the symptom experience of patients with lung cancer receiving radiotherapy. *Cancer Nursing, 38*(2), E37–E47. doi:10.1097/NCC.0000000000000150

Mahdavi, M., Ahmad, M. B., Haron, M. J., Namvar, F., Nadi, B., Rahman, M., & Amin, J. (2013). Synthesis, surface modification and characterization of biocompatible magnetic iron oxide nanoparticles for biomedical applications. *Molecules (Basel, Switzerland), 18*(7), 7533–7548. doi:10.3390/molecules18077533

Maheu, M. M., & Gordon, B. L. (2000). Counseling and therapy on the internet. *Professional Psychology, Research and Practice, 31*(5), 484–489. doi:10.1037/0735-7028.31.5.484

Mahmood, A., Kedia, S., Wyant, D. K., Ahn, S., & Bhuyan, S. S. (2019). Use of mobile health applications for health-promoting behavior among individuals with chronic medical conditions. *Digital Health, 5*. Advance online publication. doi:10.1177/2055207619882181

Malinauskas, R., Dumciene, A., Sipaviciene, S., & Malinauskiene, V. (2018). *Relationship between emotional intelligence and health behaviours among university students: The predictive and moderating role of gender.* Academic Press.

Malone, E. R., Oliva, M., Sabatini, P. J. B., Stockley, T. L., & Siu, L. L. (2020). Molecular profiling for precision cancer therapies. *Genome Medicine, 12*(1), 8. doi:10.118613073-019-0703-1 PMID:31937368

Maniruzzaman, Kumar, Nishithkumar, Abedin, Islam, Suri, El-Baz, & Suri. (2017). Comparative approach for classification of diabetes mellitus data: machine learning paradigm. *Computer Method and Program in Biomedicine, 152*, 23-34.

Manj, R. Z. A., Chen, X., Rehman, W. U., Zhu, G., Luo, W., & Yang, J. (2018). Big Potential from Silicon-Based Porous Nanomaterials: In Field of Energy Storage and Sensors. *Frontiers in Chemistry, 6*, 539. doi:10.3389/fchem.2018.00539

Manogaran, G., Shakeel, P. M., Hassanein, A. S., Kumar, P. M., & Babu, G. C. (2018). Machine Learning Approach-Based Gamma Distribution for Brain Tumor Detection and Data Sample Imbalance Analysis. *IEEE Access: Practical Innovations, Open Solutions, 7*, 12–19. doi:10.1109/ACCESS.2018.2878276

Manson, A., Myers, J., Billinger, S., Ward, J., Parker, W., Hamilton-Reeves, J., Michel, C., & Maliski, S. L. (2019). Feasibility of an intervention for men on androgen deprivation therapy: A research protocol. *Research in Nursing & Health, 42*(5), 324–333. doi:10.1002/nur.21977

Mantere, T., Kersten, S., & Hoischen, A. (2019). Long-read sequencing emerging in medical genetics. *Frontiers in Genetics, 10*, 426. doi:10.3389/fgene.2019.00426 PMID:31134132

Maraci. (2017). *Flutter*. Retrieved from https://wmaraci.com/nedir/flutter

Marino, M. M., Rienzo, M., Serra, N., Marino, N., Ricciotti, R., Mazzariello, L., Leonetti, C. A., Ceraldi, M. P., Casamassimi, A., Capocelli, F., Martone, G., & Caracciolo, A. L. (2020). Mobile screening units for the early detection of breast cancer and cardiovascular disease: A pilot telemedicine study in Southern Italy. *Telemedicine Journal and e-Health, 26*(3), 286–293. doi:10.1089/tmj.2018.0328

Market Analysis Report. (2019). *Internet of Things (IoT) in Healthcare Market Size, Share & Trends Analysis Report By Component (Service, System & Software), By Connectivity Technology (Satellite, Cellular), By End Use (CRO, Hospital & Clinic), By Application, And Segment Forecasts, 2019 – 2025.* Author.

Markozannes, G., Tzoulaki, I., Karli, D., Evangelou, E., Ntzani, E., Gunter, M. J., Norat, T., Ioannidis, J. P., & Tsilidis, K. K. (2016). Diet, body size, physical activity and risk of prostate cancer: An umbrella review of the evidence. *European Journal of Cancer (Oxford, England), 69*, 61–69. doi:10.1016/j.ejca.2016.09.026

Martinez, J. C., & Otley, C. C. (2001). The management of melanoma and nonmelanoma skin cancer: A review for the primary care physician. *Mayo Clinic Proceedings, 76*(12), 1253–1265. doi:10.4065/76.12.1253 PMID:11761506

Martins, A., Ramalho, N., & Morin, E. (2010). A comprehensive meta-analysis of the relationship between emotional intelligence and health. *Personality and Individual Differences, 49*(6), 554–564. doi:10.1016/j.paid.2010.05.029

Massard, C., Michiels, S., Ferte, C., Le Deley, M. C., Lacroix, L., Hollebecque, A., Verlingue, L., Ileana, E., Rosellini, S., Ammari, S., Ngo-Camus, M., Bahleda, R., Gazzah, A., Varga, A., Postel-Vinay, S., Loriot, Y., Even, C., Breuskin, I., Auger, N., ... Soria, J.-C. (2017). High-throughput genomics and clinical outcome in hard-to-treat advanced cancers: Results of the MOSCATO 01 trial. *Cancer Discovery*, *7*(6), 586–595. doi:10.1158/2159-8290.CD-16-1396 PMID:28365644

Mayer, J. D., & Salovey, P. (1993). *The intelligence of emotional intelligence.* Academic Press.

Mcguire, S. (2015). *World Cancer report 2014.* World Health Organization, International Agency for Research on Cancer, Who Press.

McNabb, K. (2004). Operations I Nursery operations. Encyclopedia of Forest Sciences, 649-657. doi:10.1016/b0-12-145160-7/00001-6

Mechael, P. (2012). mHealth Alliance: A history of mobile & mHealth. *mHealthinsight.* https://mhealthinsight.com/2012/11/24/mhealth-alliance-a-history-of-mobile-mhealth/

Medical News Today. (2020). *What to know about cancer.* Retrieved from https://www.medicalnewstoday.com/articles/323648

Medicine. (2019). *Dünyada Diyabet Hastasi.* Retrieved from https://www.aa.com.tr/tr/saglik/dunyada-diyabet-hastasi-sayisi-2045te-629-milyona-ulasacak/1643626

Medium. (2018) *Flutter.* Retrieved from https://medium.com/@halilozel1903/dart-programlama-dili-eeafb64ad300

Mendonca, A. M., & Campilho, A. (2011). Segmentation of retinal blood vessels by combining the detection of centerlines and morphological reconstruction. *IEEE Transactions on Medical Imaging*, *25*(9), 1200–1213p. doi:10.1109/TMI.2006.879955 PMID:16967805

Menzies, S. W., Ingvar, C., Crotty, K. A., & McCarthy, W. H. (1996). Frequency and morphologic characteristics of invasive melanomas lacking specific surface microscopic features. *Archives of Dermatology*, *132*(10), 1178–1182. doi:10.1001/archderm.1996.03890340038007 PMID:8859028

Meshgi, M. A., Kriechbaum, M., Biswas, S., Holmes, J. D., & Marschner, C. (2016). Synthesis of indium nanoparticles at ambient temperature; simultaneous phase transfer and ripening. *Journal of Nanoparticle Research*, *18*(12), 363. doi:10.100711051-016-3683-8

Metsker, Bolgova, Yakovlev, Funkner, & Kovalchuk. (2017). Pattern based mining in E HR for complex clinical process analysis. Elsevier Journal, 119, 197-206.

Metzger Filho, O., Ignatiadis, M., & Sotiriou, C. (2011). Genomic Grade Index: An important tool for assessing breast cancer tumor grade and prognosis. *Critical Reviews in Oncology/Hematology*, *77*(1), 20–29. doi:10.1016/j.critrevonc.2010.01.011 PMID:20138540

Meyer, D., & Wien, F. T. (2015). Support vector machines. *The Interface to libsvm in package e1071, 28.*

Meystre, S. M., Savova, G. K., Kipper-Schuler, K. C., & Hurdle, J. F. (2008). *Extracting information from textual documents in E HR.* IMIA Yearbookof Medical Informatics.

Middleton, R. G., Thompson, I. M., Austenfeld, M. S., Cooner, W. H., Correa, R. J., Gibbons, R. P., Miller, H. C., Oesterling, J. E., Resnick, M. I., Smalley, S. R., & Wasson, J. H. (1995). Prostate Cancer Clinical Guidelines Panel Summary report on the management of clinically localized prostate cancer. The American Urological Association. *The Journal of Urology*, *154*(6), 2144–2148. doi:10.1016/S0022-5347(01)66718-1

Mikolajczak, M., Luminet, O., & Menil, C. (2006). Predicting resistance to stress: Incremental validity of trait emotional intelligence over alexithymia and optimism. *Psicothema*, *18*, 79–88. PMID:17295962

Millar, E. K., Graham, P. H., O'Toole, S. A., McNeil, C. M., Browne, L., Morey, A. L., ... Nasser, E. (2009). Prediction of local recurrence, distant metastases, and death after breast-conserving therapy in early-stage invasive breast cancer using a five-biomarker panel. *Journal of Clinical Oncology*, *27*(28), 4701–4708. doi:10.1200/JCO.2008.21.7075 PMID:19720911

Millot, F., Rifflet, J. C., Sarou-Kanian, V., & Wille, G. (2002). High-Temperature Properties of Liquid Boron form Contactless Techniques. *International Journal of Thermophysics*, *23*(5), 1185–1195. doi:10.1023/A:1019836102776

Min-Dianey, K. A. A., Zhang, H. C., Brohi, A. A., Yu, H., & Xia, X. (2018). Optical spectrea of composite silver-porous silicon (Ag-pSi) nanostructure based periodical lattice. *Superlattices and Microstructures*, *115*, 168–176. doi:10.1016/j.spmi.2018.01.028

Mirkovic, J., Kaufman, D. R., & Ruland, C. M. (2014). Supporting cancer patients in illness management: Usability evaluation of a mobile app. *JMIR mHealth and uHealth*, *2*(3), e33. doi:10.2196/mhealth.3359

Mishel, M. H., Belyea, M., Germino, B. B., Stewart, J. L., Bailey, D. E., Robertson, C., & Mohler, J. (2002). Helping patients with localized prostate carcinoma manage uncertainty and treatment side effects: Nurse-delivered psychoeducational intervention over the telephone. *Cancer*, *94*(6), 1854–1866. doi:10.1002/cncr.10390

Misra, S., Lewis, T. L., & Aungst, T. D. (2013). Medical application use and the need for further research and assessment for clinical practice: Creation and integration of standards for best practice to alleviate poor application design. *JAMA Dermatology*, *149*(6), 661–662. https://pubmed.ncbi.nlm.nih.gov/23783150/. doi:10.1001/jamadermatol.2013.606 PMID:23783150

Mistry, I., Tanwar, S., Tyagi, S., & Kumar, N. (2020). Blockchain for 5G-Enabled IoT for Industrial Automation: A Systematic Review, Solutions, and Challenges. *Mechanical Systems and Signal Processing*, *135*, 1–19. doi:10.1016/j.ymssp.2019.106382

Mitchell, A. J., Chan, M., Bhatti, H., Halton, M., Grassi, L., Johansen, C., & Meader, N. (2011). Prevalence of depression, anxiety, and adjustment disorder in oncological, haematological, and palliative-care settings: A meta-analysis of 94 interview-based studies. *The Lancet. Oncology*, *12*(2), 160–174. doi:10.1016/S1470-2045(11)70002-X

Mittal, M., Tanwar, S., Agarwal, B., & Goyal, L. M. (Eds.). (2019). *Energy Conservation for IoT Devices: Concepts, Paradigms and Solutions, Studies in Systems, Decision and Control*. Springer Nature Singapore Pte Ltd. doi:10.1007/978-981-13-7399-2

Mogensen, M., & Jemec, G. B. (2007). Diagnosis of nonmelanoma skin cancer/keratinocyte carcinoma: A review of diagnostic accuracy of nonmelanoma skin cancer diagnostic tests and technologies. *Dermatologic Surgery*, *33*(10), 1158–1174. doi:10.1097/00042728-200710000-00003 PMID:17903149

Mohammed, Y. H., Holmes, A., Haridass, I. N., Sanchez, W. Y., Studier, H., Grice, J. E., Benson, H. A. E., & Roberts, M. S. (2019). Support for the safe use of zinc oxide nanoparticles sunscreens: Lack of Skin Penetration or Cellular Toxicity After Repeated Application in Volunteers. *The Journal of Investigative Dermatology*, *139*(2), 308–315. doi:10.1016/j.jid.2018.08.024

Mookiah, M. R. K., Rajendra-Acharya, U., Martis, R. J., Chua, K. C., Lim, C. M., Ng, E. Y. K., & Laude, A. (2013). Evolutionary Algorithm Based Classifier Parameter Tuning for Automatic Diabetic Retinopathy Grading: A Hybrid Feature Extraction Approach. *Knowledge-Based Systems*, *39*, 9–22. doi:10.1016/j.knosys.2012.09.008

Morales, I. J. C., Pupiales, S. K. N., Criollo, A. C. U., & Montalvo, P. D. R. (2017). Wearable Textile for Accident Prevention for Babies in Crawl Phase. *Proceedings of the International Conference on Information Systems and Computer Science (INCISCOS)*, 66–72. 10.1109/INCISCOS.2017.55

Morash, M., Mitchell, H., Beltran, H., Elemento, O., & Pathak, J. (2018). The Role of Next-Generation Sequencing in Precision Medicine: A Review of Outcomes in Oncology. *J Pers Med., 17*(8), 30.

Mosa, A. S., Yoo, I., & Sheets, L. (2012, Jul 10). A systematic review of health care apps for smartphones. *BMC Med Inform Dec Mak.* https://bmcmedinformdecismak.biomedcentral.com/articles/10.1186/1472-6947-12-67

Mottet, N., Bellmunt, J., & Briers, E. (2016). *Guidelines on prostate cancer.* https://uroweb.org/wp-content/uploads/EAU-Guidelines

Mukherjee, S. (2019, October). Genomics-Guided Immunotherapy for Precision Medicine in Cancer. *Cancer Biotherapy & Radiopharmaceuticals, 34*(8), 487–497. doi:10.1089/cbr.2018.2758 PMID:31314580

Murfin, M. (2013). Know your apps: An evidence-based approach to the evaluation of mobile clinical applications. *The Journal of Physician Assistant Education: the Official Journal of the Physician Assistant Education Association, 24*(3), 38–40. doi:10.1097/01367895-201324030-00008 PMID:24261171

Mursalin, M., Zhang, Y., Chen, Y., & Chawla, N. V. (2017). Automated epileptic seizure detection using improved correlation-based feature selection with random forest classifier. *Neurocomputing, 241*, 204–214. doi:10.1016/j.neucom.2017.02.053

Murugavel, A. M., & Ramakrishnan, S. (2011). Wavelet domain approximate entropy-based epileptic seizure detection. *The 5th International Conference on Information Technology.*

Musen, M. A., Middleton, B., & Greenes, R. A. (2014). Clinical Decision-Support Systems. In E. H. Shortlife & J. J. Cimino (Eds.), *Biomedical Informatics Springer* (pp. 643–674). doi:10.1007/978-1-4471-4474-8_22

Nacht, M., Ferguson, A. T., Zhang, W., Petroziello, J. M., Cook, B. P., Gao, Y. H., ... Madden, S. L. (1999). Combining serial analysis of gene expression and array technologies to identify genes differentially expressed in breast cancer. *Cancer Research, 59*(21), 5464–5470. PMID:10554019

Naeem, Z. (2014). Health risks associated with mobile phones use. *International Journal of Health Sciences, 8*(4), V–VI. doi:10.12816/0006077 PMID:25780365

Nagler, R. H., Gray, S. W., Romantan, A., Kelly, B. J., DeMichele, A., Armstrong, K. et al. (2010). Differences in information seeking among breast, prostate, and colorectal cancer patients: results from a population-based survey. *Patient Educ. Couns., 81*, S54-S62.

Naharro-Abellán & Lobo-Valbuena. (2020). Clinical Decision Support Systems: Future or Present in ICU? *ICU Management & Practice, 19*(4).

Nahata, H., & Singh, S. P. (2020). Deep Learning Solutions for Skin Cancer Detection and Diagnosis. In *Machine Learning with Health Care Perspective* (pp. 159–182). Springer. doi:10.1007/978-3-030-40850-3_8

Nanton, V., Appleton, R., Loew, J., Ahmed, N., Ahmedzai, S., & Dale, J. (2017). Men don't talk about their health, but will they CHAT? The potential of online holistic needs assessment in prostate cancer. *BJU International, 121*(4), 494–496. doi:10.1111/bju.14114

Naqvi, S. A., Zafar, M. F., & Haq, I. U. (2015). Referral System for Hard Exudates in Eye Fundus. *Computers in Biology and Medicine, 64*, 217–235. doi:10.1016/j.compbiomed.2015.07.003 PMID:26231313

Narayanan, D. L., Saladi, R. N., & Fox, J. L. (2010). Ultraviolet radiation and skin cancer. *International Journal of Dermatology, 49*(9), 978–986. doi:10.1111/j.1365-4632.2010.04474.x PMID:20883261

National Cancer Institute. (n.d.). https://www.cancer.gov/cancertopics

National Institutes of Health Consensus Development Panel. (2001). National Institutes of Health Consensus Development Conference statement: adjuvant therapy for breast cancer, November 1–3, 2000. *JNCI Monographs, 2001*(30), 5-15.

Nattestad, M., Goodwin, S., Ng, K., Baslan, T., Sedlazeck, F. J., Rescheneder, P., Garvin, T., Fang, H., Gurtowski, J., Hutton, E., Tseng, E., Chin, C.-S., Beck, T., Sundaravadanam, Y., Kramer, M., Antoniou, E., McPherson, J. D., Hicks, J., McCombie, W. R., & Schatz, M. C. (2018). Complex rearrangements and oncogene amplifications revealed by long-read DNA and RNA sequencing of a breast cancer cell line. *Genome Research, 28*(8), 1126–1135. doi:10.1101/gr.231100.117 PMID:29954844

Neville, J. A., Welch, E., & Leffell, D. J. (2007). Management of nonmelanoma skin cancer in 2007. *Nature Clinical Practice. Oncology, 4*(8), 462–469. doi:10.1038/ncponc0883 PMID:17657251

Ngoy, J. M., Wagner, N., Riboldi, L., & Bolland, O. (2014). A CO_2 capture technology using multi-walled carbon nanotubes with polyaspartamide surfactant. *Energy Procedia, 63*, 2230–2248. doi:10.1016/j.egypro.2014.11.242

Nguyen, N. S., Gautam, D., & Hee, Y. H. (2016). Nickel/cobalt oxide-decorated 3D graphene nanocomposite electrode for enhanced electrochemical detection of urea. *Biosensors & Bioelectronics, 77*, 372–377. doi:10.1016/j.bios.2015.09.046

Nicolaou, N., & Georgiou, J. (2012). Detection of epileptic electroencephalogram based on permutation entropy and support vector machines. *Expert Systems with Applications, 39*(1), 202–209. doi:10.1016/j.eswa.2011.07.008

Niedermeyer, E., & da Silva, F. L. (Eds.). (2005). *Electroencephalography: basic principles, clinical applications, and related fields*. Lippincott Williams & Wilkins.

Niemeijer, M., Staal, J., Ginneken, B. v., Loog, M., Abramoff, M. D., Fitzpatrick, J., & Sonka, M. (2004). Comparative study of retinal vessel segmentation methods on a new publicly available database. SPIE Med. Imag., 5370, 648–656.

Niesters, H. G., Rossen, J. W., Van der Avoort, H., Baas, D., Benschop, K., Claas, E. C., Kroneman, A., Van Maarseveen, N., Pas, S., Van Pelt, W., Rahamat-Langendoen, J. C., Schuurman, R., Vennema, H., Verhoef, L., Wolthers, K., & Koopmans, M. (2013). Laboratory-based surveillance in the molecular era: The TYPENED model, a joint data-sharing platform for clinical and public health laboratories. *Eurosurveillance, 18*(4). Advance online publication. doi:10.2807/ese.18.04.20387-en PMID:23369392

Niewolny, D. (2013). *How the Internet of Things Is Revolutionizing Healthcare*. Freescale Semiconductors.

Noda, K., Yamaguchi, Y., Nakadai, K., Okuno, H. G., & Ogata, T. (2015). Audio-visual speech recognition using deep learning. *Applied Intelligence, 42*(4), 722–737. doi:10.100710489-014-0629-7

Nsubuga, P., White, M. E., Thacker, S. B., Anderson, M. A., Blount, S. B., Broome, C. V., Chiller, T. M., Espitia, V., Imtiaz, R., Sosin, D., Stroup, D. F., Tauxe, R. V., Vijayaraghavan, M., & Trostle, M. (2006). *Public Health Surveillance: A Tool for Targeting and Monitoring Interventions. Disease Control Priorities in Developing Countries* (2nd ed.). Oxford University Press.

O'Neill, M. C. (1991). Training back-propagation neural networks to define and detect DNA-binding sites. *Nucleic Acids Research, 19*(2), 313–318. doi:10.1093/nar/19.2.313 PMID:2014171

Ocak, H. (2009). Automatic detection of epileptic seizures in EEG using discrete wavelet transform and approximate entropy. *Expert Systems with Applications, 36*(2), 2027–2036. doi:10.1016/j.eswa.2007.12.065

Ogundele, I.O., Popoola, O.L., Oyesola, O.O., & Orija, K.T. (2018). A review on data mining in health care. *International Journal of Advanced Research in Computer Engineering & Technology, 7*(9).

Ojha, N. K., Zyryanov, G. V., Majee, A., Charushin, V. N., Chupakhin, O. N., & Santra, S. (2017). Copper nanoparticles as inexpensive and efficient catalyst: A valuable contribution in organic synthesis. *Coordination Chemistry Reviews, 353*, 1–57. doi:10.1016/j.ccr.2017.10.004

Okur, E., & Turkan, M. (2018). A survey on automated melanoma detection. *Engineering Applications of Artificial Intelligence, 73*, 50–67. doi:10.1016/j.engappai.2018.04.028

Oliveira, R. B., Mercedes Filho, E., Ma, Z., Papa, J. P., Pereira, A. S., & Tavares, J. M. R. (2016). Computational methods for the image segmentation of pigmented skin lesions: A review. *Computer Methods and Programs in Biomedicine, 131*, 127–141. doi:10.1016/j.cmpb.2016.03.032 PMID:27265054

Olsson, C. E., Alsadius, D., Pettersson, N., Tucker, S. L., Wilderäng, U., Johansson, K. A., & Steineck, G. (2015). Patient-reported sexual toxicity after radiation therapy in long-term prostate cancer survivors. *British Journal of Cancer, 113*(5), 802–808. doi:10.1038/bjc.2015.275

Oquab, M., Bottou, L., Laptev, I., & Sivic, J. (2014). Learning and transferring mid-level image representations using convolutional neural networks. In *Proceedings of the IEEE conference on computer vision and pattern recognition* (pp. 1717-1724). 10.1109/CVPR.2014.222

Orhan, U., Hekim, M., & Ozer, M. (2011). EEG signals classification using the K-means clustering and a multilayer perceptron neural network model. *Expert Systems with Applications, 38*(10), 13475–13481. doi:10.1016/j.eswa.2011.04.149

Osei, D. K., Lee, J. W., Modest, N. N., & Pothier, P. K. (2013). Effects of an online support group for prostate cancer survivors: A randomized trial. *Urologic Nursing, 33*(3), 123–133. doi:10.7257/1053-816X.2013.33.3.123

Osheroff, J. A., & Teich, J. (2012). Improving Outcomes with Clinical Decision Support: An Implementer's Guide (2nd ed.). Chicago: Healthcare Information and Management Systems Society (HIMSS).

Osheroff, J. A., Teich, J. M., Middleton, B., Steen, E. B., Wright, A., & Detmer, D. E. (2007). A Roadmap for National Action on Clinical Decision Support. *Journal of the American Medical Informatics Association, 14*(2), 141–145. doi:10.1197/jamia.M2334 PMID:17213487

Ozdalga, E., Ozdalga, A., & Ahuja, N. (2012, September 27). The smartphone in medicine: A review of current and potential use among physicians and students. *Journal of Medical Internet Research, 14*(5), e128. doi:10.2196/jmir.1994 PMID:23017375

Ozkan, I. A., & Koklu, M. (2017). Skin Lesion Classification using Machine Learning Algorithms. *International Journal of Intelligent Systems and Applications in Engineering, 5*(4), 285–289. doi:10.18201/ijisae.2017534420

Pagliari, C., Sloan, D., Gregor, P., Detmer, D., Kahan, J. P., Oortwijn, W., & MacGillivray, S. (2005). What is eHealth (4): A scoping exercise to map the field. *Journal of Medical Internet Research, 7*(1), 9. doi:10.2196/jmir.7.1.e9

Pandey. (2016). Data mining techniques for medical data: a review. *International Conference on Signal Pricessing, Comm., Power and Embedded Sys (SCOPES).*

Panditharadhyula, R., & Kumar, P. (2018). Impact of Biographical Variables and Social Networking Platforms on Emotional Intelligence among Adolescents. *International Journal of Scientific Research (Ahmedabad, India), 7*(5), 1320–1326.

Panigrahi, G. K., Praharaj, P. P., Kittaka, H., Mridha, A. R., Black, O. M., Singh, R., Mercer, R., van Bokhoven, A., Torkko, K. C., Agarwal, C., Agarwal, R., Abd Elmageed, Z. Y., Yadav, H., Mishra, S. K., & Deep, G. (2019). Exosome proteomic analyses identify inflammatory phenotype and novel biomarkers in African American prostate cancer patients. *Cancer Medicine*, *8*(3), 1111–1123. doi:10.1002/cam4.1885

Parahoo, K., McDonough, S., McCaughan, E., Noyes, J., Semple, C., Halstead, E. J., Neuberger, M. M., & Dahm, P. (2015). Psychosocial interventions for men with prostate cancer: A Cochrane systematic review. *BJU International*, *116*(2), 174–183. doi:10.1111/bju.12989

Park, J., & Ryu, Y. U. (2014). FM: fibromyalgia: chronic pain: text mining to identify clinical distinctions and patient concerns. International Medical Journal of Experimental and Clinical Research.

Patel, D., Narmawala, Z., Tanwar, S., & Singh, P. K. (2018). A Systematic Review on Scheduling Public Transport Using IoT as Tool. In B. Panigrahi, M. Trivedi, K. Mishra, S. Tiwari, & P. Singh (Eds.), *Smart Innovations in Communication and Computational Sciences. Advances in Intelligent Systems and Computing* (Vol. 670, pp. 39–48). Springer. doi:10.1007/978-981-10-8971-8_4

Peden, M., McGee, K., & Sharma, G. (2002). *The Injury Chartbook: A Graphical Overview of the Global Burden of Injuries*. World Health Organization.

Pelletier, S. G. (2012). Explosive growth in health care apps raises oversight questions. *AAMC Reporter*. Available at https://www.aamc.org/newsroom/reporter/october2012/308516/health-care-apps.html

Perdana, N. R., Mochtar, C. A., Umbas, R., & Hamid, A. R. (2016). The risk factors of prostate cancer and its prevention: A literature review. *Acta Medica Indonesiana*, *48*(3), 228–238.

Perego, P., Andreoni, G., Zanini, R., & Bellù, R. (2014) Wearable Biosignal Monitoring System For Newborns. *Proceedings Of The 4th International Conference On Wireless Mobile Communication and Healthcare—Transforming Healthcare Through Innovations in Mobile and Wireless Technologies (MOBIHEALTH)*, 271–274. 10.4108/icst.mobihealth.2014.257403

Pereira-Azevedo, N. M., & Venderbos, L. (2018). eHealth and mHealth in prostate cancer detection and active surveillance. *Translational Andrology and Urology*, *7*(1), 170–181. doi:10.21037/tau.2017.12.22

Pereira-Azevedo, N., Osório, L., Fraga, A., & Roobol, M. J. (2017). Rotterdam Prostate Cancer Risk Calculator: Development and usability testing of the mobile phone app. *JMIR Cancer*, *3*(1), e1. doi:10.2196/cancer.6750

Perer, A. (2012). Healthcare analytics for clinical and non-clinical settings. *Proceedings of CHI Conference*.

Petrides, K. V. (2011). *Ability and trait emotional intelligence*. Academic Press.

Petrides, K. V. (2010). Trait emotional intelligence theory. *Industrial and Organizational Psychology: Perspectives on Science and Practice*, *3*(2), 136–139. doi:10.1111/j.1754-9434.2010.01213.x

Piercey, D. G., & Klapoetke, T. M. (2010). Nanoscale Aluminium Metal Oxide (Thermite) Reactions for Application in Energetic Materials. *Central European Journal of Energetic Materials*, *7*(2), 115–129.

Polat, K., & Güneş, S. (2007). Classification of epileptiform EEG using a hybrid system based on decision tree classifier and fast Fourier transform. *Applied Mathematics and Computation*, *187*(2), 1017–1026. doi:10.1016/j.amc.2006.09.022

Polat, K., & Güneş, S. (2008). Principles component analysis, fuzzy weighting pre-processing and artificial immune recognition system based diagnostic system for diagnosis of lung cancer. *Expert Systems with Applications*, *34*(1), 214–221. doi:10.1016/j.eswa.2006.09.001

Pope, Z., Lee, J. E., Zeng, N., Lee, H. Y., & Gao, Z. (2019). Feasibility of smartphone application and social media intervention on breast cancer survivors' health outcomes. *Translational Behavioral Medicine*, *9*(1), 11–22. doi:10.1093/tbm/iby002

Prasad, T. N. V. K. V., Sudhakar, P., Sreenivasulu, Y., Latha, P., Munaswamy, V., Reddy, K. R., Sreeprasad, T. S., Sajanlal, P. R., & Pradeep, T. (2012). Effect of nanoscale Zinc Oxide Particles on the Germination, Growth and Yield of Peanut. *Journal of Plant Nutrition*, *35*(6), 905–927. doi:10.1080/01904167.2012.663443

Prasad, V. K., Bhavsar, M., & Tanwar, S. (2019). Influence of monitoring: Fog and Edge Computing", Scalable Computing. *Practice and Experience*, *20*(2), 365–376. doi:10.12694cpe.v20i2.1533

Puech, P., Betrouni, N., Viard, R., Villers, A., & Leroy, X. (2007). Prostate cancer computer-assisted diagnosis software using dynamic contrast-enhanced MRI. In *29th Annual International Conference of the IEEE Engineering in Medicine and Biology Society* (pp. 5567-5570). IEEE. 10.1109/IEMBS.2007.4353608

Quanbeck, A., Gustafson, D. H., Marsch, L. A., Chih, M. Y., Kornfield, R., McTavish, F., Johnson, R., Brown, R. T., Mares, M. L., & Shah, D. V. (2018). Implementing a mobile health system to integrate the treatment of addiction into primary care: A hybrid implementation-effectiveness study. *Journal of Medical Internet Research*, *20*(1), e37. doi:10.2196/jmir.8928

Quénel, N., Wafflart, J., Bonichon, F., de Mascarel, I., Trojani, M., Durand, M., Avril, A., & Coindre, J. M. (1995). The prognostic value of c-erbB2 in primary breast carcinomas: A study on 942 cases. *Breast Cancer Research and Treatment*, *35*(3), 283–291. doi:10.1007/BF00665980 PMID:7579499

Ragab, D. A., Sharkas, M., Marshall, S., & Ren, J. (2019). Breast cancer detection using deep convolutional neural networks and support vector machines. *PeerJ*, *7*, e6201. doi:10.7717/peerj.6201 PMID:30713814

Raja, U., Mitchell, T., Day, T., & Hardin, J. M. (2008). Text mining in healthcare, applications and opportunities. *Journal of Healthcare Information Management*, *22*(3), 52–56. PMID:19267032

Rajput, D. S., & Gaur, R. (2017). *An IoT Framework for Healthcare Monitoring System*. LAP LAMBERT Academic Publishing.

Ranger, T., & Slack, P. (Eds.), *Epidemics and ideas: essays on the historical perception of pestilences* (pp. 149–173). Cambridge University Press. doi:10.1017/CBO9780511563645

Rastogi, A., Tripathi, D.K., Yadav, S., Chauhan, D.K., Ghorbanpour, M.Z.M., El-Sheery, N.I., & Brestic, M. (2019). Applications of silicon nanoparticles in agriculture. *Biotech*, *9*(90), 1-11.

Rathod, A. (n.d.). Why mHealth is Beneficial for Patients. *Referralmd*. https://getreferralmd.com/2019/04/why-mhealth-is-beneficial-for-patients/

Rauschert, S., Raubenheimer, K., Melton, P. E., & Huang, R. C. (2020). Machine learning and clinical epigenetics: A review of challenges for diagnosis and classification. *Clinical Epigenetics*, *12*(1), 1–11. doi:10.118613148-020-00842-4 PMID:32245523

Revathi, M. (2014). Survey on medical text mining. *International Journal of Computers and Applications*.

Riazul Islam, S., Daehan Kwak, Humaun Kabir, M., Hossain, M., & Kyung-Sup Kwak. (2015). The Internet of Things for Health Care: A Comprehensive Survey. *IEEE Access: Practical Innovations, Open Solutions*, *3*, 678–708. doi:10.1109/ACCESS.2015.2437951

Richards, S., Aziz, N., Bale, S., Bick, D., Das, S., Gastier-Foster, J., Grody, W. W., Hegde, M., Lyon, E., Spector, E., Voelkerding, K., & Rehm, H. L. (2015). Standards and guidelines for the interpretation of sequence variants: A joint consensus recommendation of the American College of Medical Genetics and Genomics and the Association for Molecular Pathology. *Genetics in Medicine*, *17*(5), 405–423. doi:10.1038/gim.2015.30 PMID:25741868

Ries, L. A., Harkins, D., Krapcho, M., Mariotto, A., Miller, B. A., Feuer, E. J., ... Hayat, M. (2006). *SEER cancer statistics review, 1975-2003*. Academic Press.

Rincon, E., Monteiro-Guerra, F., Rivera-Romero, O., Dorronzoro-Zubiete, E., Sanchez-Bocanegra, C. L., & Gabarron, E. (2017). Mobile phone apps for quality of life and well-being assessment in breast and prostate cancer patients: Systematic review. *JMIR mHealth and uHealth*, *5*(12), e187. doi:10.2196/mhealth.8741

Ringwald, J., Gerstner, L., Junne, F., Ziser, K., Schäffeler, N., Wallwiener, M., Hautzinger, M., Bäuerle, A., Brucker, S., Zipfel, S., & Teufel, M. (2019). Mindfulness and skills based distress reduction in oncology: Das Webbasierte Psychoonkologische Make It Training. *Psychotherapie, Psychosomatik, Medizinische Psychologie*, *69*(9-10), 407–412. doi:10.1055/a-0835-6905

Robbins, P., Pinder, S., De Klerk, N., Dawkins, H., Harvey, J., Sterrett, G., Ellis, I., & Elston, C. (1995). Histological grading of breast carcinomas: A study of interobserver agreement. *Human Pathology*, *26*(8), 873–879. doi:10.1016/0046-8177(95)90010-1 PMID:7635449

Roberts, A. L., Potts, H. W., Koutoukidis, D. A., Smith, L., & Fisher, A. (2019). Breast, prostate, and colorectal cancer survivors' experiences of using publicly available physical activity mobile apps: Qualitative study. *JMIR mHealth and uHealth*, *7*(1), e10918. doi:10.2196/10918

Rodríguez, M., Alfonso, P., MacGregor, J., Kanagarajah, K., Patel, S., & Schlagenhauf, D. (2020). Going global – Travel and the 2019 novel coronavirus. *Travel Medicine and Infectious Disease*, *33*. Advance online publication. doi:10.1016/j.tmaid.2020.101578 PMID:32044389

Rong, G. Y., Cao, Q. D., Hong, Z. S., Tan, Y. Y., Chen, S. D., Jin, H. J., Tan, K. S., Wang, D. Y., & Yan, Y. (2020). The origin, transmission and clinical therapies on coronavirus disease 2019 (COVID-19) outbreak – an update on the Status. *Military Medical Research*, *7*(1), 11. doi:10.118640779-020-00240-0 PMID:32169119

Roobol, M. J., van Vugt, H. A., Loeb, S., Zhu, X., Bul, M., Bangma, C. H., van Leenders, A. G. L. J. H., Steyerberg, E. W., & Schröder, F. H. (2012). Prediction of prostate cancer risk: The role of prostate volume and digital rectal examination in the ERSPC risk calculators. *European Urology*, *61*(3), 577–583. doi:10.1016/j.eururo.2011.11.012

Rosenholm, J. M., Zhang, J., Linden, M., & Sahlgren, C. (2016). Mesoporous silica nanoparticles in tissue engineering- a prospective. *Nanomedicine (London)*, *11*(4), 391–402. doi:10.2217/nnm.15.212

Roth, A. J., Weinberger, M. I., & Nelson, C. J. (2008). Prostate cancer: Psychosocial implications and management. *Future Oncology (London, England)*, *4*(4), 561–568. doi:10.2217/14796694.4.4.561

Rout, S. S., Verma, A., Choudhary, A. K., Sharma, K., & Chawla, P. (2020). Convolution Neural Networks for Plant Disease Identification. *International Journal of Engineering Research and Applications*. www.ijera.com

Rout, S. K., & Biswal, P. K. (2020). An efficient error-minimized random vector functional link network for epileptic seizure classification using VMD. *Biomedical Signal Processing and Control*, *57*, 101787. doi:10.1016/j.bspc.2019.101787

Rowland, S. P., Fitzgerald, J. E., Holme, T., Powell, J., & McGregor, A. (2020). What is the clinical value of mHealth for patients? *NPJ Digital Medicine*, *3*(1), 4. doi:10.103841746-019-0206-x

Rubino, F. (2008). Is type 2 diabetes an operable intestinal disease? A Provocative Yet Reasonable Hypothesis. *Diabetes Care*, *31*(Suppl. 2), S290–S296. doi:10.2337/dc08-s271 PMID:18227499

Ruland, C. M., Andersen, T., Jeneson, A., Moore, S., Grimsbo, G. H., Borosund, E., & Ellison, M. C. (2013). Effects of an Internet support system to assist cancer patients in reducing symptom distress a randomized controlled trial. *Cancer Nursing*, *36*(1), 6–17. doi:10.1097/NCC.0b013e31824d90d4

Ruland, C. M., Maffei, R. M., Borosund, E., Krahn, A., Andersen, T., & Grimsbø, G. H. (2013). Evaluation of different features of an eHealth application for personalized illness management support: Cancer patients' use and appraisal of usefulness. *International Journal of Medical Informatics*, *82*(7), 593–603. doi:10.1016/j.ijmedinf.2013.02.007

Ruparelia, J. P., Chatterjee, A. K., Duttagupta, S. P., & Mukherji, S. (2008). Strain specificity in antimicrobial activity of silver and copper nanoparticles. *Acta Biomaterialia*, *4*(3), 707–716. doi:10.1016/j.actbio.2007.11.006

Russakovsky, O., Deng, J., Su, H., Krause, J., Satheesh, S., Ma, S., ... Berg, A. C. (2015). Imagenet large scale visual recognition challenge. *International Journal of Computer Vision*, *115*(3), 211–252. doi:10.100711263-015-0816-y

Russell, S., & Norvig, P. (2003). Artificial Intelligence: A Modern Approach (2nd ed.). Prentice Hall.

Russell, S. J., & Norvig, P. (2016). *Artificial Intelligence: A Modern Approach*. Pearson Education Limited.

Ryan, T., Chester, A., Reece, J., & Xenos, S. (2014). The uses and abuses of Facebook: A review of Facebook addiction. *Journal of Behavioral Addictions*, *3*(3), 133–148. doi:10.1556/JBA.3.2014.016 PMID:25317337

Sadiq, M., Chowdhury, B., Chandrasekaran, N., & Mukherjee, A. (2009). Antimicrobial sensitivity of Escherichia coli to alumina nanoparticles. *Nanomedicine; Nanotechnology, Biology, and Medicine*, *5*(3), 282–286. doi:10.1016/j.nano.2009.01.002

Saeed, K., & Khan, I. (2014). Preparation and properties of single-walled carbon nanotubes/poly (butylene terephthalate) Nano composites. *Iranian Polymer Journal*, *23*(1), 53–58. doi:10.100713726-013-0199-2

Sahin, N., & Alpaslan, N. (2020). SegNet Mimarisi Kullanılarak Cilt Lezyon Bölütleme Performansının İyileştirilmesi. *Avrupa Bilim ve Teknoloji Dergisi*, 40-45.

Saikia, C., Das, M. K., Ramteke, A., & Maji, T. K. (2016). Effect of crosslinker on drug delivery properties of curcumin loaded starch coated iron oxide nanoparticles. *International Journal of Biological Macromolecules*, *93*, 1121–1132. doi:10.1016/j.ijbiomac.2016.09.043

Saini, A., Hou, J., & Zhou, W. (2014). Breast cancer prognosis risk estimation using integrated gene expression and clinical data. *BioMed Research International*, *2014*, 2014. doi:10.1155/2014/459203 PMID:24949450

Saini, A., Hou, J., & Zhou, W. (2014). RRHGE: A novel approach to classify the estrogen receptor based breast cancer subtypes. *TheScientificWorldJournal*, *2014*, 2014. doi:10.1155/2014/362141 PMID:24563630

Saladi, R. N., & Persaud, A. N. (2005). The causes of skin cancer: A comprehensive review. *Drugs of Today (Barcelona, Spain)*, *41*(1), 37–54. doi:10.1358/dot.2005.41.1.875777 PMID:15753968

Salama, P., Spiegel, P., Talley, L., & Waldman, R. (2004). Lessons learned from complex emergencies over past decade. *Lancet*, *364*(9447), 1801–1813. doi:10.1016/S0140-6736(04)17405-9 PMID:15541455

Salovey, P., Mayer, J., & Caruso, D. (2004). Emotional intelligence: Theory, findings, and implications. *Psychological Inquiry*, *15*(3), 197–215. doi:10.120715327965pli1503_02

Santa Mina, D., Guglietti, C. L., Alibhai, S. M., Matthew, A. G., Kalnin, R., Ahmad, N., Lindner, U., & Trachtenberg, J. (2014). The effect of meeting physical activity guidelines for cancer survivors on quality of life following radical prostatectomy for prostate cancer. *Journal of Cancer Survivorship: Research and Practice*, *8*(2), 190–198. doi:10.100711764-013-0329-z

Satapathy, S. K., Dehuri, S., & Jagadev, A. K. (2017). ABC optimized RBF network for classification of EEG signal for epileptic seizure identification. *Egyptian Informatics Journal*, *18*(1), 55–66. doi:10.1016/j.eij.2016.05.001

Satici, S. A. (2018). Facebook addiction and subjective well-being: A study of the mediating role of shyness and loneliness. *International Journal of Mental Health and Addiction*.

Schaffert, R., Dahinden, U., Hess, T., Bänziger, A., Kuntschik, P., Odoni, F., Spörri, P., Strebel, R. T., Kamradt, J., Tenti, G., Mattei, A., Müntener, M., Subotic, S., Schmid, H.-P., & Rüesch, P. (2018). Evaluation of a prostate cancer E health tutorial: Development and testing of the website prostata-information. *Der Urologe. Ausg. A*, *57*(2), 164–171. doi:10.100700120-017-0552-8

Schapira, M. M., Nattinger, A. B., Katz, D. A., & Lawrence, W. (1997). Information seeking and satisfaction with treatment decision in patients with clinically localized prostate cancer. *Medical Decision Making*, *17*, 544.

Scheffer, I. E., Berkovic, S., Capovilla, G., Connolly, M. B., French, J., Guilhoto, L., ... Nordli, D. R. (2017). ILAE classification of the epilepsies: Position paper of the ILAE Commission for Classification and Terminology. *Epilepsia*, *58*(4), 512–521. doi:10.1111/epi.13709 PMID:28276062

Schover, L. R., Canada, A. L., Yuan, Y., Sui, D., Neese, L., Jenkins, R., & Rhodes, M. M. (2012). A randomized trial of internet-based versus traditional sexual counseling for couples after localized prostate cancer treatment. *Cancer*, *118*(2), 500–509. doi:10.1002/cncr.26308

Schutte, N. S., & Malouff, J. M. (2011). Emotional intelligence mediates the relationship between mindfulness and subjective well-being. *Personality and Individual Differences*, *50*(7), 1116–1119. doi:10.1016/j.paid.2011.01.037

Schwarzer, G., Vach, W., & Schumacher, M. (2000). On the misuses of artificial neural networks for prognostic and diagnostic classification in oncology. *Statistics in Medicine*, *19*(4), 541–561. doi:10.1002/(SICI)1097-0258(20000229)19:4<541::AID-SIM355>3.0.CO;2-V PMID:10694735

Scurrey, S., Garland, S. N., Thoms, J., & Laing, K. (2019). Evaluating the experience of rural individuals with prostate and breast cancer participating in research via telehealth. *Rural and Remote Health*, *19*(3), 5269. doi:10.22605/RRH5269

SEER Cancer Statistics Review 1975-2013. (n.d.). *National Cancer Institute, Bethesda, MD*. Available from: https://seer.cancer.gov/csr/1975_2015/

Segal, C., Holve, E., Sabharwal, R., & Seer, C. X. (2013). *Collecting and using patient-reported outcomes (PRO) for comparative effectiveness research (CER) and patient-centered outcomes research (PCOR): Challenges and opportunities.* http://citeseerx.ist.psu.edu/viewdoc/download?doi=10.1.1.831.9388&rep=rep1&type=pdf

Sesan. (2019). *Oftalmoskop Vitalitaet VM-P110*. Retrieved from https://www.denizlermedikal.com/oti-oct-goz-cihazi/Foster

Shaban-Nejad, A., Lavigne, M., Okhmatovskaia, A., & Buckeridge, D. L. (2016). (in press). PopHR: A knowledge-based platform to support integration, analysis and visualization of population health data. *Annals of the New York Academy of Sciences*. PMID:27750378

Shah, S., & Singh, M. (2012). Comparison of A Time Efficient Modified K-Mean Algorithm with K-Mean and K-Medoids algorithm. *International Conference on Communication Systems and Network Technologies*. 10.1109/CSNT.2012.100

Shaikh, N. (n.d.). Implementing AI in wearable health apps for better tomorrow. *Peerbits.* https://www.peerbits.com/blog/wearable-healthcare-apps-solutions-for-better-tomorrow.html

Shamsadin, S., Pourpak, Z., Folkerts, G., Garssen, J., Moin, M., Adcock, I. M., Movassaghi, M., Ardestani, M. S., Moazzeni, S. M., & Mortaz, E. (2016). Conjugated alpha-alumina nanoparticle with vasoactive intestinal peptide as a nono-drug in treatment of allergic asthma in mice. *European Journal of Pharmacology*, *791*, 811–820. doi:10.1016/j.ejphar.2016.10.014

Sharma, A., Sharma, R., Sharma, V. K., & Shrivatava, V. (2014). Application of Data Mining–A Survey Paper. *Int. J. Comput. Sci. Inf. Technol.*, *5*(2), 2023–2025.

Sharma, G., Krug, E., & Lozano, R. (2000). Injury: A leading cause of the burden of disease. *Injury Control and Safety Promotion*, *7*(4), 261–267. doi:10.1076/icsp.7.4.261.7399

Sharma, M., Pachori, R. B., & Acharya, U. R. (2017). A new approach to characterize epileptic seizures using analytic time-frequency flexible wavelet transform and fractal dimension. *Pattern Recognition Letters*, *94*, 172–179. doi:10.1016/j.patrec.2017.03.023

Sharma, R., & Pachori, R. B. (2015). Classification of epileptic seizures in EEG signals based on phase space representation of intrinsic mode functions. *Expert Systems with Applications*, *42*(3), 1106–1117. doi:10.1016/j.eswa.2014.08.030

Sheilla Freeda, D., & Lilly Florence, M. (2017). An overview of disease analysis using association rule mining. IJSER, 8(4).

Shen, L., Margolies, L. R., Rothstein, J. H., Fluder, E., McBride, R., & Sieh, W. (2019). Deep learning to improve breast cancer detection on screening mammography. *Scientific Reports*, *9*(1), 1–12. doi:10.103841598-019-48995-4 PMID:31467326

Shensa, A., Escobar-Viera, C. G., Sidani, J. E., Bowman, N. D., Marshal, M. P., & Primack, B. A. (2017). Problematic social media use and depressive symptoms among US young adults: A nationally-representative study. *Social Science & Medicine*, *182*, 150–157. doi:10.1016/j.socscimed.2017.03.061 PMID:28446367

Shiferaw, S., Workneh, A., Yirgu, R., Dinant, G. J., & Spigt, M. (2018). Designing mHealth for maternity services in primary health facilities in a low-income setting - lessons from a partially successful implementation. *BMC Medical Informatics and Decision Making*, *18*(1), 96. doi:10.118612911-018-0704-9

Shin, W. G., Calder, S., Ugurlu, O., & Girshick, S. L. (2011). Production and characterization of boron nanoparticles synthesized with a thermal plasma system. *Journal of Nanoparticle Research*, *13*(12), 7187–7191. doi:10.100711051-011-0633-3

Shi, Q., Smith, T. G., Michonski, J. D., Stein, K. D., Kaw, C., & Cleeland, C. S. (2011). Symptom burden in cancer survivors 1 year after diagnosis: A report from the American Cancer Society's Studies of Cancer Survivors. *Cancer*, *117*(12), 2779–2790. doi:10.1002/cncr.26146

Shlens, J. (2014). *A tutorial on principal component analysis.* arXiv preprint arXiv:1404.1100

Shull, P. B., & Damian, D. D. (2015). Haptic Wearables As Sensory Replacement, Sensory Augmentation And Trainer—A Review. *Journal of Neuroengineering and Rehabilitation*, *12*(1), 595. doi:10.118612984-015-0055-z PMID:26188929

Silveira, M., Nascimento, J. C., Marques, J. S., Marçal, A. R., Mendonça, T., Yamauchi, S., Maeda, J., & Rozeira, J. (2009). Comparison of segmentation methods for melanoma diagnosis in dermoscopy images. *IEEE Journal of Selected Topics in Signal Processing*, *3*(1), 35–45. doi:10.1109/JSTSP.2008.2011119

Simon, R. (2003). Diagnostic and prognostic prediction using gene expression profiles in high-dimensional microarray data. *British Journal of Cancer*, *89*(9), 1599–1604. doi:10.1038j.bjc.6601326 PMID:14583755

Singh, K., & Landman, A. B. (2017). Mobile Health. *Key Advances in Clinical Informatics.* https://www.sciencedirect.com/topics/medicine-and-dentistry/mobile-health

Singh, V., & Verma, K. (2018). Metals from cell to environment: connecting metallomics with other omics. *Open Journal of Plant Science, 3*(1), 1-14

Singh, A., Kim, B. K., Mackeyev, Y., Rohani, P., Mahajan, S. D., Swihart, M. T., Krishan, S., & Prasad, P. N. (2019). Boron-Nanoparticles loaded folic acid functionalized liposomes to achieve optimum boron concentration for boron Neutron capture Therapy of Cancer. *Journal of Biomedical Nanotechnology, 15*(8), 1714–1723. doi:10.1166/jbn.2019.2800

Sinthanayothin, C., Boyce, J. F., Cook, H. L., & Williamson, T. H. (1999). Automated localisation of the optic disc, fovea and retinal blood vessels from digital colour fundus images. Br. J. Ophtalmol., 83, 902–910.

Sinthanayothin, C., Boyce, J. F., Cook, H. L., & Williamson, T. H. (1999). Automated location of the optic disc, fovea, and retinal blood vessels from digital color fundus images. *The British Journal of Ophthalmology, 83*(8), 902–910. doi:10.1136/bjo.83.8.902 PMID:10413690

Siuly, S., Alcin, O. F., Bajaj, V., Sengur, A., & Zhang, Y. (2018). Exploring Hermite transformation in brain signal analysis for the detection of epileptic seizure. *IET Science, Measurement & Technology, 13*(1), 35–41. doi:10.1049/iet-smt.2018.5358

Siuly, S., Li, Y., & Zhang, Y. (2016). Electroencephalogram (EEG) and Its Background. In *EEG Signal Analysis and Classification* (pp. 3–21). Springer. doi:10.1007/978-3-319-47653-7_1

Smart, E. (2019). Tourism and Hospitality Management. *International Conference on Computer, Information and Telecommunication Systems (IEEE CITS-2019),* 237-241.

Snijder, E. J., Van der Meer, Y., Zevenhoven-Dobbe, J., Onderwater, J. J., Van der Meulen, J., Koerten, H. K., & Mommaas, A. M. (2006). Ultrastructure and origin of membrane vesicles associated with the severe acute respiratory syndrome coronavirus replication complex. *Journal of Virology, 80*(12), 5927–5940. doi:10.1128/JVI.02501-05 PMID:16731931

Sofi, G. N., Sofi, J. N., Nadeem, R., Shiekh, R. Y., Khan, F. A., Sofi, A. A., Bhat, H. A., & Bhat, R. A. (2012). Estrogen receptor and progesterone receptor status in breast cancer in relation to age, histological grade, size of lesion and lymph node involvement. *Asian Pacific Journal of Cancer Prevention, 13*(10), 5047–5052. doi:10.7314/APJCP.2012.13.10.5047 PMID:23244108

Soleimani-Roozbahani, F., Ghatari, A. R., & Radfar, R. (2019). Knowledge discovery from a more than a decade studies on healthcare big data systems: a scientometrics study. Journal of Big Data, 6.

Somers, T. J., Abernethy, A. P., Edmond, S. N., Kelleher, S., Wren, A. A., & Sams, G. P. (2015). A pilot study of a mobile health pain coping skills training protocol for patients with persistent cancer pain. *Journal of Pain and Symptom Management, 50*(4), 553–558. doi:10.1016/j.jpainsymman.2015.04.013

Song, L., Tatum, K., Greene, G., & Chen, R. C. (2017). eHealth literacy and partner involvement in treatment decision making for men with newly diagnosed localized prostate cancer. *Oncology Nursing Forum, 44*(2), 225–333.

Song, Y., Crowcroft, J., & Zhang, J. (2012). Automatic epileptic seizure detection in EEGs based on optimized sample entropy and extreme learning machine. *Journal of Neuroscience Methods, 210*(2), 132–146. doi:10.1016/j.jneumeth.2012.07.003 PMID:22824535

Sood, S., Mbarika, V., Jugoo, S., Dookhy, R., Doarn, C. R., Prakash, N., & Merrell, R. C. (2007). What is telemedicine? A collection of 104 peer-reviewed perspectives and theoretical underpinnings. *Telemedicine Journal and e-Health, 13*(5), 573–590. doi:10.1089/tmj.2006.0073

Sopharak, A., Uyyanonvara, B., & Barman, S. (2013). Simple Hybrid Method for Fine Microaneurysm Detection from Non-dilated Diabetic Retinopathy Retinal Images. *Computerized Medical Imaging and Graphics*, *37*(5), 394–402. doi:10.1016/j.compmedimag.2013.05.005 PMID:23777979

Sotiriou, C., Neo, S. Y., McShane, L. M., Korn, E. L., Long, P. M., Jazaeri, A., Martiat, P., Fox, S. B., Harris, A. L., & Liu, E. T. (2003). Breast cancer classification and prognosis based on gene expression profiles from a population-based study. *Proceedings of the National Academy of Sciences of the United States of America*, *100*(18), 10393–10398. doi:10.1073/pnas.1732912100 PMID:12917485

Sotiriou, C., Wirapati, P., Loi, S., Harris, A., Fox, S., Smeds, J., ... Desmedt, C. (2006). Gene expression profiling in breast cancer: Understanding the molecular basis of histologic grade to improve prognosis. *Journal of the National Cancer Institute*, *98*(4), 262–272. doi:10.1093/jnci/djj052 PMID:16478745

Spulber, I., Chen, Y. M., Papi, E., Anastasova Ivanova, S., Bergmann, J., McGregor, A. H., & Georgiou, P. (2015). Live Demonstration: Wearable Electronics For A Smart Garment Aiding Rehabilitation. *Proceedings of the IEEE International Symposium on Circuits and Systems (ISCAS)*. 10.1109/ISCAS.2015.7169045

Sridhar, G., Masho, S. W., Adera, T., Ramakrishnan, V., & Roberts, J. D. (2010). Association between family history of prostate cancer. *J. M. H.*, *7*, 45–54.

Srinivasan, V., Eswaran, C., & Sriraam, N. (2007). Approximate entropy-based epileptic EEG detection using artificial neural networks. *IEEE Transactions on Information Technology in Biomedicine*, *11*(3), 288–295. doi:10.1109/TITB.2006.884369 PMID:17521078

Statista. (2019). *Number of apps available in leading app stores as of 3rd quarter 2019*. https://www.statista.com/statistics/276623/number-of-apps-available-in-leading-app-stores/

Steinke-Lange, V., & Holinski-Feder, E. (2019, August). Genetic Screening and Personalized Prevention in Colorectal Cancer. *Visceral Medicine*, *35*(4), 226–230. doi:10.1159/000501941 PMID:31602383

Sternberg, R. J. (Ed.). (2000). *Handbook of intelligence*. Cambridge University Press. doi:10.1017/CBO9780511807947

Stockley, T. L., Oza, A. M., Berman, H. K., Leighl, N. B., Knox, J. J., Shepherd, F. A., Chen, E. X., Krzyzanowska, M. K., Dhani, N., Joshua, A. M., Tsao, M.-S., Serra, S., Clarke, B., Roehrl, M. H., Zhang, T., Sukhai, M. A., Califaretti, N., Trinkaus, M., Shaw, P., ... Bedard, P. L. (2016). Molecular profiling of advanced solid tumors and patient outcomes with genotype-matched clinical trials: The Princess Margaret IMPACT/COMPACT trial. *Genome Medicine*, *8*(1), 109. doi:10.118613073-016-0364-2 PMID:27782854

Stolz, W. (1994). ABCD rule of dermatoscopy: A new practical method for early recognition of malignant melanoma. *European Journal of Dermatology*, *4*, 521–527.

Stornetta, A., Guidolin, V., & Balbo, S. (2018). Alcohol-derived acetaldehyde exposure in the oral cavity. *Cancers (Basel)*, *10*(1), 20. doi:10.3390/cancers10010020 PMID:29342885

Stroetmann, K. A. (2013). Achieving the integrated and smart health and wellbeing paradigm: A call for policy research and action on governance and business models. *International Journal of Medical Informatics*, *82*(4), e29–e37. doi:10.1016/j.ijmedinf.2012.05.008

Subasi, A. (2007). EEG signal classification using wavelet feature extraction and a mixture of expert model. *Expert Systems with Applications*, *32*(4), 1084–1093. doi:10.1016/j.eswa.2006.02.005

Subramaniam,, M., & Ganesh,, B. (2014). Origin and Applications of Internet of Things. *CSI Communications*, *38*(1).

Sun, W., Cai, Z., Li, Y., Liu, F., Fang, S., & Wang, G. (2018). Data processing and text mining technologies on E-medical records. Hindawi Journal of Health Care Engineering.

Sun, W., Cai, Z., Liu, F., Fang, S., & Wang, G. (2017). A survey of data mining technology on electronic medical records. *IEEE: 19th International Conference on E-Health and Networking, Conference-19.*

Sun, Y., Babbs, C. F., & Delp, E. J. (2006, January). A comparison of feature selection methods for the detection of breast cancers in mammograms: adaptive sequential floating search vs. genetic algorithm. In *2005 IEEE Engineering in Medicine and Biology 27th Annual Conference* (pp. 6532-6535). IEEE.

Sundaravadivel, P., Kougianos, E., Mohanty, S. P., & Ganapathiraju, M. K. (2018). Everything You Wanted to Know about Smart Health Care: Evaluating the different technologies and components of the Internet of Things for better healthcare. *IEEE Consumer Electronics Magazine*, *7*(1), 18–28. doi:10.1109/MCE.2017.2755378

Sundberg, K., Wengström, Y., Blomberg, K., Hälleberg-Nyman, M., Frank, C., & Langius-Eklöf, A. (2017). Early detection and management of symptoms using an interactive smartphone application (Interaktor) during radiotherapy for prostate cancer. *Supportive Care in Cancer*, *25*(7), 2195–2204. doi:10.100700520-017-3625-8

Süral, I., Griffiths, M. D., Kircaburun, K., & Emirtekin, E. (2019). Trait Emotional Intelligence and Problematic Social Media Use Among Adults: The Mediating Role of Social Media Use Motives. *International Journal of Mental Health and Addiction*, *17*(2), 336–345. doi:10.100711469-018-0022-6

Suvarchala, S. B., & Nageswararao, R. (2011). Carcinoma breast-histopathological and hormone receptors correlation. *J Biosci Tech*, *2*(4), 340–348.

Syeda, F. U. B., & Begum, I. (2017). Smart Health Care Solutions Using IOT, International Journal and Magazine of Engineering, Technology. *Management and Research*, *4*(3), 10–15.

Tamilvanan, A., Balamurugan, K., Ponappa, K., & Madhan, K. B. (2014). Copper Nanoparticles: Synthesis Strategies, Properties and Multifunctional Application. *International Journal of Nanoscience*, *13*(2), 143001–143022. doi:10.1142/S0219581X14300016

Taneja, A., & Arora, A. (2018). Recommendation research trends: Review, approaches and open issues. *International Journal of Web Engineering and Technology*, *13*(2), 123–186. doi:10.1504/IJWET.2018.092831

Tan, T. Y., Zhang, L., Lim, C. P., Fielding, B., Yu, Y., & Anderson, E. (2019). Evolving ensemble models for image segmentation using enhanced particle swarm optimization. *IEEE Access: Practical Innovations, Open Solutions*, *7*, 34004–34019. doi:10.1109/ACCESS.2019.2903015

Tanwar, S., Thakkar, K., Thakor, R., & Singh, P. K. (2018). M-Tesla-Based Security Assessment in Wireless Sensor Network. In *International Conference on Computational Intelligence and Data Science (ICCIDS 2018)*. NorthCap University.

Tanwar, S., Tyagi, S., & Kumar, N. (Eds.). (2019b). Multimedia Big Data Computing for IoT Applications: Concepts, Paradigms and Solutions. Intelligent Systems Reference Library. Springer Nature Singapore Pte Ltd.

Tanwar, S., Tyagi, S., & Kumar, S. (2017). The Role of Internet of Things and Smart Grid for the Development of a Smart City. *Intelligent Communication and Computational Technologies (Lecture Notes in Networks and Systems: Proceedings of Internet of Things for Technological Development, IoT4TD, 19*, 23-33.

Tanwar, S., & Parekh, K. (2019). Blockchain-based Electronic Healthcare Record System for Healthcare 4.0 Applications. *Journal of Information Security and Applications*, *50*, 1–14.

Tanwar, S., Tyagi, S., & Kumar, N. (Eds.). (2019a). *Security and Privacy of Electronics Healthcare Records*. IET Book Series on e-Health Technologies.

Tanwar, S., Vora, J., Kanriya, S., Tyagi, S., Kumar, N., Sharma, V., & You, I. (2019). Human Arthritis Analysis in Fog Computing Environment using Bayesian Network Classifier and Thread Protocol. *IEEE Consumer Electronics Magazine*, *9*(1), 88–94. doi:10.1109/MCE.2019.2941456

Tate, A. (n.d.). Does mHealth Improve The Patient-Provider Connection? *Referralmd.* https://getreferralmd.com/2019/09/does-mhealth-improve-the-patient-provider-connection/

Tawfik, N. S., Youssef, S. M., & Kholief, M. (2016). A hybrid automated detection of epileptic seizures in EEG records. *Computers & Electrical Engineering*, *53*, 177–190. doi:10.1016/j.compeleceng.2015.09.001

Telikani, A., Gandomi, A. H., & Shahbahrami, A. (2020). A survey of evolutionary computation for association rule mining. Information Science Under Elsevier Journal, 524, 318-352.

Thacker, S. B. (2000). Historical development. In S. M. Teutsch & R. E. Churchill (Eds.), *Principles and Practice of Public Health Surveillance* (2nd ed., pp. 1–16). Oxford University Press.

Thacker, S. B., & Berkelman, R. L. (1988). Public Health Surveillance in the United States. *Epidemiologic Reviews*, *10*(1), 164–190. doi:10.1093/oxfordjournals.epirev.a036021 PMID:3066626

Thacker, S. B., & Stroup, D. F. (1998). Foreword. *Deciphering Global Epidemics*, *xix-xx*, xix–xx. Advance online publication. doi:10.1017/CBO9780511549489.001

Thara, D. K., PremaSudha, B. G., & Xiong, F. (2019). Auto-detection of epileptic seizure events using deep neural network with different feature scaling techniques. *Pattern Recognition Letters*, *128*, 544–550. doi:10.1016/j.patrec.2019.10.029

The Medical Futurist. (2019). *How Digital Health Technology Can Help Manage The Coronavirus Outbreak.* https://medicalfuturist.com/how-digital-health-technology-can-help-manage-the-coronavirus-outbreak/

Thomas, E., Rathore, I., & Tarafdar, J. (2017). Bioinspired Production of Molybdenum Nanoparticles and Its Effect on Chickpea (Cicer arietinum L). *Journal of Bionanoscience.*, *11*(2), 1–7. doi:10.1166/jbns.2017.1425

ThorndikeE. L. (n.d.). https://en.wikipedia.org/wiki/E._L._Thorndike

Tiwari, A. K., Pachori, R. B., Kanhangad, V., & Panigrahi, B. K. (2016). Automated diagnosis of epilepsy using key-point-based local binary pattern of EEG signals. *IEEE Journal of Biomedical and Health Informatics*, *21*(4), 888–896. doi:10.1109/JBHI.2016.2589971 PMID:27416609

Tolias, Y. A., & Panas, S. M. (1998). A fuzzy vessel tracking algorithm for retinal images based on fuzzy clustering. IEEE Trans. Med. Imag., 17(2), 263–273.

Tomari, Razali, Zakaria, & Nurshazwani. (2015). *An empirical framework for automatic red blood cell morphology identification and counting.* Academic Press.

Tran, C., Dicker, A., Leiby, B., Gressen, E., Williams, N., & Jim, H. (2020). Utilizing digital health to collect electronic patient-reported outcomes in prostate cancer: Single-arm pilot trial. *Journal of Medical Internet Research*, *22*(3), e12689. doi:10.2196/12689

Trindade, I. G., Machado da Silva, J., Rui, M., Pereira, M., Lucas, J., Oliveira, L., Valentim, B., Barreto, J., & Santos Silva, M. (2016). Design and Evaluation of Novel Textile Wearable Systems for the Surveillance of Vital Signals. *Sensors (Basel)*, *16*(10), 1573. doi:10.339016101573 PMID:27669263

Trinh, L., Arbour-Nicitopoulos, K. P., Sabiston, C. M., Berry, S. R., Loblaw, A., Alibhai, S. M., Jones, J. M., & Faulkner, G. E. (2018). RiseTx: Testing the feasibility of a web application for reducing sedentary behavior among prostate cancer survivors receiving androgen deprivation therapy. *The International Journal of Behavioral Nutrition and Physical Activity, 15*(1), 124. doi:10.118612966-018-0757-2

Tsaousis, I., & Nikolaou, I. (2005). Exploring the relationship of emotional intelligence with physical and psychological health functioning. *Stress and Health, 21*(2), 77–86. doi:10.1002mi.1042

Tyson, M. D., Penson, D. F., & Resnick, M. J. (2017). The comparative oncologic effectiveness of available management strategies for clinically localized prostate cancer. *Urologic Oncology, 35*(2), 51–58. doi:10.1016/j.urolonc.2016.03.021

Tzallas, A. T., Tsipouras, M. G., & Fotiadis, D. I. (2007). Automatic seizure detection based on time-frequency analysis and artificial neural networks. *Computational Intelligence and Neuroscience, 2007*, 80510. doi:10.1155/2007/80510 PMID:18301712

Ullah, I., Hussain, M., & Aboalsamh, H. (2018). An automated system for epilepsy detection using EEG brain signals based on deep learning approach. *Expert Systems with Applications, 107*, 61–71. doi:10.1016/j.eswa.2018.04.021

University of Bonn Department of Epileptology. (2001). *EEG time series data* [Data file]. Available from http://epileptologie-bonn.de/cms/front_content.php?idcat=193&lang=3&changelang=3

University of Iowa Carver College of Medicine. (2019). *Diabetic Retinopathy: From One Medical Student to Another.* https://webeye.ophth.uiowa.edu/eyeforum/tutorials/Diabetic-Retinopathy-Med-Students/Classification.htm

Ünver, H. M., & Ayan, E. (2019). Skin lesion segmentation in dermoscopic images with combination of YOLO and grabcut algorithm. *Diagnostics (Basel), 9*(3), 72. doi:10.3390/diagnostics9030072 PMID:31295856

Vachon, D. (2005). Father of modern epidemiology. *Old News, 16*(8), 8–10.

Valderas, J., Kotzeva, A., Espallargues, M., Guyatt, G., Ferrans, C., Halyard, M. Y., Revicki, D. A., Symonds, T., Parada, A., & Alonso, J. (2008). The impact of measuring patient-reported outcomes in clinical practice: A systematic review of the literature. *Quality of Life Research: An International Journal of Quality of Life Aspects of Treatment, Care and Rehabilitation, 17*(2), 179–193. doi:10.100711136-007-9295-0

Van Bogaert, D., Hawkins, R., Pingree, S., & Jarrard, D. (2012). The development of an eHealth tool suite for prostate cancer patients and their partners. *The Journal of Supportive Oncology, 10*(5), 202–208. doi:10.1016/j.suponc.2012.02.003

van den Bergh, R. C., Roemeling, S., Roobol, M. J., Roobol, W., Schröder, F. H., & Bangma, C. H. (2007). Prospective validation of active surveillance in prostate cancer: The PRIAS study. *European Urology, 52*(6), 1560–1563. doi:10.1016/j.eururo.2007.05.011

Van IJzendoorn, D. G., Szuhai, K., Briaire-de Bruijn, I. H., Kostine, M., Kuijjer, M. L., & Bovée, J. V. (2019). Machine learning analysis of gene expression data reveals novel diagnostic and prognostic biomarkers and identifies therapeutic targets for soft tissue sarcomas. *PLoS Computational Biology, 15*(2), e1006826. doi:10.1371/journal.pcbi.1006826 PMID:30785874

van Tol-Geerdink, J. J., Leer, J. W., van Oort, I. M., van Lin, E. J., Weijerman, P. C., Vergunst, H., Witjes, J. A., & Stalmeier, P. F. (2013). Quality of life after prostate cancer treatments in patients comparable at baseline. *British Journal of Cancer, 108*(9), 1784–1789. doi:10.1038/bjc.2013.181

van Vugt, H. A., Roobol, M. J., Busstra, M., Kil, P., Oomens, E. H., de Jong, I. J., Bangma, C. H., Steyerberg, E. W., & Korfage, I. (2012b). Compliance with biopsy recommendations of a prostate cancer risk calculator. *BJU International, 109*(10), 1480–1488. doi:10.1111/j.1464-410X.2011.10611.x van Vugt, H. A., Roobol, M. J., van der Poel, H. G., van Muilekom, E. H. A. M., Busstra, M., Kil, P., Oomens, E. H., Leliveld, A., Bangma, C. H., Korfage, I., & Steyerberg, E. W. (2012b). Selecting men diagnosed with prostate cancer for active surveillance using a risk calculator: A prospective impact study. *BJU International*, *110*(2), 180–187. doi:10.1111/j.1464-410X.2011.10679.x

Van't Veer, L. J., Dai, H., Van De Vijver, M. J., He, Y. D., Hart, A. A., Mao, M., ... Schreiber, G. J. (2002). Gene expression profiling predicts clinical outcome of breast cancer. *Nature, 415*(6871), 530-536.

Varghese, D. P., & Tintu, P. B. (2015). A Survey on Health Data using Data Mining Techniques. *Int. Res. J. Eng. Technol.*, *2*(7), 56–2395.

Varol, A. B., & İşeri, İ. (2019). Lenf Kanserine İlişkin Patoloji Görüntülerinin Makine Öğrenimi Yöntemleri ile Sınıflandırılması. *Avrupa Bilim ve Teknoloji Dergisi*, 404-410.

Venderbos, L. D., & Roobol, M. J. (2017). m-PRIAS: An e-health technology for men on active surveillance for prostate cancer. *Quality of Life Research: An International Journal of Quality of Life Aspects of Treatment, Care and Rehabilitation*, *26*(1), 99.

Venkateswaran, V., & Klotz, L. H. (2010). Diet and prostate cancer: Mechanisms of action and implications for chemoprevention. *Nature Reviews. Urology*, *7*(8), 442–453. doi:10.1038/nrurol.2010.102

Ventola, C. L. (2014). Mobile Devices and Apps for Health Care Professionals: Uses and Benefits. *PMC: US National Library of Medicine National Institutes of Health, 39*(5), 356–364. https://www.ncbi.nlm.nih.gov/pmc/articles/PMC4029126/

Ventola, C. L. (2014). Mobile devices and apps for health professionals: Uses and benefits. *P&T*, *39*(5), 356–364.

Viers, B. R., Lightner, D. J., & Rivera, M. E. (2015b). Are Patients Willing to Engage in Telemedicine for Their Care: A Survey of Preuse Perceptions and Acceptance of Remote Video Visits in a Urological Patient Population. *Urology*, *85*(6), 1233–1239. doi:10.1016/j.urology.2014.12.064

Villaveces, A., Peck, M., & Price, G. (2010). Process evaluation of emergency department use of an electronic data collection tool that incorporates the international classification of external causes of injury (ICECI) into the US national burn repository. *Injury Prevention*, *16*(Supplement 1), A73–A73. doi:10.1136/ip.2010.029215.266

Vineet, K., & Sudesh, K. Y. (2009). Plant mediated synthesis of silver and gold nanoparticles and their applications. *Journal of Chemical Technology and Biotechnology (Oxford, Oxfordshire)*, *84*(2), 151–157. doi:10.1002/jctb.2023

Viswanathan, G. A., Seto, J., Patil, S., Nudelman, G., & Sealfon, S. C. (2008). Getting started in biological pathway construction and analysis. *PLoS Computational Biology*, *4*(2), e16. doi:10.1371/journal.pcbi.0040016 PMID:18463709

Vohra, J., Kaneriya, S., Tanwar, S., & Tyagi, S. (2019). Standardising the use of Duplex Channels in 5G-WiFi Networking for Ambient Assisted Living. *IEEE Conference on Communications (IEEE ICC-2019),* 1-6.

Volodina, K. V., Anvir, D., & Vinogradov, V. V. (2017). Alumina nanoparticle-assisted enzyme refolding: A versatile methodology for proteins renaturation. *Scientific Reports*, *7*(1), 1458. doi:10.103841598-017-01436-6

Vora, J., Devmurari, P., Tanwar, S., Tyagi, S., Kumar, N., & Obaidat, M. S. (2018). Blind Signatures Based Secured E-Healthcare System. *International Conference on Computer, Information and Telecommunication Systems (IEEE CITS-2018),* 177-181.

Vora, J., Tanwar, S., Verma, J. P., Tyagi, S., Kumar, N., Obaidat, M. S., & Rodrigues, J. P. C. (2018). BHEEM: A Blockchain-based Framework for Securing Electronic Health Records. *IEEE Global Communications Conference (IEEE GLOBECOM-2018),* 1-6.

Vora, J., Kanriya, S., Tanwar, S., Tyagi, S., Kumar, N., & Obaidat, M. S. (2019). TILAA: Tactile Internet Based Ambient Assistant Living In Fog Environment. *Future Generation Computer Systems, 98*, 635–649. doi:10.1016/j.future.2019.01.035

Vora, J., Tanwar, S., Tyagi, S., Kumar, N., & Rodrigues, J. P. C. (2019). HRIDaY: Ballistocardiogram-based Heart Rate Monitoring Using Fog Computing. *IEEE Global Communications Conference (GLOBECOM-2019, 209*, 1-6.

Vosgerau, S., Urbanski, D., Kollenbach, P., Schöne, M., Gedamke, M., Donatz, V., Bültmann, O., & Amelung, V. (2017). Easipro3-Enhancing satisfaction with prostate cancer treatment decision with the mobile health program Prostana: A multicenter randomized controlled trial. Easipro3. *Value in Health, 20*(9), A504. doi:10.1016/j.jval.2017.08.598

Wallace, S., Clark, M., & White, J. (2012, August 24). 'It's on my iPhone': attitudes to the use of mobile computing devices in medical education, a mixed-methods study. *BMJ Open.* https://bmjopen.bmj.com/content/2/4/e001099

Wallentin, J., Anttu, N., Asoli, D., Huffman, M., Aberg, I., Magnusson, M.H., Siefer, G., Fudd-Kailuweit, P., Dimroth, F., Witzigmann, B., Xu, H.Q., Samuelson, L., Deppert, K., & Borgstrom, M.T. (2013). In P Nanowire Array Solar Cells Achieving 13.8% Efficiency by Exceeding the Ray Optics Limit. *Science.*

Walsh, D. M., Moran, K., Cornelissen, V., Buys, R., Cornelis, N., & Woods, C. (2018). Electronic health physical activity behavior change intervention to self-manage cardiovascular disease: Qualitative exploration of patient and health professional requirements. *Journal of Medical Internet Research, 20*(5), e163. doi:10.2196/jmir.9181

Walter, T., & Klein, J. C. (2001). Segmentation of color fundus images of the human retina: Detection of the optic disc and the vascular tree using morphological techniques. Lecture Notes in Computer Science, 282–287.

Wang, W., Pullum, T., & Kishor, S. (2019). The demographic and health surveys (DHS). Encyclopedia of Gerontology and Population Aging, 1-5. doi:10.1007/978-3-319-69892-2_969-1

Wang, J., Wang, Y., Wei, C., Yao, N. A., Yuan, A., Shan, Y., & Yuan, C. (2014). Smartphone interventions for long-term health management of chronic diseases: An integrative review. *Telemedicine Journal and e-Health, 20*(6), 570–583. doi:10.1089/tmj.2013.0243

Wang, Q., De Baets, L., Timmermans, A., Chen, W., Giacolini, L., Matheve, T., & Markopoulos, P. (2017). Motor Control Training for the Shoulder with Smart Garments. *Sensors (Basel), 17*(7), 1687. doi:10.339017071687 PMID:28737670

Wang, Y., Klijn, J. G., Zhang, Y., Sieuwerts, A. M., Look, M. P., Yang, F., ... Jatkoe, T. (2005). Gene-expression profiles to predict distant metastasis of lymph-node-negative primary breast cancer. *Lancet, 365*(9460), 671–679. doi:10.1016/S0140-6736(05)17947-1 PMID:15721472

Watermann, A., & Brieger, J. (2017). Mesoporous Silica Nanoparticles as Drug Delivery Vehicles in Cancer. *Nanomaterials (Basel, Switzerland), 7*(7), 189. doi:10.3390/nano7070189

Weigelt, B., Peterse, J. L., & Van't Veer, L. J. (2005). Breast cancer metastasis: Markers and models. *Nature Reviews. Cancer, 5*(8), 591–602. doi:10.1038/nrc1670 PMID:16056258

Whaite, E. O., Shensa, A., Sidani, J. E., Colditz, J. B., & Primack, B. A. (2018). Social media use, personality characteristics, and social isolation among young adults in the United States. *Personality and Individual Differences, 124*, 45–50. doi:10.1016/j.paid.2017.10.030

White, H. (1989). Learning in artificial neural networks: A statistical perspective. *Neural Computation, 1*(4), 425–464. doi:10.1162/neco.1989.1.4.425

WHO publications. (1993). Article. *International Journal of Epidemiology, 22*(6), 1212–1212. doi:10.1093/ije/22.6.1212

Wilczewska, A. Z., Niemirowicz, K., Markiewicz, K. H., & Car, H. (2012). Nanoparticles as drug delivery systems. *Pharmacological Reports*, *64*(5), 1020–1037. doi:10.1016/S1734-1140(12)70901-5

Wilder, B. (2012). *Cloud Architecture Patterns: Develop Cloud-Native Applications*. O'Reilly.

Wild, S., Roglic, G., Green, A., Sicree, R., & King, H. (2004). Global Prevalence of Diabetes: Estimates for the Year 2000 and projections for 2030. *Diabetes Care*, *2004*(27), 1047–1053. doi:10.2337/diacare.27.5.1047 PMID:15111519

Wilson & Keilthe. (1999). *MIT encyclopaedia of the cognitive sciences*. MIT Press.

Wilson, K. M., Giovannucci, E. L., & Mucci, L. A. (2012). Lifestyle and dietary factors in the prevention of lethal prostate cancer. *Asian Journal of Andrology*, *14*(3), 365–374. doi:10.1038/aja.2011.142

Wong, C. S., & Law, K. S. (2002). The effects of leader and follower emotional intelligence on performance and attitude: An exploratory study. *The Leadership Quarterly*, *13*(3), 243–274. doi:10.1016/S1048-9843(02)00099-1

Woodruff, B. A. (2006). Interpreting mortality data in humanitarian emergencies. *Lancet*, *367*(9504), 9–10. doi:10.1016/S0140-6736(05)67637-4 PMID:16399135

Wootten, A. C., Abbott, J. A., Meyer, D., Chisholm, K., Austin, D. W., Klein, B., McCabe, M., Murphy, D. G., & Costello, A. J. (2015). Preliminary results of a randomized controlled trial of an online psychological intervention to reduce distress in men treated for localized prostate cancer. *European Urology*, *68*(3), 471–479. doi:10.1016/j.eururo.2014.10.024

World Health Organisation. (2014). *Electromagnetic fields and public health: mobile phones*. https://www.who.int/news-room/fact-sheets/detail/electromagnetic-fields-and-public-health-mobile-phones

World Health Organization (WHO). (2019). *Epilepsy: a public health imperative*. World Health Organization.

World Health Organization (WHO). (2020). *Coronavirus disease (COVID-19) Pandemic*. https://www.who.int/emergencies/diseases/novel-coronavirus-2019

World Health Organization (WHO). (2020). *Epilepsy*. Retrieved from https://www.who.int/news-room/fact-sheets/detail/epilepsy

World Health Organization Report. (2020a). *How common is skin cancer?* Retrieved from https://www.who.int/uv/faq/skincancer/en/index1.html

World Health Organization Report. (2020b). *Canser*. Retrieved from https://www.who.int/news-room/fact-sheets/detail/cancer

World Health Organization. (1999). *Definition, Diagnosis, and Classification of Diabetes Mellitus and Its Complications. Part 1: Diagnosis and Classification of Diabetes Mellitus*. World Health Organization.

World Health Organization. (2018). *Global tuberculosis report 2018*. WHO.

World Health Organization. (n.d.). *Infection prevention and control during health care when COVID-19 is suspected*. https://www.who.int/publications-detail/infection-prevention-and-control-during-health-care-when-novel-coronavirus-(ncov)infection-is-suspected-20200125

World Health Statistics 2005. (2005). WHO.

Wu, Q., Wang, X., Liao, C., Wei, Q., & Wang, Q. (2015). Microgel coating of magnetic nanoparticles via enzyme-mediated free-radical polymerization for colorimetric detection of glucose. *Nanoscale*, *7*(40), 16578–16582. doi:10.1039/C5NR05716G

Wu, R., Wang, D. P., Kumar, V., Zhou, K., Adrian, W. K. L., Lee, P. S., & Lou, J. (2015). MOFs-derived copper sulfides embedded within porous carbon octahedra for electrochemical capacitor applications. *Chemical Communications*, *15*(51), 3109–3112. doi:10.1039/C4CC09065A

Wyatt, J. C. (2000). Decision Support Systems. *Journal of the Royal Society of Medicine*, *93*(12), 629–633. doi:10.1177/014107680009301206 PMID:11193060

Wynn, R., Adams, K., Kowalski, R. L., Shivega, W. G., Ratwani, R. M., & Miller, K. E. (2018). R. The Patient in Precision Medicine: A Systematic Review Examining Evaluations of Patient-Facing Materials. *Journal of Healthcare Engineering*, *2018*, 1–10. doi:10.1155/2018/9541621 PMID:30250657

Xiong, M., Fang, X., & Zhao, J. (2001). Biomarker identification by feature wrappers. *Genome Research*, *11*(11), 1878–1887. doi:10.1101/gr.190001 PMID:11691853

Yanan, Y., Meisong, G., Mengwei, Y., Weitong, L., & Jingbo, H. (2016). Nickel nanoparticle-modified electrode for ultrasensitive electrochemical detection of insulin. *Biosensors & Bioelectronics*, *77*, 215–219. doi:10.1016/j.bios.2015.09.036

Yanez, B., McGinty, H. L., Mohr, D. C., Begale, M. J., Dahn, J. R., Flury, S. C., Perry, K. T., & Penedo, F. J. (2015). Feasibility, acceptability, and preliminary efficacy of a technology-assisted psychosocial intervention for racially diverse men with advanced prostate cancer. *Cancer*, *121*(24), 4407–4415. doi:10.1002/cncr.29658

Yang, W., Li, Z., Lan, Y., Ma, J., Jin, L., Lai, S., Liao, Y., Lv, W., Sun, Q., Wang, J. (2017). China Infectious Diseases Automated-Alert and Response System (CIDARS). *Early Warning for Infectious Disease Outbreak*, 131-161.. doi:10.1016/B978-0-12-812343-0.00007-2

Yassin, N. I., Omran, S., El Houby, E. M., & Allam, H. (2018). Machine learning techniques for breast cancer computer aided diagnosis using different image modalities: A systematic review. *Computer Methods and Programs in Biomedicine*, *156*, 25–45. doi:10.1016/j.cmpb.2017.12.012 PMID:29428074

Yates, L. R., Seoane, J., Le Tourneau, C., Siu, L. L., Marais, R., Michiels, S., Soria, J. C., Campbell, P., Normanno, N., Scarpa, A., Reis-Filho, J. S., Rodon, J., Swanton, C., & Andre, F. (2018). The European Society for Medical Oncology (ESMO) precision medicine glossary. *Annals of Oncology: Official Journal of the European Society for Medical Oncology*, *29*(1), 30 35. doi:10.1093/annonc/mdx707 PMID:29140430

Yavuz, E., Kasapbaşı, M. C., Eyüpoğlu, C., & Yazıcı, R. (2018). An epileptic seizure detection system based on cepstral analysis and generalized regression neural network. *Biocybernetics and Biomedical Engineering*, *38*(2), 201–216. doi:10.1016/j.bbe.2018.01.002

Yıldız, O. (2019). Melanoma detection from dermoscopy images with deep learning methods: A comprehensive study. *Journal of the Faculty of Engineering and Architecture of Gazi University*, *34*(4), 2241–2260.

Yoo, J. H. (2013, June 26). The meaning of information technology (IT) mobile devices to me, the infectious disease physician. *Infection & Chemotherapy*, *45*(2), 244–251. doi:10.3947/ic.2013.45.2.244 PMID:24265976

Yun, W. L., Rajendra Acharya, U., Venkatesh, Y. V., Chee, C., Min, L. C., & Ng, E. Y. K. (2008). Identification of Different Stages of Diabetic Retinopathy Using Retinal Optical Images. *Information Sciences*, *178*(1), 106–121. doi:10.1016/j.ins.2007.07.020

Yusuff, H., Mohamad, N., Ngah, U. K., & Yahaya, A. (2012). Breast cancer analysis using logistic regression. *International Journal of Research and Reviews in Applied Sciences*, *10*(1), 14–22.

Zainuddin, Z., Huong, L. K., & Pauline, O. (2013). Reliable epileptic seizure detection using an improved wavelet neural network. *The Australasian Medical Journal*, *6*(5), 308–314. doi:10.4066/AMJ.2013.1640 PMID:23745153

Zelefsky, M. J., Lee, W. R., Zietman, A., Khalid, N., Crozier, C., Owen, J., & Wilson, J. F. (2013). Evaluation of adherence to quality measures for prostate cancer radiotherapy in the United States: Results from the Quality Research in Radiation Oncology (QRRO) Survey. *Practical Radiation Oncology*, *3*(1), 2–8. doi:10.1016/j.prro.2012.01.006

Zhang, G., Shen, X., Chen, S., Liang, L., Luo, Y., Yu, J., & Lu, J. (2019). DSM: A Deep Supervised Multi-Scale Network Learning for Skin Cancer Segmentation. *IEEE Access: Practical Innovations, Open Solutions*, *7*, 140936–140945. doi:10.1109/ACCESS.2019.2943628

Zhang, H., Yu, C. Y., Singer, B., & Xiong, M. (2001). Recursive partitioning for tumor classification with gene expression microarray data. *Proceedings of the National Academy of Sciences of the United States of America*, *98*(12), 6730–6735. doi:10.1073/pnas.111153698 PMID:11381113

Zhang, M. M., Yang, H., Jin, Z. D., Yu, J. G., Cai, Z. Y., & Li, Z. S. (2010). Differential diagnosis of pancreatic cancer from normal tissue with digital imaging processing and pattern recognition based on a support vector machine of EUS images. *Gastrointestinal Endoscopy*, *72*(5), 978–985. doi:10.1016/j.gie.2010.06.042 PMID:20855062

Zhang, X. W., Zou, Y. J., Yan, H., Wang, B., Chen, G. H., & Wong, S. P. (2000). Electrical properties and annealing effects on the stress of RF-sputtered c-BN films. *Materials Letters*, *45*(2), 1110–1115. doi:10.1016/S0167-577X(00)00086-0

Zhang, X., & Chutatape, O. (2005). Top-down and Bottom-up Strategies in Lesion Detection of Background Diabetic Retinopathy. *IEEE Computer Society Conference on Computer Vision and Pattern Recognition (CVPR'05)*, *2*, 422-428.

Zhang, Z. Q., & Song, S. C. (2016). Thermosensitive/superparamagnetic iron oxide nanoparticle-loaded nano capsule hydrogels for multiple cancer hyperthermia. *Biomaterials*, *106*, 13–23. doi:10.1016/j.biomaterials.2016.08.015

Zheng, B., Yoon, S. W., & Lam, S. S. (2014). Breast cancer diagnosis based on feature extraction using a hybrid of K-means and support vector machine algorithms. *Expert Systems with Applications*, *41*(4), 1476–1482. doi:10.1016/j.eswa.2013.08.044

Zhou, B. P., & Hung, M. C. (2003, October). Dysregulation of cellular signaling by HER2/neu in breast cancer. *Seminars in Oncology*, *30*, 38–48. doi:10.1053/j.seminoncol.2003.08.006 PMID:14613025

Zhou, C., Lai, C., Zhang, C., Zeng, G., Huang, D., Cheng, M., Hu, L., Xiong, W., Chen, M., Wang, J., Yang, Y., & Jiang, L. (2018). Semiconductor /boron nitride composites: Synthesis, properties, and photocatalysis applications. *Applied Catalysis B: Environmental*, *238*, 6–18. doi:10.1016/j.apcatb.2018.07.011

Zhou, L., Rzeszotarski, M. S., Singerman, J., & Chokreff, J. M. (1994). The detection and quantification of retinopathy using digital angiograms. *IEEE Transactions on Medical Imaging*, *13*(4), 619–626p. doi:10.1109/42.363106 PMID:18218540

Ziegler, M. (2015). *The Black Death and the future of the plague*. Pandemic Disease in the Medieval World. doi:10.2307/j.ctvmd83jc.14

Zolbanin, Delen, & Zadeh. (2015). Predicting overall survivability in comorbidity of cancers: a data mining approach. *Decision Support Systems, 74*, 150-161.

Zou, J., Huss, M., Abid, A., Mohammadi, P., Torkamani, A., & Telenti, A. (2019). A primer on deep learning in genomics. *Nature Genetics*, *51*(1), 12–18. doi:10.103841588-018-0295-5 PMID:30478442

About the Contributors

Divakar Yadav is presently working as an Associate Professor at NIT, HAMIRPUR, Gorakhpur. Prior to Join MMMUT he worked at Jaypee Institute of Information Technology, Noida from 2005 to 2016 as Associate Professor. He did his B.Tech. in Computer Sc. & Engg., M.Tech. in Information Technology, PhD in Computer Science & Engineering. He spent one year 2011-2012 at University of Carlos-III as Post Doc Fellow. He guided 4 PhD scholars and 17 M.Tech. dissertations. His research interests are Information Retrieval, Soft-computing, Machine Learning and Data Mining. He published more than 70 research papers in reputed International journals and conferences. He is also reviewer/ committee member of various International Journals and Conferences.

Jorge Morato is a professor of Information Science in the Computer Sc. Dept. at Carlos III University of Madrid, in 1999 he obtained a PhD in Library Science from the same university. He is head of the research group GigaBD. He is principal investigator of the National R&D program with a project about readability on the Web, and PI of several projects in biomedicine (e.g. CIE-10). Besides, he has collaborated in several international and European projects. He is the author of more than one hundred publications, thirty of them indexed in ISI and Scopus. His field of research is knowledge organization, linguistics, and information publication and retrieval on the Web.

* * *

Lennox Anderson-Jackson holds the Caribbean Diploma in Diagnostic Radiological Science from the University of the West Indies Mona, Kingston, Jamaica; A Bachelor of Science degree with honors in Diagnostic Medical Sonography from Weber State University in Ogden, Utah, USA; A Master of Science degree in Counselling and Consulting Psychology from the International University of the Caribbean, Kingston, Jamaica. Presently Mr. Anderson-Jackson is pursuing the MPhil / PhD in Chemical Pathology at the University of the West Indies, Mona, Kingston, Jamaica. He has over 28 years of experience in the field of radiological science and has worked in 4 countries including Jamaica, United States of America, Cayman Islands and Anguilla. He worked in several Government hospitals and Private hospitals and clinics in Jamaica including: Kingston Public Hospital (1991), Bustamante Hospital for Children, Cornwall Regional Hospital, Montego Bay Hospital, Radiology West (2003-2013), Royale Imaging Centre (2009-2013) and Reddy's Medical Centre. He also worked as a Clinical Ultrasound Instructor at the School of Medical Radiation Technology, University of the West Indies, Mona, Jamaica in collaboration with Michner Institute in Canada (2004-2008). Mr. Anderson-Jackson is presently the CEO and chief Medical Ultrasound Practitioner and Radiographer at the LYL Ultrasound Centre in

Lucea, Hanover, Jamaica. He is a member of Who's Who amongst Students of American Universities and Colleges (Edition 1999). He was also a nominee for Crystal Crest Scholar of the year for Weber State University (1997). A Member of the Profession Supplementary to Medicine, Jamaica. He has been involved in some published articles as author and co-author. Mr. Anderson-Jackson was honoured in 2011 with the Distinguished Alumni Award by the Rusea's Old Student Association (ROSA) for achievements in the field of Science and Research.

Komal Kumar Bhatia is working as Professor in Department of Computer Engineering at J. C. Bose University of Science and Technology has a work experience of 19 years. He received his B.E., M.Tech. and Ph.D. degrees in Computer Engineering in 2001, 2004 and 2009 respectively. He has guided seven Ph.Ds and guiding five Ph.D. scholars. He has also guided more than sixty M.Tech. Dissertations. He has published more than hundred research papers in reputed journals and conferences and his areas of interests are Information Retrieval Systems, Hidden Web and Web Mining. Currently, he is also working as Dean, Faculty of Informatics & Computing and Chairman of Department of Computer Engineering. He is also member of several Professional bodies at National/International level.

Jabari Brown is a Medical Technologist in the Department of Pathology, The University of the West Indies. Mona Campus, Kingston Jamaica. He Graduated from the University of Technology, Jamaica with a Bachelor of Science Degree in Medical Technology. His area of research interest includes endocrine function and disorders, and effectiveness of modern treatment regimen.

Ali Çevik is a 4th year bachelor of engineering student for computer engineering at Ondokuz Mayıs University.

Vandana Chauhan has a graduate and masters in Biotechnology. My research interest is Medical microbiology, Cancer Biology, Nanotechnology and biomedical Sciences. I had worked at Indian Institute of Technology, Kharagpur, West Bengal. My research work include study on self assembly of nano-liposome in vas deferens for prostate cancer prevention. Also I worked for artificial heart development program in a DST project. At present i am working as Assistant Professor at Amity Institute of Biotechnology, Amity University, Uttar Pradesh.

İrem Çınar is a 4th year bachelor of engineering student for computer engineering at Ondokuz Mayıs University.

Sercan Demirci received the B.S. degree in (high honors) in computer engineering from Eastern Mediterranean University, Famagusta, North Cyprus, in 2008, the M.S. degree in 2010, and the Ph.D. degree in information technology from the International Computer Institute in Ege University, Izmir, Turkey, in 2018. He is an Assistant Professor with the Computer Engineering Department, Ondokuz Mayıs University, Samsun, Turkey. His research interests include P2P networks, live streaming, wireless sensor networks, cognitive radio networks, and optimization problems in communication networks.

Manish K. Dwivedi, Ph.D. scholar in the Department of Biotechnology, Indira Gandhi National Tribal University, Amarkantak, Madhya Pradesh has completed his M.Phil. and M.Sc. in Biochemistry from Awadesh Pratap Singh University, Rewa, MP. He has been awarded gold medals during M.Sc. and

M. Phil. His areas of interest are infectious disease biology and drug development. He has published several national and international papers.

Can Eyupoglu received the B.Sc. degree with high honor in Computer Engineering and Minor degree in Electronics Engineering from Istanbul Kültür University, Turkey in 2012, the M.Sc. and Ph.D. degrees with high honor in Computer Engineering from Istanbul University in 2014 and 2018, respectively. From 2013 to 2019, he was a Research Assistant with the Computer Engineering Department, Istanbul Commerce University. He is currently an Assistant Professor with the Computer Engineering Department, Air Force Academy, National Defence University, Istanbul, Turkey. His current research interest includes machine learning, data mining, bioinformatics, neural networks, image processing, big data privacy and natural language processing.

Yogita Gigras is currently working as a Assistant Professor in the NorthCap University. Area of Specialization is soft computing,Cyber Security.

Usha Gupta is a Research Scholar CSE, FET, MRIIRS.

Svenja Kohler is in their final year medical student at University of Lübeck in Germany and future resident in the Department of Haematology and Oncology at the University Clinic Lübeck. Passionate and keen researcher in the field of human genetics.

Monika Lamba is a PhD Scholar at The Northcap University. Working as a visiting faculty in reputed institutions for the past 3.5 years. My area of interest is data mining, pattern recognition, and machine learning.

Rosy Madaan is a PhD in Computer Engineering department from YMCA University of Science & Technology, Faridabad. She has completed her B.E. from M.D. University in CSE department in 2005. In 2010, she completed M.Tech., in Computer Engineering from YMCA University of Science & Technology, Faridabad. She has total of 10 years teaching experience. She has worked in various engineering colleges and currently she is working as an Associate Professor in MRIIRS, Faridabad. Her areas of interest are information retrieval, search engines, crawlers and question answering systems.

Donovan McGrowder holds Bachelor of Science (Honours) and Doctor of Philosophy (PhD) degrees in Biochemistry and Chemistry, and Biochemistry respectively from the University of the West Indies, Mona, Kingston, Jamaica. Dr. McGrowder also holds a Master of Science degree from University of Westminster, London, UK and a Master of Arts in Psychology and Counselling from St. Stephens College, Alberta Canada. He also has post-graduate training and experience in Clinical Biochemistry and Molecular Biology. Dr. McGrowder joined the staff of The University of the West Indies, Mona in 2001 as Research Fellow in the Department of Basic Medical Sciences – Biochemistry Section and was promoted to Lecturer in 2003 and Senior Lecturer in 2009. He is also Consultant of Chemical Pathology at the University Hospital of the West Indies. He is Fellow of the Institute of Biomedical Science, UK, Fellow of the Royal Society of Tropical Medicine and Hygiene, UK, and Member of the Institute of Health Promotion and Education, UK.

Fabian Miller is a Lecturer, Researcher and the Head of Department of Physical Education at The Mico University College; he has participated in research in the Medical field and Sport Science field. He has worked on research in sport services in the CARIFORUM region which aim was to establish regional policies for sport services for the member states involved and to establish sport services as a viable industry in the region. His current research is aimed to establish Biological Passports of College/ University Athletes who compete in Sprinting and Long Distance events. Mr. Miller also published peer reviewed journal articles and book chapters. He co-authored the manuscript titled "Prostate Specific Antigen Testing in a Tertiary Teaching Hospital" and co-authored the book chapter titled "Dietary Antioxidants in the Chemoprevention of Prostate Cancer. Mr. Miller is a graduate from G.C Foster College where he completed a Diploma in Education and a Bachelors Degree in Physical Education and Sport, he went on to pursue and complete his Masters of Science in Physical Education at The University of Technology, Jamaica and he is currently a PhD student in Biotechnology, Faculty of Science and Technology, University of the West Indies, Mona. Mr. Miller is a board member of the Social and Human Sciences Advisory Committee of Jamaica National Commission for UNESCO (Period of 2016-2019).

Geetika Munjal has a teaching experience of more than 12 years in various esteemed institutions.She has completed a project titled 'Phylogenetic model for cancer classification' funded by the Department of Science and Technology. Her current areas of research include Data Mining, Pattern Recognition, Machine Learning, Image Processing and Deep Learning. She has guided around 20 B.Tech projects, 10 M.Tech thesis.

Suvashish Pandey is a sophomore Bachelor of Technology graduate student specialized in Biotechnology from Vellore Institute of Technology. I am always fueled with passion for learning new things, considering myself as 'forever student' and love doing interdisciplinary research and implement them for improving humanity. I have worked on various projects like Immunological characterization of recombinant galectin of human lymphatic filariid Brugia Malayi as novel Vaccine candidate and evolution of immune response elicited by chitosan and liposomes as adjuvants, image diagnosis using AI, and other microbiology and food related projects.

Shreyans Pathak attended Jaypee Institute of Information Technology for a bachelor's degree in Computer Science and Engineering Major.

Ritu Punhani is working as an Assistant Professor in Department of IT in Amity University, Noida, having 20 years of experience in education as well as industry.

Rahul Rustagi is a student from Department of Information Technology, Amity University, Noida.

Durmuş Özkan Şahin received a Bachelor degree in Computer Engineering from Süleyman Demirel University Isparta in 2013 and the Master degree in Computer Engineering from Ondokuz Mayıs University Samsun in 2016. Currently, he is a doctorate student in Computational Sciences. His research interests include machine learning, text mining, information retrieval, and mobile malware analysis.

Sonia Saini is working as a faculty in Amity Institute of Information Technology, Amity University, Noida, having 15 years of experience.

Kamlesh Sharma is currently working as a Associate Professor, MRIIRS, Faridabad, India (more than 12 years teaching experience). MCA, M. Tech from MDU University and Ph. D. in Computer Science and Engineering from Lingaya`s University, India. She is Supervising 2 Ph. D. scholars. Supervised and Guided research projects of M. Tech, B.Tech and application based projects for different competitions. She is also associated with two research projects related to health recommender system and NLP. She has published more than 40 research papers in field of NLP, IOT, Bigdata, Green Computing and Data Mining. Her research area "Natural Language Processing" is based on innovative idea of reducing the mechanized efforts and adapting the software to Hindi dialect. Adopted innovative teaching methodology like role play, case studies, simulation, presentations, live projects, smart classrooms technologies and combined these with regular lecture method to make the overall teaching learning process more effective.

Prashant Kumar Singh, Assistant Professor, Department of Biotechnology, Indira Gandhi National Tribal University, Amarkantak, Madhya Pradesh has eleven years of research and seven years of teaching experience. He obtained his Ph.D. degree from JNU, New Delhi while working at CSIR-CDRI, Lucknow. His areas of research interest are Infectious disease biology and drug development. He has several research publications and research projects to his credit.

Vijeta Singh is a professional Biotech Biologist with over 10 years of research and 6 years of research and teaching experience in plant biotechnology and environmental science. Strong molecular, biochemical and plant tissue culture skills with the ability to multitask in a busy environment. Self-motivated with ability to work independently and as a team.

Manju Priya Sundaramurthy is working as Professor in Department of CS, CA & IT, Karpagam Academy of Higher Education. She has about 15 yrs of teaching experience . She has received the Ph.D Degree in Computer Science from Karpagam Academy of Higher Education in 2014. She has published more than 40 papers in various National/International Journals. Her research interest includes Wireless Sensor Network, Network Security, and IoT.She has published a book on the title Wireless Sensor Networks:101.

Ceyhun Tüzün is a 4th year bachelor of engineering student for computer engineering at Ondokuz Mayıs University.

Nimriti Varun is a student from Department of Information Technology, Amity University, Noida.

Cameil Wilson-Clarke is presently a Clinical Pharmacist and the Programme Director for the Doctor of Pharmacy Programme. She also is a lecturer at the Pharmacology & Pharmacy Section, Faculty of Medical Sciences, University of West Indies, Mona Campus. She has been lecturing in the field of clinical pharmacy for more than a decade. Dr. Wilson-Clarke achieved her Doctor of Pharmacy (Pharm. D) at the Ohio State University, Columbus Ohio USA. She also holds a Master of Arts in Teaching, at the University of the West Indies, Mona. Her areas of focus are Sickle Cell Disease, Oncology, Diabetes Research/Education, Medicinal Cannabis and Pharmacovigilance. Currently she is involved in clinical trials research in sickle cell disease and medicinal cannabis.

Index

F

G

H

I

K

L

M

N

P

R

S

T

W

www.ingramcontent.com/pod-product-compliance
Lightning Source LLC
LaVergne TN
LVHW080536300926
849162LV00007B/1616